Narrative Means to Sober Ends

THE GUILFORD FAMILY THERAPY SERIES

Michael P. Nichols, Series Editor

Narrative Means to Sober Ends

Treating Addiction and Its Aftermath

JONATHAN DIAMOND

Foreword by David Treadway

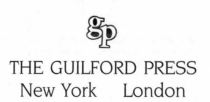

THE GUILFORD PRESS
New York   London

Library of Congress Cataloging-in-Publication Data

Diamond, Jonathan, Ph.D.
    Narrative means to sober ends : treating addiction and its aftermath/
Jonathan Diamond.
        p. cm.—(The Guilford family therapy series)
    Includes bibliographical references and index.
    ISBN 1-57230-566-5 (hc.)   ISBN 1-57230-835-4 (pbk.)
    1. Substance abuse—Patients—Rehabilitation. 2. Letter writing—
Therapeutic use. 3. Substance abuse—Treatment. I. Title. II. Series.
RC564.D535 2000
616.86′06—dc21   00-026074

All of the stories and voices in this book are derived from the author's clinical experience
in private practice and in various hospitals, clinics, and treatment programs. Names,
places, and other details contained in these materials have been altered to protect the
privacy and anonymity of the individuals to whom they refer. Therefore, any client or
story found in this book that corresponds to an actual person living or dead is inadvertent
and purely coincidental.

The following publishers have generously given permission to reprint from the following
works:

"Vowel" by Nina Cassian, translated by Brenda Walker and Andrea Deletan, from *Life
Sentence: Selected Poems*, edited by William Jay Smith. Copyright 1990 by Nina Cassian.
Published in the United States by W. W. Norton & Company, Inc. Published in the United
Kingdom by Anvil Press Poetry. Used by permission of the publishers.

Section XXXV of "Horatians" from *Nights That Make the Night: Selected Poems of
Vicent Andrés Estellés*. Translation copyright 1992 by David H. Rosenthal. Reprinted by
permission of Persea Books, Inc. (New York).

In memory of my father,
Malcolm L. Diamond;
and my aunt,
Susan Reingold Oshins

About the Author

Jonathan Diamond, PhD, received his doctorate from Smith College School of Social Work, his MSW from the University of Connecticut, and his postgraduate training in marital and family therapy at the Brattleboro Family Institute in Brattelboro, Vermont. His previous experience includes establishing and directing outpatient substance abuse and inpatient dual diagnosis treatment programs for children, adolescents, adults, and their families. Dr. Diamond has been teaching and training in the fields of addiction and psychotherapy for the past 15 years. He is currently in private practice in Northampton and Greenfield, Massachusetts.

Contents

PART III. STORIES FOR OUR TIMES

PART IV. NO CONCLUSIONS

Foreword

Dear Jon,

It's 6 A.M. I'm sitting in my backyard as a murky humid dawn unfolds. The traffic noise is beginning to drown out the birds. I just finished your book. Your last sentence made me laugh out loud.

In another hour I will be in the chair again, privileged to be bearing witness to the rich mix of misery, courage, and mystery that my clients bring to me every day. Having just read your work, I feel renewed and ready. Undoubtedly, it will seem like a very good idea to suggest letter writing to most of the folks I see today. Then I thought I would start by writing to you.

As you may have already surmised, this is a somewhat unconventional foreword, but *Narrative Means to Sober Ends* is no ordinary book. From the first few pages, I knew I was reading something special. I could tell you were a creative and courageous therapist, and that you'd written a book that truly reflects your exciting ideas, clinical acumen, and passionate commitment.

Narrative Means to Sober Ends is about stories—yours and your clients'. Through being completely present to each of your clients in the therapeutic moment and then in your telling of it, you convey the elusive essence of therapy in full flight. In story after story, you reveal the complexity of integrating psychodynamic and addictions theory on the one hand, and narrative and family system therapy on the other, while maintaining the precious individuality of each client and each therapy relationship. Your book reveals the art and mystery of therapy. It captures the bird on the wing.

Job well done.

It's been odd reading your final draft this week because while you have written luminously about the magic of therapy and the healing power of recovery, I've been slogging through one of those times when it seems like all my substance-abusing clients are referrals from what some Alcoholic Anonymous folks call "the shoe department" (i.e., the loafers, sneakers, slippers, and heels). There's Sam, who after doing great for months, has landed in jail for drinking while driving. Ellen is sneaking sips of cooking sherry while claiming to be completely sober. One of my Georges was once again slipping while staving off his wife with lame promises about maybe starting to attend AA meetings in the fall. Then my other George is also back to drinking and told his furious wife yesterday, "Sometimes a guy's got to do what a guy's got to do."

It's been one of those weeks when my 30 years of work in the addictions field feels like 29 too many.

On the other hand, reading *Narrative Means to Sober Ends* has been like going to an AA gathering. In any meeting, amid the telling of bottle stories and drunkalogues, there's always a renewal of hope and possibility—stories of people whose lives have been shattered but who somehow pick up the pieces and start over. Your book is similarly inspiring. On page after page, your belief in your clients shows through, and your willingness to go the extra mile or two or three comes through, too.

I believe, as you do, that addicts are folks looking for a spiritual home who have shown up at the wrong address. For us therapists, treating addicted people can often feel as though we practice at the wrong address, only to discover we've found our spiritual home. Addictions therapy is truly a spiritual practice. Your book reminds me that our work is an act of faith.

Good stories beget good stories. I thought I would share with you and your readers one of the stories that I draw on when I'm having one of those bad weeks with the folks from the shoe department. As this book does throughout, the story of Sister Mary Catherine and the Johnson family reminds me to hang in there and keep on keeping on.

Leroy Johnson sat huddled up in the chair with his head hanging down toward his chest as if it were too heavy to hold up straight. His body seemed frail and shrunken underneath his black and gold New Orleans Saints warm-up jacket and his baggy khaki pants. He looked like a man of 80, even though the chart in my lap said he was 42. He had been let out of the hospital to come to this interview. He was flanked by his son, Jamal, and his daughter, Jamalya. The chart said she was 13 and he was 11. They sat protectively close to their father. Jamal held his left hand, and Jamalya held his right. It looked like they were holding on for dear life.

Mrs. Jeanette Johnson sat across from her husband. With her back straight, hands folded primly in her lap, she had her eyes firmly fixed on me. She seemed to be on the edge of her seat, waiting for me, the expert doctor from up North, to say something that might save her family. Next to her sat the caseworker, Sr. Mary Catherine. She was a freshly minted social worker who looked at me with the same eager anticipation as Mrs. Johnson.

The Johnsons were Sr. Mary Catherine's first case. She didn't know enough about therapy to be discouraged by the family, even though 100% of the relatives on both sides of the family were alcoholics. The case was referred to her because the kids weren't going to school. They were staying home to take care of the house because their parents were usually too drunk to take care of much of anything.

Sr. Mary Catherine had started visiting the family 9 months earlier. At first Mr. Johnson wouldn't even speak to the "evil white lady from the city," but she sat in the kitchen and listened to Mrs. Johnson complain and sip bourbon. Apparently she was the first person that ever sat and listened to Mrs. Johnson. The kids would hover around while Mrs. Johnson and Sr. Mary Catherine talked. Sr. Mary Catherine decided to try intervening directly, and set to cleaning the kitchen with the kids while their mom smoked and chatted. On the third visit, when Sr. Mary Catherine went over to the sink, Mrs. Johnson got up and began to help, and so she, the kids, and Sr. Mary Catherine started cleaning together.

Sr. Mary Catherine didn't make a big deal of it directly when Mrs. Johnson stopped drinking at their cleaning sessions. She didn't even make a big deal of it when Mrs. Johnson decided that the kids needed to go back to school and that she ought to stop drinking entirely so she could take care of Mr. Johnson.

Meanwhile, Mr. Johnson had begun to sit in on the family clean-up sessions with his quart size bottle of Tiger Rose. He just watched suspiciously while his newly energetic wife and kids worked alongside of the "social worker lady from the city." Of course Sr. Mary Catherine had not been trained to believe that her commitment and generosity might be labeled as overfunctioning and being codependent. She decided to take the family on an outing to McDonald's, and it turned out that it was the first time that the whole family had ever gone to a restaurant together.

As Sr. Mary Catherine's visits continued, everyone seemed to be doing better except Mr. Johnson, who seemed to be determined to drink himself to death. Sr. Mary Catherine initiated a family discussion right in front of him about what they all would do if Mr. Johnson died. Apparently there was a lot of weeping because they all still loved him, but they also said that if they had to, they'd go on without him, and Mrs. Johnson even said, "And I'm not about to use his passing as an excuse to go back to that evil drink." Mr. Johnson got peeved at the whole meeting and muttered that it was like attending his own funeral.

As he got worse, Mr. Johnson was not only drinking around the clock but also refusing to eat, and the kids started skipping school again to check up on him. Mrs. Johnson and Sr. Mary Catherine didn't know what to do, so one day when he was passed out on the sofa, they just called an ambulance and the emergency medics took him off to the hospital where he had been for the 5 days before I met with the whole family.

There they were in front of me while an audience of clinicians watched on closed-circuit TV in the auditorium next door. I didn't know what to do. I felt like a beginning social worker myself. I remembered asking Sr. Mary Catherine how she had been able to work so well with these folks, and she said, "I just try to look at them through the Lord's eyes." I didn't know much about that idea back then, but I decided that I was just going to try and get to know this family and make room for each of their stories and all their unspoken stories.

Everyone seemed appropriately centered on Mr. Johnson as the identified patient, but it seemed to distance him from the rest of the family, so I decided to talk to him on a dad-to-dad level about raising teenagers. I asked him to describe what he was most proud of about his kids, and he mumbled some words back in a barely audible whisper. Jamalya kept reporting what he was saying. My efforts didn't seem to go anywhere, and the interview kind of meandered. Toward the end, I asked 13-year-old Jamalya what she was going to do to help her dad when he got out of the hospital. She answered, "Well, Dr. Trailways, you just got to love him from the bottom of the well, that's all."

I was very moved by just being with this family, and so I asked them if they would all write me a few lines about how they were doing a year from the date of the interview. Sure enough, a year later, I got a letter from Sr. Mary Catherine in which she had taken dictation from each of the family members. Everyone reported that they were doing better. But I always reread in particular what Jamalya said: "You would be so proud of my dad. He hasn't had a drink since the hospital and right now he's out mowing the lawn."

I've saved that letter just as you've saved those of your clients, and I'm sure they have saved yours. I treasure the Johnsons' story just as you clearly treasure the stories of so many of the people you have touched and been touched by. It is the privilege of our work.

Narrative Means to Sober Ends captures the heart of a good man doing good work with good people suffering a terrible disease. And yet behind the elegant theoretical formulations and inspired creative techniques, I hear Jamalya's simple message: "You just got to love from the bottom of the well, that's all."

Thanks for the gift you've given all of us, Jon. And as they say, just keep on coming back.

DAVID TREADWAY, PhD
Director, Treadway Training Institute
Weston, Massachusetts

Acknowledgments

The first people I wish to thank are a group of authors, most of whom I have never met—David Berenson, Stephanie Brown, Claudia Bepko, JoAnne Krestan, and David Treadway—pioneers in the fields of addiction, individual, and family therapy, whose writing and research were inspirational to me and created a literary home for this book.

I thank next four writers and therapists in particular who have influenced my thinking and contributed to the lifeblood of this project. Lynn Hoffman has served throughout my career as a friendly editor. The intellectual debt I and this book owe her is priceless. Her steady guidance and mentoring over the years has shaped my writing from a " 'Diamond' in the rough" to a more refined expression of my own voice. Needless to say, I take full responsibility for any parts of the book that still need buffing up. Michael White, upon whose work many of my ideas are based, has taken an unwavering stand against exploitation and patriarchy in a field that often refuses to take responsibility for its own prejudices, values, and beliefs. His voice is a refreshing one that has made a difference in how I and many others have gone about the practice of social work and therapy. Dusty Miller is an author and therapist whose gentle spirit and powerful voice are providing a generation of women survivors with a safe and protective presence in their therapy and recovery. Her writing serves as a role model for clinicians trying to help clients on their sojourn from pain and hurt to truth and healing. Her vision and astute guidance came at a crucial time as I wrote this book and gave me the confidence to see it through to completion. And last, a special embrace for Roget Lockard, who has given his conceptual wisdom about addiction and sobriety so generously to this book. Roget shares his intellect with the same reckless abandon as he shares his recovery—I hope the way I have chosen to "pass it on" does it justice.

My colleagues have generously given their time and energy to me and the book: Ruth Anderson-Zaber, Doug Arey, Mary Brown, Ken Epstein, Jean Footit, Susan Gulick, Richard Feinberg, Jim Jones, Meryl Joseph of South Hawk Studios, Lauren Kaplan, Diane Kurinsky, Sarah Lockard, Susan Loud, Emma Morgan, Samuel Muri, Bob Oldenberg, Carol Owen, Hugh Rosen, Sally Ann Roth, Karen Rowe, Shanti Shapiro, Suzanne Slater, Julie Weissman, and Adrienne Wolmark all read parts of the manuscript and provided invaluable feedback. Martha Sweezy gave to each word and each turn of phrase a patient, thoughtful, and critical reading. Frank Marotta provided me with an enthusiastic introduction to Roy Schafer's work that I still enjoy. Herb Bernstein, Gerry Schamess, Kathy Rees, Bob Shilkret, Jim Sackstedder, Cecilia Jones, and Ed Hanna—exceptional teachers and writers all—read earlier incarnations of my ideas and encouraged me to develop them further, while Joan Laird's rigorous critique of the book in one of its past lives made it a better piece of scholarship and writing. Above all, I offer heartfelt thanks to my partner at Osgood Street Associates, Prudence Grand. Her voice can be heard and her presence felt in every clinical story herein.

A special thank you as well to another group of professionals: Leslie Fraser of Words on Wing for serving as midwife to the project, helping me safely guide it from cyberspace into print; Carol Edelstein for providing both the manuscript and me with a healing dose of her writer's TLC; Leslie Breed for helping me negotiate the business end of writing; Eileen Seymore and Fern Kolakoski for recognizing that it takes more than literary credit to write a book; Kitty Moore, Senior Editor at The Guilford Press, for taking a chance on both the book and me; David Treadway for convincing her it was a risk worth taking and for a letter I will treasure always; Michael Nichols, editor of The Guilford Family Therapy Series, for bringing his tough, insightful criticism to the book; Guilford's exceptionally talented production and marketing staff; and finally, Lyra Johnson, the "childcare goddess," who gave me the greatest gift of all—time.

A writer once said, "Some day I hope to have the kind of life where I have nothing to think about but writing. Where I don't have to scribble my poems on the back of a delicatessen bill. Where if I file the darn thing under bills I'm out of a poem and if I file it under poems the delicatessen man has me in a tight place." I'd like to credit the author of these words, but I copied them on the back of a napkin, which I have since misplaced;

however, the sentiments expressed in the writer's comments resonate deeply for me. Until I'm able to have a "writer's life," I'll have to continue relying on a group of people whose love and encouragement help me to create space for writing in the life I have now. They are: Pru, Anemone, Jan, Cal, Richard, Ken, Ann, Hannah, Dean, "News," Nancy, Taylor, Silvia, Jeff, Amilia, Andrea, James, Pan, Debbie, Dianne, Paul, Lloyd, Mouf, Rob, Theo, Adrienne, Gesher, Samuel, Gerry, my brother Michael, Jennifer, Jamie, Beth, Scott, Amy, Boo, E. J., Judy, JoJo, Ray, Doug, Lauren, Mal, Joyce, Grandma Bess, and Uncle Henry.

To Jon, Karen, Jacob, and Leah for always being there.

To Denise for her strength and fortitude during a time when we both really needed it.

To my mother for her writer's DNA, her generosity, and her unconditional love and support. To my father, a great philosophic thinker, who instilled in me a passion for life and learning and gave so generously of his writings and ideas. As he didn't want credit as author or clinician, I can only thank him as a parent. Reading and editing earlier drafts of the text as he did was a loving thing to do and, apropos of the book's main tenets, a splendid reauthoring of Freud's reading of Greek myth that presents all father and son relations as a constant struggle for power and control. I miss you, Dad.

To Caryn Markson for lending her compassionate thoughts and insights to the book and for helping me find the protective presence needed to carry me through the process. To my sons, Julian and Oliver, and their "orange" posse—Cajun, Calla, Jazz, and Blues—who made sure, protected or not, the adventure never got boring!

To Dana, my best friend and partner in all matters of the heart— thank you. Not just for her love and all the intangible contributions she's made to our life while I pursued this project, but for her critical observations of both my writing and the contents of the book and her steadfast refusal to be easily impressed.

Finally, to all my clients, past and present, a special word of gratitude for sharing your stories of strength, hope, and recovery, and for the gift you've given me by allowing me to share them with others.

Prologue

A few hours later I took my leave of Dr. Bob . . . The wonderful, old broad smile was on his face as he said almost jokingly, "Remember, Bill, let's not louse this thing up. Let's keep it simple!"
—*ALCOHOLICS ANONYMOUS COMES OF AGE*

Why another volume on a subject that already accounts for so many titles on the shelves of therapists' offices and in the psychology and recovery sections of bookstores and libraries? Despite the myriad texts, articles, journals, and primers on alcoholism and recovery—not to mention diaries, short stories, novels, and memoirs—I find that some of the ways I think about addiction that are particularly successful in my practice as well as helpful to me personally are not represented in this literature. For the therapists who work with them daily, addicts and alcoholics are an endless source of uncertainty and frustration—but also of exhilaration, insight, and hope. The problems addictions pose demand some of our best thinking and most dexterous manipulations, as well as our greatest leaps of faith.

This book offers readers a different sort of narrative about addiction and trauma. The book's most humble objective is to showcase a collection of letters and stories intended to help alcoholics, addicts, and their therapists explore alternative solutions to substance abuse issues. In its most grand design, *Narrative Means to Sober Ends* is about the kind of therapy offered people suffering from addiction and trauma in the 20th century and the kind of healing and recovery we need in the 21st. This is a book about how we make sense of people's stories and provide sense to them. Think of *Narrative Means to Sober Ends* as a basic text for a different kind of literacy project for psychotherapy and recovery, a project to reimagine and enact therapy as operations of language, thought, compassion, and heart.

This is also a book about the politics and culture of therapy and recovery and the diverse sociocultural processes of which they are made. This book is about how therapists affect people not only through the clinical interventions we use but by generating the images and metaphors we use in our conversations with clients.

SITUATING MYSELF

> There is no private life which is not determined by a wider public life.
>
> —GEORGE ELIOT

I first began using letter writing in my work in 1986 in groups I ran for substance-abusing teens and children from alcoholic and drug-addicted families. When working with problems of addiction I often ask clients to write "good-bye" letters to alcohol or their drug of choice. One of my clients, a 14-year-old girl named Miranda, wrote the following letter*:

Miranda's Good-Bye Letter to Drugs and Alcohol

~~Dear~~ Narcotics, Pot (acid, alcohol) etc.

>   thanks for all You've done for me. You've helped me forget my problems, You've made me feel good, You've made me see the world in a whole new perspective, You've made me fail out of my freshman year, You've made me Ruin the lining of my esophagus and stomach. You've made the Relationship with my Parents go down hill, You've given me a who gives a shit attitude—i've gotten fucked up Emotionally and Physically. (Relationship wise also) I've gotten used by abusing you: even after all those complaints I don't want to give you up Because i'll be alone.

Miranda

---

*Although the letters presented have been typed to make them more readable, visually they have been reproduced as close to their original form—including punctuation, capitalization, etc.—as possible.

Miranda's story will be explored in more depth in subsequent chapters. My reason for including her letter here is to offer an example of this type of work, as well as to honor the humanness and the sacredness of the therapeutic relationships we engage in and practice our ideas upon.

At the time of my therapy with Miranda I drew my ideas from therapeutic approaches to addictions which, along with Alcoholics Anonymous (AA) and other 12-step programs, have a rich history of using writing as a tool for recovery. In 1989 I participated in a postgraduate externship in marriage and family therapy with Lynn Hoffman and Bill Lax at the Brattleboro Family Institute. Hearing about my work with these adolescents, Lynn suggested I look into the ideas of family therapist Michael White, as he, with coauthor David Epston, had developed an entire clinical approach organized around letter writing and correspondence—what they aptly call narrative or reauthoring therapy. The match was a good one.

In addition to being a very soulful communication, Miranda's letter harnesses the spirit of collaboration, the construction of reality through language—that is, the power of naming and putting our experience into words—and the intersection of personal and cultural oppressions (in the form of her addiction) that have become the cornerstones of narrative and other postmodern therapies. The exercise also creates a ritual that helps my clients and me honor the primacy of their relationship with drugs and alcohol and explore the specific role chemicals—and other problems or habits—play in their lives. In Miranda's case, the letter also helped us assess her ability to let go of her addiction.

White and Epston use "therapeutic letters" to help fashion their own and their clients' experiences of therapy according to less "problem-saturated" descriptions of their lives. In their correspondence White and Epston (1991) invite clients to "externalize" the problems they're up against, a process "that encourages persons to objectify and, at times, to personify the problems that they experience as oppressive" (p. 147).

Following White's lead, I find that letter writing seems to create some distance between clients and their dilemmas. Encouraging people to define their values and sense of self, separate from problems, often leads to a shift in perspective from "I am the problem" to "I am up against a problem." I also appreciate what an important and powerful tool the act of writing itself can be for people in therapy. Writing helps clients like Miranda—recovering from abuse, addiction, and abandonment—struggle to reclaim their bodies and their histories by gradually fitting images and then names to their traumatic experiences. From the standpoint of medicine and pharmacology, Miranda's letter, and other narrative techniques employed in this book, might be viewed as a kind of "narrabuse"* that helped her access her own creative voice as an antidote to alcohol, narcotics, and other self-destructive habits.

Another dimension of therapy draws me to this work. Clients suffering from alcoholism and addiction don't just get over "symptoms" and "problems" in a traditional or conventional sense; rather, their lives appear to be transformed in the midst of incredibly desperate circumstances and overwhelming odds. There is an expression in AA that captures the same sentiment: "An addict," the saying goes, "is a person with a spiritual calling who shows up at the wrong address." It is my hope that this book and the ideas it holds will help some of its readers (and their therapists) who feel lost in the world of alcoholism and addiction regain their sense of direction and find their way home.

David Epston offers the following story of why writing a letter seemed so natural an extension of therapy for him—a mystery, he said, he had been trying to solve for some time. On visiting the town in Canada where he grew up, he met with his mother's best friend, Dorothy, who said she had kept every letter his mother ever wrote her:

> I was confused by this revelation as, for the life of me, I could not recall my mother ever writing Dorothy a letter. After all, they spent hours on the phone every day and were neighbors. "Didn't you know?" she asked me. "She wrote me a letter after every phone call! She said she wanted to get it down. She said that talk wasn't enough." (Epston, 1994, p. 63)

Letters, says Epston, ought to be moving experiences, doorways through which everyone can enter the family's story and be touched by the bravery, the pain, and even the humor of the narrative. Miranda's letter created an entrance for me into her life, it closed the gap she experienced between herself and others—bridging her world and ours. Writing (and "externalizing problems" in this fashion) helps people connect with the larger culture. It brings them from silent isolation into language and community restoring—and restorying—their faith in themselves and their future. I also find, in my own and my clients' therapy, that writing inspires another kind of hope more introspective in nature. Journal and

---

*A play on the name of the prescription medication Antabuse, which, when combined with alcohol, makes the person violently ill. This medication is requested by some alcoholics who use it in early recovery as a means of buying themselves more time to think before picking up a drink.

letter writing serves as a kind of hope chest where the most precious parts of ourselves can be placed for safekeeping.

This last point suggests further common ground between addiction treatment and narrative practices. Therapy is never just a collection of stories about our clients. They are stories about ourselves as well. Ours is always both a professional and a personal journey. Miranda's and the many other people's experiences gathered in this volume—painful as they are—are stories of clinical reflection and spiritual growth. They describe many different roads to sobriety, including the path I have traveled to cope with growing up in a violent and alcoholic family, and how my decision to become a therapist and the way I practice my profession is intimately connected to my own recovery.

NARRATING THE UNCONSCIOUS

A question asked of Michael White and other presenters at every family therapy gathering I've attended is, "Do you believe in the unconscious?" For me the answer is simple, like Starhawk, who, when asked if she believes in the goddess, replied that she believes in the goddess the same way she believes in rocks. She doesn't "believe" in either god or rocks— she connects with them. I do not believe in the unconscious; I connect with it. The unconscious, writes Metzger (1992), is like a plumb line running through all our worlds: "Every time we speak, write, or act, we sacrifice completeness. Given that things will be omitted, moments will be truncated, experiences will, at best, be rendered partially, we learn to communicate through silences and absences as well as through disclosure" (p. 33). Psychoanalyst Christopher Bollas describes the unconscious as a kind of spirit place wrapped in language. In this sense, and from the standpoint of literary theory, we are all authors of our own inner worlds and idioms—creators of our own psychic genres.

The trouble with psychotherapy is not its belief in the unconscious; it is its need to diagnose it. The language of psychopathology and the language of psychotherapy are not the same. "Borderline" and "narcissistic personality disorder," "codependency," "enmeshed families"— these terms function as linguistic straitjackets that bind us and deprive us of our personhood. Psychotherapy, it seems to me, is more about mystery and wonder—matters of the heart and soul—and our language should reflect those practices.

Reading about alcoholism and addiction in the psychoanalytic literature leaves one with the feeling that when Narcissus looked into the pool of water and saw his reflection looking back, from the standpoint of psychodynamic theory he must have been staring into a glass of bourbon. Psychoanalytic theory sees all addiction as masking an underlying characterological disorder of narcissism. This stripping of people's addiction narratives and healing stories of their personal contexts, of whatever makes them truly unique, reflects what Walker Percy called "cow paths"—the narrow ruts of language and thought that characterize psychiatric and other professional mental health training.

According to postmodern and narrative perspectives, the tragedy of psychotherapy has been the ways in which people's stories are categorized and arranged like aisles in a supermarket. In the latter approach, words and behaviors have significance in terms of the categories and the systems in which they're placed, as opposed to their relevance to the therapeutic relationship and meaning they have to the client. In a narrative approach to therapy, the many commonalities found among alcoholics are better thought of as the common outcomes of alcoholism rather than as antecedent conditions or the result of an alcoholic personality.

While expressing a clear preference for the lexicon of narrative family therapy over psychoanalytic forms of discourse, I believe neither approach has exclusive rights to compassionate or dehumanizing methods of practice. Listening, caring, relationship, and affect are the heart of a narrative approach to addiction: listening to people's stories; expecting competence; respecting differences; and, when people's stories break apart, recognizing the pain and suffering, and searching for health within the broken fragments. In other words, we have faith and trust that conversations and stories can be healing for both therapist and client. The postmodern lens and packaging in which narrative therapy comes enable therapists and clients to gain freedom from constraints that limit conversation, preclude listening, and lead toward diagnosis rather than growth.

When we are consulting with people, all theories about therapy—including the narrative ideas presented here—do violence to our relationships with clients. They create distance between us by dividing us into observers and subjects. This leaves many of us in the helping professions in a quandary. We need our theories and stories about therapy. More like flotation devices than navigational equipment, they help us stay afloat and remain calm in the face of great pain and injustice. Postmodern family therapists say we can engage in this kind of conversation and hold onto our theories about therapy if we need to, so long as we make ourselves more aware of what socially, and in fact morally and ethically, we are doing in our talk. It is a clinical version of the judgment of Solomon: those of us willing to give them up are awarded the privilege of keeping them. The challenge is to allow ourselves space to engage with psychological wisdom and thinking without forgetting the harm done, historically, by our psychological theories and language practices, to the people we are trying to help.

These explorations remind us just how artificial are the boundaries and different languages we use to distinguish one form of practice from another. In actuality, there are no such entities as narrative, social constructionist, deconstructive, or postmodern therapies. Like Sigmund Freud's typography of the mind—the id, ego, and superego—these are imaginary paper worlds we create that shape our thinking about therapy and help us make sense of our own and our clients' experiences. Therapy is always about a relationship between two people (or parties)—it is not a technique. Theories have meaning and purpose only to the extent that they serve to deepen and strengthen those relationships.

"Models" and theories about therapy are, as a whole, more helpful to authors trying to write about therapy than those of us trying to practice it. People look to "second-generation" books and practitioners for integration and synthesis and to help them make connections among different approaches, as well as the application of them to specific types of problems. I don't expect Michael White, one of narrative therapy's most well-known authors and advocates, to write about the influence of analytic ideas on his thinking as he is trying to establish a legitimate place for narrative approaches at the larger family therapy table, so to speak.[1] But most of us use some kind of psychodynamic thinking in our work—particularly object relations and attachment theory—as well as borrowing from other models and methods (e.g., Bowen's genograms, feminist interventions and approaches to gender issues advocated by the Women's Family Therapy Project, and the multicultural thinking of Monica McGoldrick and others). Many of these ideas are compatible with one another and not just the obvious matches like narrative therapy and feminism. As therapists we don't want to feel as if we are being heretical because we find other approaches useful and draw from different models, even when we feel strong affiliations or loyalties to one particular school of thought (often the one we were first trained in). What's more, most of us were not trained in a homogeneous environment "at the feet of a master"; rather, we learned our craft from a variety of sources in a kind of "bootleg" way.

Psychoanalysts D. W. Winnicott, Christopher Bollas, Roy Schafer, and Donald Spence, whose writings bridge the gap between the personal and social worlds of experience, are the most recent additions to my narrative therapy album. These analysts, although oriented to Freud, listen to postmodern voices. Schafer (1992), along with Spence (1982), introduced the concept of narrative into psychoanalytic discourse. Their rereading of traditional psychoanalytic concepts as "interpretive storylines," rather than scientific principles, undercuts the claim to objectivity of the psychoanalyst and the therapeutic hour. These analysts join their more relational postmodern psychoanalytic feminist cousins—Jessica Benjamin and Jane Flax—who, using the lens of gender, call for an end to psychotherapy's love affair with the concept of a unified, autonomous, and independent self. Collectively, throughout the book, these therapists and their work serve as a kind of analytic reflecting team, helping me deconstruct my rendition of narrative therapy and ideas. By showcasing the work of these analysts and its application to addiction treatment, I hope to demonstrate how psychoanalytic concepts can be used in all sorts of clinical encounters in highly innovative ways, even in single—sometimes decisive—exchanges, rather than confining these ideas to the luxury of long-term psychotherapy or the slow unfolding process of an analysis.

Many perspectives on narrative and other postmodern therapies that inform my work with addictions are discussed in the following chapters and the differences between, for example, its psychodynamic and family therapy versions are explored. Rather than summarizing them here, I will share a story that captures some of my frustration with these narrative silences in the literature.

Earlier, when discussing my introduction to narrative therapy, I intended to share a conversation with my Aunt Joyce, who, after reading some of my correspondence to my parents and samples of my communications to clients, told me that I have my mother's gift for letter writing. Her comment reminded me of a year my family lived in Europe (when I was 5 and 6 years old); my mother would write home weekly, sometimes more frequently. My grandfather kept all of her letters, and when he died my mother's oldest sister returned them all to her. One of my favorite activities today is to sit on the floor of my mother's home and read through the shoe boxes full of correspondence about our family's travels. (My mother has at various times in her life threatened to write a book, *Europe by Tricycle*.)

For aesthetic reasons, I wasn't going to tell you this story. I didn't want it to interfere with David Epston's vignette about his mother's correspondence, presented earlier. Also, unlike Epston, I was not trying to solve a personal mystery of any kind. I had, as mentioned, a much more direct introduction to letter writing and other narrative practices and did not feel it necessary to say more. However, I find it amusing that for all the fuss and refutation of traditional psychoanalytic concepts, two passionate proponents of narrative therapy, Epston and I, both discovered that when writing letters in therapy, we had, unconsciously, been thinking back through our mothers.

HOW TO READ THIS BOOK

The best praise this book could ever receive was bestowed on it before it even made it into print. A number of colleagues who read earlier drafts of the manuscript said there are people they're seeing in their practices who would greatly benefit from reading all or parts of its chapters. This brought me untold delight and is acknowledgment enough for its author that the project was a worthwhile one. The following is a brief trail guide, so to speak, for therapists, clients, and other readers negotiating the book's terrain.

The book's first part fleshes out a narrative approach to addiction, what I call a "sobriety of literary merit," and describes the sorts of processes people move through in therapy and recovery. This includes ways of inviting addicts and alcoholics to explore their relationship with drugs and alcohol and take the first steps toward dismissing them from their lives; how to help people accept their situation and step out of these endless power struggles with substances and other compulsive relationships; and, finally, once they've stopped clinging to their problems and let go of their addictions, how to engage people in dialogues that can restore their broken spirits and create meaning out of their lives and experiences.

Part II, "Detoxing the Theory," introduces the concept of 12-step literacy and explains why it's such an important quality for therapists to possess, as well as how to come by it. It looks at how psychotherapists can strengthen their clients' recovery and connection to AA and other 12-step programs, as well as how certain aspects of the analytic dialogue have been telling the wrong story about addiction. Some readers may prefer to skip this part, go immediately to Part III (Chapters 7–11), and then return to this part at a later stage when they are looking for answers to questions about AA and how I apply its philosophy and methods to the therapy context.

Part III, "Stories for Our Times," looks at the application of these ideas about alcoholism and addiction in my work with families and adolescents, as well as my efforts at muddling through these places with people facing a number of other problems in therapy and recovery including trauma, incest, compulsive overeating, and other food addictions. Chapter 11, "Narrating Our Own Stories," looks at how these problems bankrupt the lives of clinicians and other concerns specific to therapists and other helping professionals who are in recovery themselves. A brief addendum found at the end of this chapter reviews some questions I am frequently asked when training and consulting on this topic.

Part IV, the book's conclusion, revisits the discussion (presented in the Introduction) about how the stories and metaphors we choose to describe alcoholism and addiction inform our work with these problems; examines the issues that arise when addiction therapy needs to be brief; as well as offers some additional thoughts on the connection between psychotherapy and writing and the use of narrative techniques in therapy.

While the book is put together like a story with a beginning, middle, and end, it does not have to be read that way. It can be used more in the fashion of a handbook if that suits the reader better. Therapists more interested in family therapy, for example, may choose to read Chapter 9 first and then go back and glean from the book's other sections ideas that assist them in understanding more about that endeavor. The introduction, "Remembering Addiction," offers a phrase book, in a manner of speaking, that will make your travels through the text more pleasant regardless of where you choose to begin. I will caution those of you who are therapists not to skip the chapter on adolescents because you don't see children in your practice or the chapter on families because you work exclusively with individuals. What's important are the relationships and patterns of addiction I describe. Each chapter has relevance regardless of the sort of therapy you practice or theoretical approach you're drawn to. As you read you can generalize to other settings, people, and problems.

For therapists interested in sharing the book's ideas with clients more directly, Parts I and III contain passages that would be most accessible and of most interest to recovering persons or individuals still struggling with an addiction, while Parts II and IV address issues that arise more frequently in conversations among therapists and other helping professionals. Scholars of AA and others more interested in 12-step culture as a whole will find Part II of particular interest as well.

The goal foremost in my mind when I wrote the book was that it be useful. Consequently, I have sacrificed theory if I did not think it had a practical application to the lives of real people and their problems. Where I have felt it necessary to discuss the writers whose work forms the philosophical underpinnings of the book's ideas, I've chosen to pay homage to their contributions rather than critique their shortcomings. This is in keeping with the overall tenor of the book in which I've tried to embrace an analytic attitude of curiosity and inquisitiveness. Where there are controversies, I will point them out and share with the reader my own interpretation and understanding of them. However, in the process of fleshing out differences and conflicts, I will avoid the tendency to demonize or villianize one participant or another in the conversation or argument because, to paraphrase Rabbi Abraham Twersky, it is not by a person's sins that you get to know him or her but by what that person celebrates.

Extensive endnotes have been used to keep the main text readable and avoid disrupting the flow of the narrative. These notations provide more detailed explanations of concepts and technical terms, expansion on additional points, as well as annotated entry points to the wider literature on psychotherapy, recovery, and philosophy from which the main text draws. While this seemed the most proficient way of allowing for varying degrees of inquiry and interest among readers, in no case are these notes essential to an adequate grasp of the book's ideas.

A Word about Language

A few remarks on my use of language and the writing process—that is, my choice of words and idiom when documenting people's stories. Therapy, like art, evokes a kind of mystery and wonder. Our job as therapists is to deepen the mystery. In order to function in the language of therapy we need to learn to live in it comfortably. As Julia Cameron (1992) observed in another context, the language of therapy is one of image and symbol. It is a wordless language even when our very art is to chase it with words. Therapy is a language of felt experience. The writing and stories found in the following chapters try to put words to these kinds of experiences—events meant to be felt, not described. As a consequence, this book speaks of passion not pathology, history not etiology; compulsions and desires take the place of dysfunction and disease, memories replace symptoms. There is little mention of family systems; instead there is discussion of mothers, daughters, fathers, and sons.

A word about pronouns. Using the word "she" doesn't solve the problem of sexist language and bias. However, in a book about therapy, where the majority of the providers and an even greater portion of the clientele are women, the issue seemed both political and pragmatic. Thus, sometimes in the text I've chosen to use "her" and "she" in place of the more customary "his" and "he" or the more cumbersome "his or her" and "he or she."

Regarding the interplay between trauma and addiction (themes addressed most comprehensively in Chapters 7 and 8), first, the decision to emphasize the story of people's addictions in this book rather than stories of trauma could easily have been reversed. The following chapters make a case that the experience of addiction is, in and of itself, a trauma of immense proportion. Further, in the "real" world, our experiences of these problems do not fit into the convenient categories that our theories prescribe for them. It is a messy process. Problems often travel in packs and clusters. When a therapist comes across problems of addiction, she is more likely, for example, to find herself also having to deal with issues of violence and abuse.

In addition, clients in therapy for posttraumatic stress disorder, dissociative experience, and other sequelae of trauma often present an array of compulsive and self-destructive behaviors (e.g., substance abuse, eating disorders, self-mutilation, and other forms of self-harm), a position supported in the literature (Gelinas, 1983; Herman, 1992; D. Miller, 1994; Pearlman & Saakvitne, 1995; Shapiro & Dominiak, 1992). Consequently, the emphasis on addiction rather than trauma stems directly from my attempt to develop a narrative perspective on addiction, not because I view one problem clinically more significant than the other.

Narrative Means to Sober Ends

Remembering Addiction

A word spoken from within the doorposts of the ancestral
home can not go astray.
—MARTIN BUBER

This is a book about passion, desire, sensual pleasure, lust, fears, pain,
and insatiable hungers. It's about a love so powerful it's paralyzing and
a need so strong it's greater than a person's will to live.

"Like drinking stars," is how some alcoholics describe the sensation
of consuming alcohol. Imagine the feeling of being able to capture and
hold the entire Milky Way in your hand, this is what the addict feels she
is losing every time she puts down her bottle—marijuana, cocaine, heroin, pills, or food. In a personal account of her own struggle with addiction, author Caroline Knapp (1996) says that alcohol illuminated a
calmer and gentler piece of her soul. Addiction, surmises Geneen Roth in
When Food Is Love (1991), is the act of wrapping ourselves around an
activity, a substance, or a person in order to pretend we have love in our
lives. It helps people believe they are surviving, even thriving. It helps
them tolerate an enormous pain they are denying.

Perhaps this explains, in part, why, in spite of the best efforts of
substance abuse counselors, individual and family therapists, partial
hospitalization programs, residential treatment centers, public health of-
ficials, and policymakers, we are losing the so-called war on drugs.
When clinicians and mental health researchers pull out drug and alcohol
assessment tools that try to measure the severity of a person's problem,
they are missing the point. They are trying to measure something that
cannot be measured and defies the logic of standard psychological instruments. If medical research ever develops a scientific approach to ad-

diction, it will not be a science of genes, neurotransmitters, biochemistry, or brain waves, it will be a science of desire.

We might get closer to the mark if these tools were to ask questions like the following: (1) What do you do if the only way to sate your craving for crack cocaine is to leave your baby unattended in a hot car with the windows sealed on an 80-degree day in the summer in a neighborhood occupied by gangs, drug dealers, and prostitutes? (2) Your doctor warns you that having another drink—even one beer—means losing your kidneys and starting dialysis immediately; do you follow her advice or go out and enjoy a six-pack because you realize you're going to die soon? Or (3) If continuing to ingest alcohol and refuse treatment meant severing your relationship to your only daughter and not being invited to her wedding, would you seek help or pour yourself a drink to ease the pain and suffering experienced from the impending loss of connection to your child?

These are not extreme examples, although the dilemmas they propose may seem unfathomable to anyone who hasn't felt their life controlled by or at the mercy of an addiction over which he or she was powerless. In fact, most of us wouldn't consider these real choices or serious questions at all—they are beyond anything we can comprehend. However, addicts have a different center of gravity, one that tends to organize itself along two axes: control and sensation (i.e., the maximization of pleasurable sensations and the avoidance of painful ones).

As a consequence, people suffering from addiction make lousy candidates for psychotherapy. One day a college professor remarked to Martin Buber that Freud is reported to have answered a question about the meaning of life by saying, work and love. Buber laughed and said that was good but not complete. He would say: work, love, faith, and humor.[1] This sort of badinage is not likely to uncover the meaning of life, but the terms "work, love, faith, and humor" do go a long way toward describing peoples' experience of therapy. In my view, a crucial omission from this list is "courage."

Therapy is courageous work, which requires letting go of control—having faith in oneself and others—and allowing oneself to experience a number of uncomfortable feelings, many quite painful. Addicts and alcoholics embrace a lifestyle that avoids pain at all costs, seek immediate gratification, and tend to rely on—put their faith in—chemicals more than people. In other words, for those who are addicted recovery means abandoning the very things that sustain them. This makes it difficult for therapists who treat addiction. I've always felt that if I haven't learned something during a client's therapy, chances are the client hasn't either. The upheaval and chaos created by addiction makes for a challenging learning environment. Understandably, the task does not generate a great deal of enthusiasm, and where it exists it is often short lived and quickly replaced by pessimism, cynicism, and burnout.

My main objective in writing this book is to counter the therapeutic nihilism surrounding problems of alcoholism and addiction. Clinicians are all too willing to work with people in recovery but often dread taking on clients who are active addicts and alcoholics trying to change or who "want to want to change." Furthermore, many therapists don't share their colleagues' enthusiasm for collaborating with persons in recovery. They find the celebratory nature and testimonial style of some AA gatherings off-putting, and too dissonant with the more quiet and reserved sensibilities of psychotherapy. It's as if AA inherited all of people's strength, hope, and recovery, and psychotherapy their grief and pain. In treating addiction it is crucial to understand the amount of loss and suffering endured in the process of recovery—loss of jobs, homes, friendships, family relations, and other AA members. For every alcoholic whose sobriety results in his or her reconnecting with others there are five others whose stories are punctuated by abandonment, cutoffs, and death because of the way alcoholism and drug abuse continues to ravage their families and their lives. Persons in AA need to emphasize hope and celebrate one another's successes in order to counter the intense feelings of loss stemming from the knowledge of how many comrades and loved ones will not make it and eventually fall prey to the "disease" of addiction.

My wish for therapists who pick up this book is that after reading it they will approach these problems, and the people who struggle with them, with more hope and less dread. I hope that they will come to see compulsive drinking as an outward manifestation of the alcoholic's inner anguish. For alcoholics, addicts, and their friends and family members, it's my hope that the fear and trepidation with which they often approach therapy and recovery will be replaced with a renewed sense of faith in themselves, other human beings, and the possibilities of their lives.

BORDER CROSSINGS: COMMITMENTS OF A POSTMODERN PSYCHOTHERAPIST

Everywhere I go I find a poet has been there before me.
—SIGMUND FREUD

In his groundbreaking essay, "The Cybernetics of 'Self': A Theory of Alcoholism," Gregory Bateson (1972a) uses the challenges addiction and recovery pose us to call for a new understanding of mind, self, human relationships, and power. Bateson describes the alcoholic as having adopted an unusually disastrous variant of "the strange dualistic epistemology characteristic of Occidental civilization" (p. 321); he warns of the dangers this kind of "cause-and-effect" thinking can pose alcoholics and nonalcoholics alike. These problems or paradoxes are, according to Bateson, not unique to addiction but are more evident when one is dealing with it. In a dynamic process captured in the oft-used expression "mind over matter," addicts separate their "self" or "will" from their environment in an effort to control it (Berenson, 1991). In other words, the alcoholic's attempt at arriving at solutions through drinking is simply another piece of modern drama acted out in the Cartesian theater. Except in this version of Western philosophy's longest running show, the protagonist's signature line has been changed from "I think therefore I am" to "I drink therefore I am." Counter to prevailing beliefs that alcoholics drink for all the wrong reasons, Bateson concludes that for the alcoholic drinking offers "a short cut to a more correct state of mind."

Bateson reminds us that the "logic" of addiction has puzzled psychiatrists no less than the "logic" of the "strenuous religious regime whereby the organization Alcoholics Anonymous is able to counteract the addiction" (1972a, p. 309). While Bateson looked to cybernetics and systems theory for his new epistemology, he felt the nonalcoholic world had much to learn from the ways of AA. He used AA's spiritual outlook to help him construct a view of the world more relevant to our current problems as well as to deconstruct what is wrong with our current way of thinking about humankind and nature. If, says Bateson, double binds* cause anguish and despair and destroy personal epistemological premises, then the serenity prayer, with its promotion of noncompetitive spiritual relations, heals wounds and frees a person from these maddening bonds.

Epistemology is the branch of philosophy that concerns itself with the origins, nature, methods, and limits of knowledge. This term, however, has gained colloquial currency in the family therapy field as a synonym for the word "paradigm." While Bateson showed how our culture was caught in a frenzy of biological materialism, his aforementioned article, along with his other writings, generated a frenzy of paradigmatic thinking and what I call "epistemological speak" within the mental

---

*Such double binds are, in Bateson's theory, the painful and competing contradictory messages and directives about the self that contribute to the onset of mental illness.

health professions. Unfortunately, the focus of this new wave of family systems thinking was on the tools and methods Bateson employed and, for the most part, ignored the questions and mysteries that initially captured his attention.

A Narrative Approach to Psychotherapy

The early stages of any fresh practice or discipline are always poetic. This book proposes a narrative metaphor for people's recovery and healing. A narrative approach to psychotherapy offers therapists an alternative to the dominant biological and disease metaphors for human suffering inherited from science and medicine. From the standpoint of narrative: Stories, not atoms, are the stuff that hold our lives—and our world—together. Put another way, when it comes to treating alcoholism and addiction, therapists employing narrative practices (including me) are more interested in knowing what sort of person has a disease than what sort of disease a person has.

Why is it that we invest so much time, energy and money into exploring the medical and biological aspects of addiction? Or, said another way, why are we so afraid of looking beyond the biology of addiction? Could this be a manifestation of something Bateson was trying to tell us about the "disease" itself and our will to control the experience and make it more manageable? In other words, if we describe addiction solely as a genetic illness, then we can "cure" or eliminate it. Ironically, the third of the "three C's" of the Al-Anon program—"You didn't cause it, you can't control it, and you can't *cure* it"—stands in contradiction to what is generally considered sound medical practice and the standard scientific approach to research. What is it about this simple credo practiced in quiet meditation by millions of men and women every night in church basements and community halls, in small towns and big cities in every country on every continent, that is so frightening and too much for many of us to witness?

The disease concept as embraced by AA has been a very helpful metaphor to people.* However, the way AA thinks about and employs the terms "disease" and "illness" is very different than the way these concepts are applied in medicine and science. Most notably is the manner in which AA conceptualizes addiction as a spiritual *dis*ease with

---

*Some of the many ways the disease concept has assisted people's healing and contributed to our understanding of the problems they face are discussed extensively in Chapters 4 and 6.

physical symptoms, whereas medicine looks at addiction exclusively from the standpoint of pathology.

Clearly, there are genetic profiles that lead to more successful metabolism of alcohol and higher incidents of addiction among certain groups of people. But how does this research account for the large numbers of people who share these genetic profiles and who aren't and don't become alcoholic? Further, I've known people to work hard to overcome a pronounced physiological aversion to alcohol because other aspects of their ecology conspired so strongly on behalf of their addiction.

Finally, if science were to establish the presence of a proto-alcoholic gene, what would this minute piece of DNA programming represent? DNA is a chemical template of life. Cultural conditioning and trauma leave their footprints in these molecular sands in the same way the HIV virus can create mourning rituals (e.g., the AIDS quilt and the Names Project) and can change public policy and other cultural practices. As Bernstein and Fortune (1998) observed, "Biology is not the ground on which the social gets overlaid: We and our laboratory kin are not organisms 'first' and social, cultural, or symbolic 'second.' Just as the sciences are all these things at once so are we" (p. 225). Science is not a careful construction of theories based on the laborious accumulation of neutral facts but a contingent social activity, and we mythologize and story our relationships with chemistry and biology the same as we do all other human experience or activity. Peter Kramer (1993) has us listening to Prozac, Bernie Siegel (1986) asks that we embrace our chemotherapy, and many clinicians have produced intimate biographies of mental illness in the form of their own memoirs, such as Kay R. Jamison's story (1995) of her struggle coping with bipolar depression.[2]

There is a term in medicine and epidemiology, "Koch's postulate," which refers to a set of principles clinicians use in their search for a "single unitary cause" of an illness when tracing the origins of a disease. The rationale for seeking the sole cause of an illness is the assumption that, once you discover its causative agent, you are likely to find a "single unitary solution"—that is, a so-called magic bullet treatment. The classic example is syphilis. They used to say that if you knew syphilis, you knew medicine. Called the great masquerader because it affected every organ of the body, once diagnosed, the solution for these myriad symptoms was, amazingly, a single dose of penicillin.[3]

This is the miracle of modern medicine. Its methods, scientific and objective, epitomize the zeitgeist that has colored thinking in the physical sciences from the Enlightenment to the present.[4] This is the model social science and psychotherapy try to emulate. Despite having received the Goethe Prize for literary merit and being nominated for the Nobel Prize for literature rather than medicine, Freud—the founder of psycho- analysis from which most modern psychotherapies derive—desperately sought to demonstrate the scientific character of his work.

Narrative and other postmodern perspectives undermine modern approaches to "valid" knowledge. If the example of syphilis, presented above, represents medical science's past and present, then alcoholism and addiction represent its future. If alcoholism research throughout the 20th century has shown us anything, it's this: *if you know alcoholism, you know where science and medicine are going.* Developments in the field of addictions have had a revolutionary impact on the way we prac- tice medicine and therapy and on the way we view societal problems. The problems of the alcoholic are now seen to impact upon and be influ- enced by the entire culture. One reason for this is because the potential causes for alcoholism cannot be narrowly defined within the discourse of contemporary science. In other words, there is no "magic bullet" cure. The crucial point being made here is that the phenomenon of alco- holism defies Western medicine and know-how and cannot be captured with a 20th-century mindset.

This book, like its subject matter, is a creative literary endeavor. It hopes to inspire more projects and investigations that emphasize narra- tive metaphors over biological ones for psychotherapy and other human sciences. However, neither the book nor its author advocate abandoning or ignoring biology, physiology, or brain functioning and other neuro- logical research. This would be impossible in the case of addictions, and ill-advised in any effort to understand human beings whose bodies pro- duce, every moment, thousands of chemical reactions independent of any foreign substances introduced into them.

It would be foolish to ignore the stories chemistry, neurobiology, and other sciences produce about alcoholism and addiction, because when you ignore or stay away from something you are not allowing its story to be part of the larger one. Studies that emphasize the im- portance of the mind–body connection in coping with stressful illness and psychological trauma top the best-seller lists and abound in the professional literature as well.[5] In certain stages of recovery it can be incredibly helpful to get information on the biology of addiction to cli- ents when they're ready for it.[6] This is vital work. However, it is not the focus of this book and, what's more, there are many others more qualified than me to speak to the science of addiction and plenty of primers and texts on this subject available to readers in need of them.[7] When all is said and done, I simply feel that stories have as much to tell us about human nature as theory and that when it comes to understanding addiction psychotherapy's specific contribution is more literary than scientific. The two perspectives (science and therapy) are not mutually exclusive.

Deconstructing Alcoholism

Psychiatrist and author David Berenson (1986) likens alcoholism to the story of the five blind men and the elephant, each one feeling a different part and trying to describe his discovery based solely on the evidence at hand. As is well known, one, his arm wrapped around the elephant's leg, thinks it's a tree; another, holding the trunk, believes it to be a giant snake—and so on, each of the five describing the part he's encountered but never grasping the whole picture. Similarly, how a person's condition is defined by a clinician or counselor depends on the latter's vantage point. The physician treating damage to the person's liver and esophagus or broken bones from a drunken driving accident defines it as a physical malady. The psychiatrist might respond to the depression that many alcoholics suffer with medication or therapy, without exploring the connections between the person's drinking and her feelings (maybe forgetting that alcohol itself is a depressant that suppresses the central nervous system). The social worker may see the environmental factors—unemployment, poverty, racism, homophobia, and so forth—at play in the person's life. The family therapist may trace the condition's origins to the dysfunctional patterns of communication that feed the cycle of shame and blame in which family members so often become mired. The pastoral counselor may see the condition as a spiritual crisis that has compromised the drinker's values, belief system, and self-worth. What we have here, from the standpoint of the alcoholic, are five blind theories. Collectively, they're onto something; individually, they have nothing.

It is, as Stephanie Brown (1985) observed, the rare alcoholism text that does not include a review of the most current and controversial models of addiction. Berenson's adaptation of this parable does a nice job of summarizing some of the more prominent ones as well as exposing the pitfalls of wedding ourselves to any one point of view— be it psychological, spiritual, systemic, social, or biological. Absent from this illustration is the behavioral psychologist who emphasizes conditioning principles, both in understanding the development of addiction and in its treatment. To paraphrase D. W. Winnicott, we don't just use words and language, language and words use us. Our theories condition us in the same fashion. They determine what we look for. Like the character in the old folktale, first we shoot holes in the fence, then we paint the bull's-eyes around them. Another goal of this book is to put the voice of the person before the voice of the text—that is, to privilege people's stories of addiction over our theories and methods of understanding them.

A further lesson Berenson's allegory holds for us also has to do with language, as well as the problem discussed earlier of our falling into "cause-and-effect" thinking when addressing issues of addiction. Not only Bateson but physicists, biologists, information theorists, and social scientists across many disciplines have long demonstrated how our notions about cause and effect are inaccurate and outmoded. However, in the field of addiction, as in the story of the elephant, many clinicians are still looking for "absolute" causes, trying to find out, as Berenson describes, if alcoholism is caused by an antecedent biological condition, if alcoholics are "oral dependent people," if a person's family environment causes his or her addiction, or if alcoholism is caused by a breakdown in our social institutions and supports.

As Efran, Hefner, and Lukens (1987) write, "The issue of alcoholism is neither pharmacological nor not pharmacological, neither a learned habit nor not a learned habit, neither a social protest nor not a social protest. It is all of these and none of these. . . . [A] pattern of behavior, such as problem drinking, can never be fully described in one set of language terms" (p. 44). Therapists trained differently use different paradigms, and so our language about our work is bound to be different. The language we choose to describe our respective experiences with addiction or "deviant" reality may vary, but the urge to facilitate change and transform the way we perceive our lives is the same. We all want to create conditions that let experience speak in a way that heals. The whole idea of theory and method is to get close to that experience, to honor the sacredness of the therapeutic relationship. Intimate moments of engagement Martin Buber called "I–Thou." Language and words can only hope to approximate this experience, although some come closer than others. That's why I find writing such a powerful tool. Ultimately the only authentic speech is silence. Writing is often better able to capture and express the sense of the ineffable about our work.

The idea of this book is to get close to the experience we call addiction. Consequently, this is, more than anything, a book about relationships. It is a collection of people's experiences with alcohol and drugs and I–Thou encounters in therapy and recovery. As their stories unfold a definition of addiction emerges, as well as a language that describes it.

WORKING ASSUMPTIONS

> Trying to describe the process of becoming an alcoholic is like trying to describe air. It's too big and mysterious and pervasive to be defined. Alcohol is everywhere in your life, omnipresent, and you're both aware and unaware of it almost all the time; all you know is you'd die without it, and there is no simple reason why this happens, no single moment, no physiological event that pushes the heavy drinker across a concrete line into alcoholism. It's a slow, gradual, insidious, elusive *becoming*.
>
> —CAROLINE KNAPP

In her book *Drinking: A Love Story*, Caroline Knapp (1996) describes her own process of becoming addicted—from drinking as mere social convention, a companion on the path to self-enlightenment, to viewing alcohol as the single most important relationship in her life, something she couldn't fathom living without.

The present book will not resolve the questions "What is addiction?" and "How does one become addicted?" However, it does hope to expand our understanding of the experience of addiction, and broaden our descriptions of alcoholism, substance abuse, and other addictive phenomena. Consequently, the book does not present a comprehensive theory of alcoholism and chemical dependency or new method of treatment. We already have more than we need or know what to do with. It merely attempts to locate a set of ideas about psychotherapy and narrative practices that help people address some of the problems they face in recovery—ideas that readers can easily apply to their own lives and experiences.

In addition to fleshing out a *working* definition of addiction, the remainder of this chapter presents a list of principles, biases, and assumptions that will help map out some of the landscape covered, and offer the reader a kind of glossary for a number of, what I call, "tent terms" used throughout the book.

One Addiction: The Addiction to Control

"At the heart all addictions," writes Knapp, "are driven by the same impulses and most accomplish the same goals; you just use a different substance or take a slightly different path to get there" (1996, p. 134). I have been using the terms addiction, alcoholism, and chemical dependency interchangeably because one of this book's fundamental premises is that there is *one addiction—the addiction to control*. Alcohol, marijuana, cocaine, heroin, and other (what I call) "tissue-based" substances, as well as addictive processes such as certain relationships and types of behavior (e.g., eating, gambling, or debting), all are mood-altering technologies. Certainly some of the dynamics and specific interventions will vary according to the substances abused, but the overall treatment framework will remain unchanged.

Nor, as a quick aside, is it just the "high" alcohol or chemicals provide that is hard to give up; a gesture associated with a particular drug or habit roots the experience in the addict's experience of selfhood and can be just as captivating and difficult for the person to let go of:

> I loved the sounds of drink: the slide of the cork as it eased out of the wine bottle, the distinct glug glug of booze pouring into a glass, the clatter of ice cubes in a tumbler. I loved the rituals, the camaraderie of drinking with others, the warming, melting feelings of ease and courage it gave me. . . . [D]rinking seemed as natural as breathing, an ordinary part of social convention, a simple prop. (Knapp, 1996, pp. 6–7)

The issue of control—over actions, feelings, and other people's behavior—is central to any addiction or compulsion. Alcohol and other substances help people believe they have control over events. People suffering from addiction, says Geneen Roth, cannot bear to surrender to the truth of their lack of control for fear it will bring the pain they felt when they were open to love and it wasn't there; addiction at its most fundamental is lack of love: "Our compulsions help us avoid the feeling that no one is *really* there for us. We become compulsive to put someone there for us" (1991, p. 21).

Escape from pain and the illusion of control are core issues for all addicts and persons in recovery. For the addicted person consuming alcohol (or their drug of choice) provides an extraordinary affective experience. Feelings of power, freedom, connectedness, and safety are the primary characters in this compelling drama. According to therapist Roget Lockard, "This experience is so potent and consistent that the individual prioritizes the act of drinking to provide these feelings. In effect, what has happened is the discovery of an *instrument* for the manipulation of feeling states—the discovery of a *technology of feelings management*" (1993, p. 3; emphasis added). For Miranda (the girl whose letter was presented in the Prologue), being under the influence of drugs and alcohol allowed her access to powerful feelings of anger and rage that countered cultural messages she received dictating acceptable and unacceptable ways for girls to act. Drinking and drug use also provided her with a sense of comfort and security in an otherwise unsafe world.

Once we accept the premise that alcohol and other mood-altering chemicals are a technology of feelings management, we must recognize that, like all technologies, they come with a body of laws or principles that govern people's behavior and actions when operating under their influence. The problem is that most addicts and alcoholics drink or use drugs themselves because they're tired of "playing by the rules." Alcohol provides the freedom and power to ignore social convention—to be who they want to be and feel how they want to feel. It's a rude awakening when a person discovers that the mood-altering technology they've always depended on to help them escape or feel more in control of their environment comes with its own set of rules and laws that severely restrict the consumer's choices and options for living.

A gifted and talented artisan who is also addicted to heroin cannot contemplate leaving a job she hates in order to pursue her craft because she can't be without the money she needs for her fix—even for one night. An alcoholic father wants to fulfill the promise he made to his son to spend the day at the ballpark together. However, his addiction reminds him he must stop at the bar on his way for just a couple of drinks—stopping at "just a couple" being something he's tried to do every day for many years without success. As the Chinese proverb tells us, "First the person takes a drink, then the drink takes a drink, and finally the drink takes the person." Drugs and alcohol come to represent yet another area of the alcoholic's or drug addict's life in which he or she is no longer in charge.

The road to recovery, which will occupy more pages of this book than my descriptions of people's drinking problems, takes a similar path—in which the alcoholic moves from a position of "I cannot control my drinking," through "I cannot drink," to "I can *not* drink."

More will be said about "controlled drinking" in the following chapters, but it bears comment that obviously some alcoholics are able to exercise control over their drinking on some occasions, whereas others who can no longer control their drinking could at one time. Clearly, changes in a person's ability to exert influence over his or her own use of chemicals can be explained, in part, by the natural progression of addiction or thickening of its story plot in a person's life. However, it may also be a result of the strong sense of shame associated, in our culture, with not being able to control any part of our personal world. In therapy, the emphasis on helping clients' develop self-control and belief in their ability as individuals to exert "free will" in any situation can interfere with recovery. This is especially troublesome when either the client, the therapist, or both feel that a person *should* be able to control his or her drinking and would be able to if only he or she could find the proper solution to certain problems or the right approach. Even among therapists who recognize that controlled drinking is not possible for their client and abstinence must be the goal, self-control, observes Stephanie Brown (1985), often remains the ideal and those who can't achieve it are viewed as weak or flawed.

Toward a Working Definition of Addiction

Dylan Thomas said that an alcoholic was someone you don't like who drinks as much as you do. Current metaphors and myths view the chemically dependent client as "bad" (i.e., immoral), "crazy," "stupid," or "sick." As one colleague, in recovery herself, pointed out to me, alcoholics don't do much to dispel these misconceptions and bear some responsibility for them, as they often, when under the influence, act crazily, do and say stupid things, and can—especially toward the end of their drinking—engage in bizarre and unusual behavior. However, I prefer to regard clients who are suffering from these types of troubles as blocked.

The "disease" (or biological) model can be a useful metaphor for families trying to break out of the cycles of shame and blame that grip persons facing problems with drugs and alcohol, but it does not explain the complexity of the phenomenon we call addiction. More important than how I define or label a problem is how I position myself in relation to it. Years of experience have helped me come to the understanding that I am as powerless over my clients and their drinking as they are, and I try and model that understanding in my relationships with them.

The word "addict," in Latin, means toward (*ad*) voice (*dict*), and I find that people often prefer to listen to (or move toward) that voice, rather than their own or that of the therapist.* Put another way, the alcoholic is caught in an epistemological bind:

> For those whose relationship with alcohol will eventually manifest as addictive, the use of alcohol is proving to answer a question perhaps even more fundamental than "how can I manage my feeling states?" and that is, "*who am I?*" In other words, the relationship with alcohol makes a critically significant contribution to the experience of a more adequate identity for the consumer, such that over time the use of alcohol and the experience of authentic self seem to be inseparable.

Another Voice: A Handbook on Addiction, Recovery, and the Survival of the Human Species is the title of a manuscript in preparation by addictions therapist and author Roget Lockard (1999).

For some drinkers, this "identity consolidation" aspect happens almost instantaneously; for others it accumulates gradually over varying time spans. Eventually, however, the experience of existential adequacy is absolutely contingent on the drinking of alcohol. It is this development that gives the behavior the remarkable *author*ity, as it were, to overrule common sense—if the very experience of selfhood seems at stake, then virtually all other considerations become subordinate. (Lockard, 1985a, p. 3; emphasis added)

This description of a person's alcoholic belief system has profound consequences for treatment. The implication is that people drink for good reasons. Or, as a client once explained it, "Jon, the best idea I ever had in the world was to get sober. The second best idea I ever had was to pick up a drink." These themes will be explored fully later in this book; here, I merely note that there is a false dualistic logic—which AA calls "all or nothing" or "drinking thinking"—that keeps the addict blocked, unable to see other options other than living with drinking or dying without it.

Problem Drinking versus Addiction

There is in both the psychotherapy and recovery communities much debate over the dividing line between substance abuse or problem drinking, on the one hand, and substance dependence or addiction, on the other. However, I find when it comes to drugs and alcohol we often don't know what kind of problem we're dealing with until we try to do something about it.

For the purposes of this inquiry I will keep things simple. Most of us can relate to the experience of abuse. Even a child who makes one too many unauthorized withdrawals from the cookie jar can identify with this experience, for example, the physical hangover—upset tummy and sugar headache—that reminds the child it has had one too many. A problem develops once a pattern of abuse has been established. While the frequency of a person's abuses and volume of alcohol or drugs consumed in any given episode is often relevant when we are trying to situate a person on a continuum of addiction or when we are treating their medical symptoms, it is not as important for identifying a problem. The person who drinks to the point of intoxication on every occasion that alcohol is present is in trouble regardless of how often the opportunity presents itself or how much of a given substance it takes for him or her to achieve the desired state of euphoria.

Clinicians who invest a great deal of time determining the volume and frequency of a person's consumption are missing the distinction between individual acts of drinking or drug abuse and alcoholism or addiction. The issue gets blurry when we are trying to determine when a person crosses over the invisible line from problem use to full-fledged addiction. Many find the discussion of a dividing line between substance abuse and addiction profoundly misleading. Indeed, talking about crossing over the invisible line from "problem use" to "addiction" is like talking about crossing over the invisible line between emphysema and lung cancer. They are two distinct plights, which just happen to share many experiential and circumstantial features.[8] While I agree with the supposition that substance abuse and addiction are two separate phenomena, because they present clinicians with so many common features I still find this a useful way of conceptualizing them.

Again, simplicity seems prudent, as I do not intend to spend much time arguing the minutiae of these categories, especially since this book is more concerned with how to help people who are suffering from these kinds of problems. The most useful answer to this dilemma I've found is that, for the problem drinker or drug abuser, once she's determined she has a problem with alcohol or drugs she'll stop, or at least make adjustments to prevent further problems from developing. This point is often reached when a person reaches a crossroads where the solutions to her problems provided by chemicals are overshadowed by the problems that these substances create in her life. Lockard (1985b) calls this "the point of common sense." The problem drinker who makes an effort to change is usually successful—maybe not right away, and maybe not without help, but eventually her patterns of abuse are arrested. The addict is the person who continues to use substances beyond "the point of common sense" despite her best efforts to quit or control her drinking and despite many people's best efforts to help her.

Simplifying even further we might say, along with Knapp (1996), that "when you're drinking, the dividing line between you and real trouble always manages to fall just beyond where you stand" (p. 30).

Hitting Bottom

"Hitting bottom" is another "tent term" found in most addictions therapy and treatment and is used here as well. This experience, which will be explored in more depth especially in the book's second part, consists, according to Lockard (1993), of three events that converge simultaneously in the life of an addict: (1) the intersection of pain and understanding; (2) the ownership of powerlessness; and (3) an occasion where the individual is no longer willing to live with the person he or she has become—what AA calls "deflation at depth."

Several crucial points about these ingredients: First, the person's understanding may be incorrect. People often hit bottom in a resounding and painful fashion, and then proceed to take action based on a totally mistaken understanding of their situation, such as "My life depends on learning to control my drinking better!" When a person draws this conclusion from a life-threatening experience with alcohol or drugs, recovery cannot follow. Second, powerlessness (a concept that will be discussed in more depth in Chapter 4) is manifested in different ways at different stages of recovery. The most adequate generic definition of powerlessness in this context, writes Lockard (1993), might read: "*I am powerless to achieve fulfillment through the exercise of control*" (p. 13). Third, the last point, regarding those individuals who are no longer being able to live with the persons they've become, has a spiritual quality referred to in AA as "the gift of desperation." This is for Lockard and for me the most viscerally satisfactory characterization of hitting bottom, because it captures the existential emergency at the heart of the experience: "Imagine that someone has held your head under water for the last 90 seconds or so, what are you prepared to do now on behalf of being able to breath? Well, of course, anything! Because you are feeling that your survival—the continued viability of your elemental self—is at stake" (R. Lockard, personal communication, 1999). This is the experience of people in advanced stages of addiction when they are confronted with the prospect of relinquishing their drugs—or whatever substance or experience their addiction has coalesced around. Paradoxically, this is where healing must start if their problem is to be not merely managed but transformed.

PART I

Writing for Our Lives

All suffering is bearable if it is seen as part of a story.
—Isak Dinesen

CHAPTER 1

A Sobriety
of Literary Merit

> Literature is no one's private ground; literature is common
> ground. Let us trespass freely and fearlessly and find our
> own way for ourselves.
>
> —VIRGINIA WOOLF

KAREN'S STORY: ACT I

I remember the day Karen came into my office. Fashionably dressed in
Patagonia workout gear, Karen had an athletic build from her job as a
swimming instructor at a local community center. She arrived with a
toddler in tow. Although her child seemed content in his stroller with a
bottle and was, as his mother commented, "having a good day," Karen
appeared frazzled. When she made the appointment she said she'd
wanted the entire family to come because, as she said, "They were having trouble getting along." Karen said that her family consisted of herself, her husband, their four children ages 9, 10, 12, and their new 14-
month-old baby. The oldest three, two girls and a boy, were Karen's
from a prior marriage. She said their father was no longer in their lives
and that her oldest son, Sean, seemed to be having a particularly difficult
time with his feelings about that lately. Karen felt this was creating tension between him and his stepfather and that their fighting had everyone
else on edge, left Karen feeling "depressed," and was causing "terrible
arguments" between her and her husband about how to "manage it all."
Karen was disappointed about not being able to find a strategy for getting her entire family to come to the session with her. Eventually she de-

cided to go anyway on her own with the baby so she could at least "get things started" and perhaps give me some background into the problems they were having.

Karen was able to get everyone to attend our next appointment. Theirs was clearly a very loving family. Her children seemed to genuinely care for one another and showered lots of affection on Douglas, their new baby brother. Karen and her husband, Robert, were understandably nervous, having their whole brood on display in a therapist's office, but in spite of their anxiety they were respectful of one another and the children. Karen and her husband talked about how exhausted they were all the time from mediating disputes between the kids. Robert said that no matter how hard he tried he couldn't seem to do anything right in the eyes of his oldest son who, until recently, had always gotten along with him.

Robert was the only father Sean and the girls had ever known. Their biological father was a Vietnam veteran who because of the emotional damage suffered in the war had had a severe breakdown and left the family when the kids were little. Karen's ex-husband had also been violent toward her. Karen worried about Sean being old enough to remember that. Karen had tried to maintain a relationship with her ex-husband and his family so the children could have him in their lives, but he started stalking her and her new husband and then, violating a restraining order, showed up at the children's school and became abusive and threatening toward the principal when he wouldn't let him take the kids out of class and leave the grounds with him.

Karen felt that her son was having trouble making new friends because of his anger about these experiences and the fact that the family had just moved to the area, so that Robert, a junior executive in a manufacturing company, could take a new position. Another consequence of the move was that the couple were still living out of suitcases in close quarters with their children—Karen and Robert in the living room with the 1-year-old, and the remaining children upstairs in the three bedrooms, leaving Karen and her husband with little emotional or physical space for themselves.

Compounding the family's stress was an incident several years ago in which Robert suffered a broken back in a mountain climbing accident. Karen and he had met while rock climbing and used to enjoy spending time doing physical activities of all kinds together. Robert, now "fully recovered," was in chronic pain that significantly curtailed his mobility and, doctors said, would in all likelihood remain with him throughout his life. Robert said the pain from his injury left him with little patience and accounted for his irritability with the children after a long workday. Karen feared that Robert would never be the same man and would end up leaving the marriage because of the stress and aggravations at home. In our first meeting, Karen also shared her resentment about the fact that when she and Robert married they wanted to have a baby together, but now she felt alone in raising her youngest child—a place she had already been three times over in her first marriage and did not want to return to.

Together we came up with a plan. I emphasized the need for Karen and Robert to set firmer limits on the children and make time for themselves. What we undertook, in the language of Robert's corporate culture, was a course of radical "organizational change." Karen and Robert took a bedroom for themselves (something they hadn't done sooner because they felt guilty about making the kids move), and I encouraged them to start taking daily walks together with and without the baby.

What we did was simply normalize a lot of their stress as stemming from too many people living in a small house, Robert's injury, and the oldest boy getting to an age where all sons become more curious about their fathers' lives and childhood experiences. Children at that age are looking for role models to help them with their passage into adulthood, which in their son's instance left him wondering where his father was and why he left him. What's more, he had reached an age where he was old enough to understand the circumstances surrounding his father's absence—to experience the reality and finiteness of it.

Sean and Robert came in for several sessions together to discuss the impact of these events on their relationship. Sean was able to express the loss even positive encounters between him and his stepfather stirred up. Sean perceived his relationship with Robert as a betrayal of his father, even though he acknowledged that Robert was the only "real Dad" he'd ever had and couldn't imagine his life without him. A discussion with all the children resulted in Karen and the kids talking for the first time about what the children remembered about their father and their life before Robert came along. This seemed to allay some of Karen's fears and alleviate some of her guilt about having permanently damaged her children by not leaving her first husband sooner. All of the children, the girls especially, said they were proud of their mother for having gotten out of a bad situation and looking out for them. They also made it clear that they spent more time thinking about how much better things were now than they did dwelling on the past.

Finally, in several couple's sessions, Karen and Robert aired the resentment they were feeling toward one another and expressed their concerns about the future. Karen shared her fear that if things did not improve Robert might abandon the family. That had, after all, happened to her once already. Robert responded, in ironic fashion, that he had been walking around feeling afraid that Karen might no longer want him—that she might leave him for someone else because he wasn't the same man she'd married. And, in an outcome usually reserved for journal articles and conference presentations, Robert accepted my referral to a pain management group in the hospital I was working in and stuck with it. He also agreed to see a therapist who helped him master the relaxation exercises he learned in group and also helped him develop strategies to better manage his stress at the job and in family life. Things improved dramatically. All of us considered it a successful therapy.

KAREN'S STORY: ACT II

Shortly after we stopped meeting, Karen called. She said in spite of how much improved things were she still felt depressed and wanted to come see me, this time by herself. In this meeting she confided that sometimes her husband got embarrassed by her behavior when they went out together. She said the evening always started out fine but in the end she would inevitably "cut into him" with biting sarcasm or become openly abusive and insulting. She said she became increasingly loud and boisterous when they fought, and whenever she started an argument she always created a scene. Afterward she was remorseful and apologetic, but by then the damage was done. When I asked to hear more about those incidents it turned out that alcohol played a significant role. She said she was better off when they didn't go out and drank at home instead. The best times, Karen explained, were the rare occasions when she refrained from drinking at all, but even then she always had to be sure there was alcohol in the house and became panicked if there wasn't any. Her husband sometimes picked up a six-pack of her favorite brand of beer from the package store on his way home from work so they could "party together," but on nights he didn't do that Karen would drink a six-pack of "whatever was in the house," by herself. Karen also smoked pot. She got high every morning except on the days she had to work, in which case she waited until she got home. Karen's husband didn't approve of her using marijuana. He used to smoke with her, but now that they had a new baby and were getting older he felt it was no longer worth the hassle and risk. He also felt that they were being hypocritical, given the antidrug messages they were always giving the children. Karen didn't feel good about her pot smoking either but felt that it made her less anxious without the angry side effects of drinking.

I don't know why Karen's problems with alcohol or drugs didn't come up in any of our previous conversations. Karen certainly didn't fit my idea of an addict (an attitude on my part that could only contribute to her ambivalence about disclosing her concerns about her drinking and pot smoking, decreasing the chances of their being attended to even more). I can't remember if I asked about Karen's or her husband's drinking habits or not. Sometimes even if you ask the right questions people aren't ready to answer them. Frequently, after discussing with people the problems they are ready to talk about, and if they find me a useful resource or capable ally, I find myself being invited into conversations that are more difficult for them to have. These might include their concerns about their own or a loved one's drinking, or other sources of shame and angst. But, then again, oftentimes people aren't aware there's a problem to begin with.

In Karen's case, if I had reason to inquire about her drinking habits I'm certain Karen would have said they weren't anything to be concerned about, which from her point of view, at the time, was true. Karen's husband clearly didn't think Karen's drinking was a problem either. In a subsequent session he commented that he saw the issue as one of "self-control" and "restraint" rather than seeing it as Karen having a problem with "drinking" or "alcohol." He felt they would be fine if they just made a commitment to take better physical care of themselves and wanted to help Karen do that. He was even willing to cut back with her so she wouldn't have to do it by herself. He also thought Karen was depressed about things that happened in her past and hoped therapy would help her with those troubles.

However, the next series of meetings and conversations between Karen and me did revolve around the theme of alcohol and drugs because, not surprisingly, it turned out that alcohol and drugs played a significant role in Karen's past. Many of her most painful experiences took place while she was drunk or high. Some years earlier Karen had dropped out of a group a former therapist had sent her to for her drinking because, as she put it, "I didn't feel I belonged there." Then, she said, she stopped going to therapy because of a "personality conflict" and her disagreement with her former therapist's diagnosis of her alcoholism. Karen had difficulty viewing her drinking as alcoholic or her drug use as problematic, because she was able to function at home and work and was able to stop drinking when she was pregnant. Although much of the time, when she made the effort, she was able to exercise choice about whether to drink or not, once she started, she felt compelled to finish whatever alcohol was in the house. Karen described the onset of her addiction:

"When I was 13 nobody liked me. Later it was because I had such a bad attitude, hanging out with all the delinquents and troublemakers. But then I always felt like a round peg trying to fit into a square hole. Always that phrase just fit me. I was shy, or else a total smart aleck; nobody liked me and no one wanted to be my friend. I was always the last one picked in sports. I never went to dances or even a party. Drinking was the hidden key. That was it. That was the answer. That was what was missing—that feeling of 'I'm OK' just settled over me when I drank. It felt warm.

"I was at a sleep-over and a little bottle was going around. And so I said, 'To hell with it, this is my way in,' and then I discovered that I was the best one at it. No one could drink more than me. I remember scaring the other girls. That was it. I was the best. I was the most popular person there. All my inhibitions left. I had a rush of self-confidence. I could go and do it all. The one friend I always could count on was with me.

"When I was seventeen I got into pot and other drugs, especially acid. These helped me escape and were part of an older crowd I hung out with—a more rebellious group—but it wasn't the same as alcohol. These I knew I could give up if I had to and did. But I would rather die than stop drinking. There was no question—what would be the point of living?"

Trauma and Addiction

Abused and exploited by men throughout her life, Karen's alcoholism can be appreciated as both an act of compliance and resignation—that is, a prescription for sexual abuse and trauma—and at the same time an act of passive rebellion for her. Although Karen wanted to stop drinking, she described a tremendous fear of AA and abstinence, both of which equaled the loss of herself and the loss of control.

At this juncture in treatment, I asked Karen to write a "good-bye" letter to her addiction. I suggested that she write a letter that would help her accomplish this, while honoring the primacy and self-preserving role drinking had played in her life.

Karen's Letter

A good-bye letter to alcohol:

Needing to write this letter presupposes a relationship between us. I have to be honest and say that there has been one (although I may deny it if questioned). I used you to cope during (or starting) in my teens. During our 20-year relationship we were together sometimes on a daily basis and other times much less—but I always came back to you—you of course always being faithfully available.

Now its time to say good-bye—I have high aspirations and you are unable to reach them due to your inherent characteristics. You wont miss me—I will miss you as I reach my higher goals.

This letter was followed by 3 months of successful sobriety and attendance at AA, at which point Karen relapsed. She was attending meetings erratically and had stopped going to her home group, an all-women's meeting, altogether.

I asked Karen if she would mind drafting a second communication to alcohol. She came to therapy with her letter doubling as a bookmark in a copy of Harriet Lerner's *The Dance of Anger* (1985) and proclaimed:

"I don't want to be so angry anymore. I'm angry at my anger. I used to be ashamed of my drinking. Now I feel shame about my anger, especially when it spills over and impacts on my relationship to my children. I'm angry at what it took from me my whole life. Twenty years could have been different. I was angry at the women at the meeting who had so much support and help from their families when they were kids. I'm angry at God."

Then she read me her letter:

Karen's Second Correspondence

As an excuse to have another fling with you I became angry with [my husband] and set out to show him how close we could be—on Sept. 2 we again had an affair that left me ashamed and hurt—you of course were unaffected. I don't know what, if anything, I proved to [my husband] but I proved to myself that I am addicted to the deceit that you peddle. I have been sober since and enjoy the clarity and self-respect that I have when not with you. By the grace of God, being in AA, and becoming my real self I will never again visit your den of deceit. To me you are a slow death—a rapist that takes my pride, self-respect, and future. To castrate you is my goal—you will not have power over me unless I allow it by accepting you back into my life with that first drink.

Implied in many of the interactions described in her letter was Karen's equation of abstinence and sobriety with an aggressive and hostile move against her husband and family. Karen was having a hard time with recommendations that she attend more AA meetings and put herself and her sobriety first, ideas she'd received from other women in AA. These ideas ran counter to the dictates of her female role at home and in the community, and it was important for both of us to understand how messages from the larger culture affected her treatment. Karen and I discussed how her recovery might allow her to become the subject of her own experience and to "say no" to the expectations of others without guilt and fear of rejection.[1]

This theme of needing to be able to say no, to listen to her own voice, colored Karen's experience of sexual intimacy as well. At the time, Karen described desperately wanting her body back and said that after drinking she was able to have sex without panic attacks and "flashbacks" for the first time in months. We discussed Karen's relapse from the standpoint of narration as involving, like her sexual trauma, a cast of three of what Dusty Miller calls the triadic self: a voice who says, "I don't care if this hurts you, I want to drink" (the perpetrator); a second who responds, "I don't want to drink, this is going to hurt me" (the innocent victim); and a third who says, "I know this is not good for you, but what do you want me to do? I need this" (the nonprotecting bystander).[2]

Regarding Karen's spiritual quandary—her anger at God—I suggested she might view her rage and despair as a form of prayer and "conscious contact" with her higher power—"owned and accepted, it's your friend and ally; denied, it undermines your sobriety." This was a reference to the 11th step of AA: "*Sought through prayer and meditation to improve our conscious contact with God as we understood her/him, praying only for the knowledge of her/his will and the power to carry that out.*"

Karen, who had always had a strong religious faith, often found her spiritual beliefs and values at odds with her emotional needs and desires. Understanding what the two might contribute to each other and creating opportunities for her to reconcile them, to experience them together, was an important part of the therapy and her healing.

Karen's willingness to explore AA, a short-term women's support group for survivors of sexual abuse, and an ongoing therapy group for individuals in recovery were other significant developments in her self-care. Creating a space for a "woman's voice" and perspective in her therapy and being able to come together with other alcoholics and women struggling with these issues resulted in Karen feeling less isolated and alone and created a safe environment for her to incorporate new and more positive descriptions of herself.

As John Briere (1989) reminds us, the bind for clients in all trauma-focused and shame-based therapy, which alcoholism treatment in general and Karen's therapy in particular both qualify as, is that in order to recover from injuries sustained in one or more abusive childhood relationships ultimately each of these clients must enter into what is, in some ways, an equally threatening relationship as an adult. Karen's group work had a positive effect on her individual therapy, changing the structure of our relationship from one that in certain respects paralleled the dynamics of her abuse—that is, Karen meeting alone with a man to talk about "secrets"—to a more transparent and open one.

At her 1-year sober "anniversary," Karen was the speaker at an AA meeting attended by all the members of her therapy group and her husband. The celebration marked a significant shift in her recovery and represented another important retelling of her life story.

The diversity of themes and modes of treatment represented in Karen's therapy and in this book in general, ambitious as they may seem, feel necessary. This is how addiction and the problems associated with it present to the therapist. Chemical dependency rarely unfolds in therapy in a timely fashion as a distinct or isolated problem but shows up in more complex ways, and at inopportune moments, in our work—sometimes making therapy with an already challenging family, couple, or individual that much more difficult. It is a messy process.

Information about a parent's abuse of narcotics or drunken binges may be disclosed (unexpectedly) during a quiet moment in a child's play session; a man's alcoholism might not surface until, after years of treatment for depression, he decides to try medication that causes dangerous side effects when combined with liquor; or a woman's daily marijuana habit is not discovered until the end of a therapy that focused on helping her overcome a severe trauma history. Alcohol and other drugs, as Caroline Knapp (1996) reminds us, offer people protection from the pain of self-discovery.

THE FIVE STAGES OF RECOVERY

For therapists, suffering is no abstraction. The stories people tell us are often filled with horror and misery. Because of the work we do, we often see people at their most grievous and formidable moments. People, at these times, are severely wounded. They feel fragmented, as though they are missing parts of themselves. Their situations seem hopeless and their lives beyond mending. If one sees, to paraphrase Bernie Siegel (1990), one can witness how noble and beautiful people are when they're going through these painful places and experiences. One sees their strength and wholeness. Therapy—like dreams and prayer—can create a space to hold the broken pieces for safekeeping. It allows us to speak our truth, to think things down to the bone. Writing amplifies and expands people's truths. Letters, like poems, writes Louise Gluck (1994), "do not endure as objects but as presences" (p. 128); indeed, she points out, they make our stories come alive and seem more real. And, as we learned from *The Velveteen Rabbit*, once we are real, our lives and the stories we tell about them never seem broken or ugly except to those who don't understand.

The power of language, says analyst Donald Spence, is that by putting our experiences into words we give them authenticity. Therapy, according to Spence, is about helping people find a narrative home for their words. Like a good story, interpretations are meant to help people construct narratives that give new meaning to their experience and their lives. As Spence (1982) writes, they are "designed to open up new possibilities, to bring ideas together in a new and potentially evocative combination" (p. 178). My reading of Karen's difficulty with AA and my invitation to help her quit drinking by asking her to compose a letter created a new cluster of ideas, a cluster that had probably never been expressed in exactly that way. Asking her to write the "good-bye" letter to alcohol and the follow-up letter to her relapse was an attempt to give responsibility for her decisions and choices back to her—to transform disclaimed actions into ones for which Karen would feel some accountability.

The ideas Karen's letters created, her second correspondence in particular, provided us with a new awareness of the connections in Karen's life between sex, violence, alcohol, and abuse. The letters offered us new ways of understanding these connections in Karen's past and present, as well as creating the possibility of our finding a different way to talk about them in her future.

The reason I prefer to have the people write letters to their addiction is that I find this helps me understand the particular meaning their substance use holds for them much better than a "formal" alcohol or drug assessment could do. It also allows me to collaborate with people on a course of action—a "treatment plan"—that takes into account their view of their problem and is firmly grounded in each person's experience of her relationship with chemicals. I also, when asked to write up my impressions of a client's relationship to alcohol or drugs, often prefer to do it in the form of a letter.

These letters don't always result in people ending their relationship with an addiction. Sometimes they result in a process of bargaining with it. These conversations are often of a spiritual nature, as one client wrote in a letter to alcohol: "Whenever I'm around you I find myself on my knees hugging the toilet praying, 'God, if you just get me out of this mess I will never drink that much again.' " At other times they end up writing what could only be viewed as a kind of daily affirmation for a drunk or stoned lifestyle, like this letter written to marijuana from a teenager during her stay in a drug treatment center:

Dear Ganja,

Hello old friend, what's up? It's been a long time since we last saw each other. I miss you. I want you back in my arms. Everyone here wants me to forget about you, but I won't. I miss hanging out with you, and the familiar way you made me laugh. I miss the way you cheered me up—brightening even the darkest day—and the way you made me feel so accepted all the time.

As a result of being locked up in this program, I will be unable to see you and smile at your great jokes. Hopefully I will be out soon, and we will be able to party with each other again. I can't wait to get home to see you. You bring me a kind of happiness no one else can, and I can't find anywhere else. When I get out we'll spend every minute of our day together. I will be yours and yours only, all day and all night.

Love Always,

Gwen

When asking clients to participate in such an exercise, therapists need to keep their own expectations in check and not place too much emphasis on outcome. Our training teaches us to look for results—"What's changed and how much?" However, the letters I invite clients to write and the other narrative practices I employ in my work are not prescriptions designed to bring about a certain effect. They are rituals meant to invoke a relationship and give people a renewed sense of purpose in their lives.

Letters serve their author much as a journal serves its writer or a poem the poet. In Myerhoff's words, they provide "a frame surrounding internal chaos"—a clinical hope chest—where the most cherished items are placed for safekeeping (1982b, p. 353). Collectively, the letters and stories gathered here represent an archaeology of therapy, written in what Mary Douglas (1982) would call a "grammar of agency," transforming the addict's experience from the passive to the active voice.

In all of these therapies, issues with drugs and alcohol are themes that surface in clients' stories and writings and are a primary component of the work. They're part of the person's "inner relational melodies":

> The alcoholic sings to the bottle, rages at it, mourns its passing, and brightens at its return. We personify what we are most intimately connected with. Personifying is our most fundamental mode—it is what makes us human. When we lose the capacity to personify, to, as Buber says, "speak the primary word you," when we relate to those most intimate to us in a detached way and see them only as a means to getting what we want, we have lost part of our humanity. (Jones, 1991, p. 129)

Therapy at these moments is about restoring or, from the standpoint of writing, restorying clients' capacity for concern and faith in their own humanity—a process described by analyst Hans Loewald (1980) and expanded on by Roy Schafer (1992, p. 307) as "safeguarding a future for that person."

I have always conceptualized addictions treatment, which Lockard views as a disorder of the spirit (i.e., alcoholism) and its related disorders of the heart (i.e., coalcoholism/codependency),[3] as a form of grief work. Perhaps the same argument could be made for most therapies; however, with addiction the connections are particularly strong ones, not the least of which are the stages of *denial, anger, bargaining, acceptance*, and *letting go* that individuals and families move through in recovery.

As much as I sometimes wish I did, I don't have a "model" in my head of how it's all supposed to work or come together. In its current form, what I am proposing is a tapestry or patchwork quilt of ideas about treating substance abuse that contrasts with more systematic theories of alcoholism and addiction. Following White and Epston (1990), this book proposes a sobriety of "literary merit."

The following chapters presents some of my own and my clients' letters in a way that gives readers insight into some of the common experiences people encounter in their sojourn from addiction to recovery. It will also illustrate how narrative therapy can change the way we conceptualize and think about this passage.

CHAPTER 2

Letters of Invitation
and Dismissal

No matter how badly we think life has beaten us, we still
cling to the idea that acceptance and surrender are a kind
of hopeless giving-in, a weakness of character. Not so!
Acceptance means simply admitting there are things we
cannot change. Accepting them puts an end to our futile
struggles and frees our thoughts and energy to work on
things that can be changed.
—*ONE DAY AT A TIME* (Al-Anon Book of Daily
Meditations and Readings)

Freedom is what you do with what's been done to you.
—JEAN-PAUL SARTRE

The beginning of every therapy relationship is filled with hope and dread
for the client and the therapist.[1] For individuals trying to overcome an
addiction, sitting in a therapist's office for the first time (or during an
initial appointment) might raise fears of moral judgment. This may include the fear of being seen as degenerate because they can't control
their drinking and so place alcohol before their family or career, or the
anxiety that some shameful way they feel about themselves might be revealed, or the terror that some act they committed while under the influence of drugs or alcohol might be found out. At the same time, this
dread may be offset by the hope that they may finally have found a place
where they can get help with their addiction and be at peace with themselves. The letters I ask people to craft in these initial phases of therapy

are intended to flesh out their hopes and fears in a way that will facilitate further discussion of them.

This chapter will try to answer some of the more common questions that might arise about the use of letter writing in the therapy context. However, readers more interested in these practices, in particular, and the use of writing, in general, are referred to Chapter 12, where these issues are addressed in more detail. Here I am more likely to comment on the timing of a letter, when, for example, in a specific therapy relationship such a ritual or exercise was introduced. For answers to questions such as how I know whether it's good timing or bad to introduce these concepts to a client or what I do if a person seems reluctant to try these ideas that I think would be useful, or other questions as to the politics and history of these ideas, I would refer readers to the aforementioned chapter.

By presenting my thoughts in this way, I do not mean to give readers the impression that I use writing more than talking in my consultations with people. While I do not value one practice more than the other, I use speech more than writing in my work. I talk with all people who seek my help, but I do not correspond, or introduce writing practices, with everyone I see in therapy. Words in a letter experienced outside the context of a concerned and caring relationship ring hollow. As David Treadway (1989) noted, writing a letter does not heal the wound. It simply acknowledges it. The scar remains. In my first meeting with a person struggling to overcome an addiction or any other problem, my initial remarks rarely pertain to a letter. What I find myself speaking to more often is how alone people seem with their pain, how much hurt and fear they've had to face on their own. Therapy, I explain, may not bring them immediate relief from their problems, but at least they will no longer have to face them by themselves.

HOLLY: ACID, A LOVE STORY

Holly was a 17-year-old young woman who was referred to me by her parents because she had been suspended from high school for breaking her school's drug policy. Holly was not interested in getting help or changing her relationship with chemicals, as her letter makes clear.

Holly's Good-Bye Letter to Drugs

Dear acid,

I want to thank you for the great times you've given me. When there was a boring night or day, you came along and gave me some good times. you made me laugh. you put me into a different world when I really needed it. you brought me up when I was down. I like how you only cost $15 and give me an enjoyment that lasted for a while and was just so cool. It is like something I have never experienced before. I love you!!!!

holly

As discussed in the Prologue, this exercise helps me and my client honor the important role that their relationship with drugs and alcohol holds in their lives. However, I've included Holly's correspondence here, because, in her case, in addition to giving us both a sense of what we were up against, her letter prevented me from becoming more invested in change and working harder than my client—a very demoralizing and exhausting position for me as a clinician.

Holly was more committed to doing something about her relationship with food, which she identified as causing more stress in her life than drugs. While she was clearly in trouble because of her drug use, I too was not convinced that Holly's issues with food weren't more problematic than her relationship with substances. Holly had been identified by her physician as an anorexic, and I thought she might have been using drugs, as do many young women her age, as a diuretic. (She didn't drink because, she said, "It makes me fat.") Although Holly wasn't that invested in changing her patterns of behavior around food either, with some encouragement she was at least willing to talk about them. Nor did I feel that we were ignoring her budding drug problem by talking about her weight and her eating, as many of the issues were the same: feelings of embarrassment and shame; not wanting to talk about her eating habits and concealing her behavior from others; feeling deprived and unworthy of love; and longing for a connection to someone or anything that felt safe, reliable, and within her control. Holly did not make, or see, most of these connections herself or, if she did, she didn't see their significance. However, together we developed a common language for understanding her love–hate relationship with food and her body that we eventually found applicable to some of the ways she used drugs.

One conversation in particular helped us break down some of the rigid boundaries Holly maintained between the various troubles she faced. I told Holly that she had been painfully honest with me about her eating disorder but seemed afraid of the same kind of candor in our conversations about drugs and alcohol. She worried, she said, that if "I talk to you about it you might tell my parents and they'll send me to a hospital or rehab." I asked her if that was the worst thing that she could imagine happening. When she responded yes, I reminded her that she had already been hospitalized because of her weight loss on several occasions. That even when she lied about her drug use she had, with the help of substances (that allowed her to achieve increasingly lower and more dangerous body weights), ended up in the hospital anyway. In other words, she was afraid of what had already happened. It seemed to me that the only thing she hadn't tried was making an honest assessment of her entire situation to see what, if anything, about it she might be overlooking and what could be done about it.

The theme of multiple addictions as well as the interface of addiction and other problems—what medicine calls "comorbidity"—will be taken up again later. What I mean to emphasize in Holly's case is the importance of meeting clients where they're at and working with their understanding of the problem before trying to expand their awareness to include other thoughts and ideas. Both these ideas represent sound social work practice, adapted by postmodern, narrative, and other more contemporary therapies. Together they give the reader a sense of how I try and situate myself early in treatment when confronted by a substance abuser's denial, an adolescent's sense of omnipotence and control, or a client's anger and resentment when his or her opinion about the problem and what to do about it differs from my own.

I suggested to Holly that she think of her "good-bye" letter to acid as an invitation rather than a farewell. It was an opportunity to look at what she had to gain as well as what she risked losing if she chose to end her relationship with drugs. Most of all it provided Holly with an opening to examine the way her present lifestyle seemed to feed and nourish acid while leaving her feeling physically and emotionally starved. In Holly's therapy, as with so many clients, saying good-bye to drugs and alcohol was just the beginning.

ANGELA: "RE-STORYING RELATIONSHIPS"

Angela came from a working-class Italian family of five children. Her four siblings were all accomplished doctors or lawyers. Angela, a middle manager in a construction company, felt tremendous pressure to succeed in business and achieve the same stature her brothers and sisters had obtained. Toward this end, she was also taking courses at night for her bachelor's degree. Angela said that her parents were concerned that she wasn't as bright as her siblings and told her when she was in high school that she'd better get married, as only a man could secure a safe future for her. They used this logic as a rationale for not helping Angela pay for college, although they had helped the other children. These conversations were devastating to Angela, who felt deprived of the ability to make her own future.

A year prior to our work together, Angela went on a date with one of the other managers in her division, who proceeded to sexually assault and rape her. Angela saw a rape crisis counselor but decided not to press charges. Angela did tell her supervisor and colleagues, who said that this manager had a history of harassing women employees. Her supervisor offered to transfer Angela—not her assailant—to another division if Angela no longer felt comfortable working with him.

Angela never told her family about what happened because she didn't want to upset them or give anyone the sense that she "couldn't handle things." Angela felt that her family believed nothing ever worked out for her and that this incident would just confirm their beliefs.

In a process that mirrored many of the dynamics as well as her feelings about the sexual assault, Angela kept secret from her family that she had spent the year enduring an abusive relationship with her fiancé, Edgar, whom she thought had a drinking problem. Angela cried when explaining to me that she had already called off her marriage to another man, on the actual day of the wedding, in a relationship that fell apart under similar circumstances 5 years earlier.

Angela first met Edgar after the rape. Edgar had initially been very kind to her and was, according to Angela, the reason she was able to get over that experience: "At a time when I felt horrible about my life and hated myself, Edgar came along and made me feel lovable again." Angela sought therapy to help her better understand and end her pattern of staying in relationships with alcoholic and abusive men. What she described was a desperate fear of being alone:

> "I wish someone in my family understood. There are times after a week like last week [referring to an anxiety attack in the middle of the night] when I just want to curl up in a little ball and disappear—if I could figure out a way to kill myself without anyone knowing it was suicide, without anyone getting hurt. I don't really want to kill myself, it's more like I wish that I'd never been born."

Angela and I talked about her anxiety attacks and suicidal feelings as being about her wanting to undo the past: a desire to make things that never should have happened not have happened. We talked about her not being able to make the events themselves or her feelings about them disappear, and hence her desire to make herself disappear. Suicide for Angela—and others who contemplate these choices—was not only about death or an unrelenting desire to end her life, but an effort at breaking the past's hold on her life.[2]

In a therapy session she attended with her fiancé, Edgar, he agreed to participate in a batterers' group and seek help for his drinking. However, upon completion of the group, as the couple prepared to return to therapy together, Edgar revealed that he was having an affair with another woman and intended to move in with her. Angela told her family the wedding was off.

Months later, Edgar asked Angela if she would consider taking him back. At this juncture in the therapy I asked Angela, who was extremely frustrated with herself for once again considering returning to an abusive relationship, if she would mind my asking her to draft a "good-bye" letter to her "fear of loneliness," the issue that she had identified as pushing her back into this self-destructive situation. The timing of Angela's letter came at a pivotal point in the life of her problem, and in her therapy. "It's funny," wrote Angela, "but this is the first relationship I have broken off first." The letter countered many of the painful beliefs that Angela held about herself, which kept her returning over and over again to harmful relationships:

Angela's Good-Bye to Loneliness

Dear Fear of Loneliness,

You have been an important part of my life for as long as I can remember. I don't know how you arrived or from where you arrived but I believe it's time for us to dissolve our dependency.

There were times, ~~when~~ looking back, when you were the best friend I could have. You were the reason I turned to God for strength, you were the reason I found the church full of Christian friends who care for me, and you were the reason I searched for a dog to give love to me.

However, many of the painful relationships I jumped into were your handiwork also. I looked for anything to fill the gap in my life. I would take any abuse because of you. I feel that way sometimes now, but I now realize that it is only because of my "fear of loneliness." This is why I am stopping this relationship. It's funny but this is the first relationship I have broken off first. Every other relationship's end has been initiated by the other person.

I'm sure there will be times when I feel your presence again in my life, but never again will you be a controlling factor in my decisions about relationships.

Good-bye, Angela

In a conversation about what she'd written, I asked Angela's opinion on loneliness' intentions for her—what did she feel it wanted her to do with her life and how closely were its needs aligned with her own? Angela reported that writing the letter allowed her to take more responsibility for her predicament without taking on more blame or guilt—two emotions her "fear of loneliness" seemed to thrive on. The concept of detox in recovery is usually associated with a physical process where the alcoholic's body rids itself of the noxious effects of chemicals. In psychotherapy, detox is more of an emotional process whereby clients rid themselves of the toxic effects of shame, guilt, and blame.

Angela's letter also provided both of us the opportunity to discuss the dramatic irony of her having turned in therapy to yet another man to help her end her destructive dependencies on men. It gave us both an opportunity to look at the ways in which the configuration of our relationship replicated these patterns (of looking to others for validation and approval) in other relationships in her life, as well as how she might go about changing them and recruiting others to help her.

The remainder of the year was spent working on the source or origins of Angela's loneliness and despair. Over the approximately 11-month period of our relationship, Angela used 12-step recovery groups (Al-Anon and Adult Children of Alcoholics [ACOA]) as well as women's services and other supports, along with our individual and family sessions, to help her rid herself of these unwelcome visitors: abusive men, depression, and loneliness.

Letters of invitation and dismissal are meant to help people examine their relationship with alcohol or, as in Angela's case, an alcoholic and abusive partner, with more honesty and rigor. They invite people to look at what obstacles exist in their life that might be keeping them from seeing their plight with more clarity—that is, in the language of recovery and addiction treatment, to "come to terms with their denial."

"Denial" is a term I try to avoid using because it has become such an overused and overburdened expression in addictions therapy. Denial is not a mental process unique to alcoholic experience, it is a human phenomenon. Staying with the corporeal metaphor provided earlier, from the standpoint of medicine an example of denial would be the way our body goes into shock when it has been in an accident in which the pain caused would be unbearable. In physical trauma our body shuts down, causing our blood pressure to drop and our heart rate to lessen, which keeps our heart from pumping too hard so we lose as little blood as possible. In the case of emotional trauma denial serves the same purpose. It is a way of mentally and spiritually buffering ourselves in the face of emotional tur-

moil and upheaval so great that their full weight is too painful and threatening to bear. Yet, most metaphors that describe people's experience of denial in psychotherapy and recovery involve "breaking through" their
denial or "confronting" persons with the facts of their situation.

Addiction is a shocking truth to discover about oneself, and a form of
trauma in and of itself. This explains why for Karen (see Chapter 1), or any
newly sober person, identifying at an AA meeting was both traumatizing
and liberating. Every alcoholic, and the people whose lives she touches are
traumatized when confronted by the "fact" of her addiction. However,
when wrapped in a narrative and fashioned into a story, the trauma loses
its grip on the person and gives new meaning to his or her life.

The emphasis, in therapy, on confronting people with the "facts" of
their lives so they can come to grips with "reality" or better comprehend
the "truth," stems from the proliferation of Western concepts of reason
found in most contemporary psychologies. This approach has, as White
and Epston observed, "a time-honored tradition that privileges sight
above the other senses—a tradition of 'ocularcentrism' " (1991, p. 34).
Popular expressions such as "I need to see it with my own eyes" or "Believe
what you see, not what you hear" are some of the ways this scientific code
has been disseminated among the populace at large. The introduction of a
letter or other such personal documents in therapy can capitalize on this
social bias: "In many circumstances, writing achieves unsurpassed authority from the fact that it is not heard, but seen" (p. 34). Said another way,
putting things down in "black and white" may give people's experience
more authority in their own or another's "eyes."[3]

A little more than a year after our therapy ended, Angela scheduled
another appointment. When she came in for our session she said she
hadn't slept at all the night before, or the night before that, because Edgar had been in contact with her again. He told Angela his new relationship fell apart shortly after it had started and he now realized "What a
fool I'd been to let you go." He said he loved her. He also told her he
was drinking again and that he wanted to stop, "this time for good," but
didn't think he could do it without her. Even though it had been a year
since they had seen one another he wanted to know if there was any
chance they could get back together and, if her answer was no, could
they at least get together and talk. Angela said she was a "nervous
wreck." In addition to not sleeping she couldn't eat anything either. She
said she was just starting to feel good about herself and feel as though
her life was her own again when Edgar called.

After listening to Angela's plight I asked her to wait a moment. I
went to my files and pulled out a copy of her letter to "loneliness."

Angela was surprised that I still had it. She said she'd carried the original around in her purse for months until it fell apart from wear and tear. She said she thought there might be pieces of it hanging around the bottom of her bag that were still with her, not unlike some of her feelings for Edgar. Rather than viewing these remnants as a sign she was still clinging to an abusive relationship, I suggested she look at these words, dwelling at the bottom of her purse, as compost—helping her transform events she felt ashamed of into an experience from which she could learn and grow.

Angela told me that she was terrified of giving into her fears of being alone and the whole mess starting over again. She experienced the fact that she had any feelings left for Edgar at all as a huge setback—"I feel like a total loser!" she exclaimed. Reading the letter, something written in her own hand, helped Angela remember another critical moment in her life when, in spite of her fear and self-doubt, she demonstrated great courage.

Edgar's actions and overtures toward Angela made clear that he was plagued by fears of being alone as intense as Angela's, if not more so. This was something both Angela and I recognized. She said thinking of Edgar this way gave him less power over her and made him seem more like a helpless little boy than the man to whom she'd given her heart and by whom she'd been mistreated. She said this turn of events made her feel sad and genuinely sorry for Edgar. Regardless of their meaning for Edgar, Angela and I decided to read Edgar's advances as a postcard to her from her fears of loneliness that read, "Just arrived in town yesterday, thought I might drop in. Don't know how long I'll be staying. Could use a place to crash. Do you have any plans?" Angela wrote back to "Loneliness," a correspondence she eventually transformed into a letter to Edgar—one she decided to actually send.

Angela's Letter to Edgar

Dear Edgar,

I am sorry but I am not interested. I do have plans now and they no longer include you. Even though I felt at one time that I loved you and what we had was special, I wouldn't even call it a relationship now. It was a hostage crisis. You held captive by alcohol, and me held captive by you and the hope that someday, if I hung around long enough and kept putting up with your abuse, you would love me back.

I know you are not completely to blame for this. I did not think I deserved any better, and because of my fears of being alone I have always been willing to settle for less in my relationships with men. What's even sadder is that often I didn't feel worthy of the little care or attention I did receive from you and others.

If stopping drinking for yourself isn't reason enough, then there isn't anything that I, or anyone else, can do to help you. I know you said you still love me and that I'm the only one you ever really cared about, but I don't think, if you are completely honest with yourself, that you can say you have ever cared about anyone other than yourself enough to know what it's like to love another person. As far as I can tell, alcohol is the only relationship you've ever been truly faithful to.

Even after all you put me through I don't wish you any harm. I just hope you are able to get the help you need. Of course I still have feelings for you. This makes me mad. But when we first met you did, just by being there, help me through a very difficult and painful episode in my life and I am grateful to you for that. It is hard for me to remember those times (the fun we had) because you buried my old hurts with new ones.

If you want to apologize to me (the only reason I'd ever want to hear from you again) for some of the despicable things you said about my body, my family, and my job, and the awful way you treated me, I would rather you not contact me in person. Please just put it in a letter. I probably won't write you back but would still appreciate having it. Hopefully something you write with a counselor or a sponsor while in treatment for your drinking and poor treatment of women. I won't be expecting it anytime soon.

If you want to tell me anything else about your life that is okay but I would prefer that you not. I worry that it would just give you hope that there is some possibility of our having a future together.

There is none.

Goodbye, Angela

P.S.: You didn't "let me go," I chose to leave of my own free will, and I will never settle for that kind of relationship with you, or anyone else, again.

HATE MAIL: LETTERS OF ANGER AND DENIAL

> When angry, count four; when very angry, swear.
> —MARK TWAIN

The climate surrounding conversations about denial is not always as honest as the one Angela created in her letter and therapy. More often than not these discussions generate intense amounts of anxiety and anger between the alcoholic and family members and, in turn, between the therapist and client. It is important when therapists are confronted with this kind of "hate mail," so to speak, not to respond in kind, and when (not if) we do, to take responsibility for our actions, make amends, and try and move the therapy conversation to a better place.

I recall a session with a couple at an employee-assistance program (EAP) where I worked in which the husband's drinking was out of control. He came to see me because his employer, whom he described as a "friend" as well as his "boss," insisted that he needed to "talk to someone." He was more concerned about saving his marriage than his job, explaining to me that his wife and he had been divorced once, remarried each other, and were now separated and in the final stages of divorcing again. He said his drinking had increased as a result, and he wanted to come in with her to see if there was any hope they could patch things up again. He said his wife was willing to join him at our next visit.

He was right about that—his wife did attend our next meeting. However, as we got started she made clear why she was there. She said she had no intention of stopping the divorce proceedings. She felt her husband had a very serious drinking problem, which in the past resulted in his becoming violent and battering her. While she could see how much he wanted to change and corroborated his story that he had not hit her since they'd gotten back together, recently he had been drinking heavily and had become verbally abusive again. She'd made it clear to him when they got back together that she would not tolerate that kind of behavior or way of relating to her and, as a result, they were through.

However, even when drinking he did not behave this way toward his children, she added. He was, in her eyes, a good father and she wanted to see him get whatever help he needed in order to preserve his relationship with their son and daughter. She said she came home from work the other day and found him in his truck in their driveway passed out from alcohol and knew that time was running out and she'd better act soon. That was why she agreed to come to the session that day.

I said it seemed his wife's concern was warranted, that his drinking was nearing another bottom, and if he was invested in seeing anything better or different come out of this all too familiar situation he'd found himself in again, we needed to start there. The husband proceeded to get up off the sofa, shook his fist in my face, and said "You're just another fucking spooner!" and stormed out of the office, leaving me shaking in my chair and his wife sitting with me in silence. I offered her a referral to women's services and a therapist. She thanked me and said she had all the numbers—indicating that while she did not feel the need to use them now she had used them before—which was the reason she was leaving him again, this time for good.

Later that week my supervisor received a complaint from this man's company about my handling of the situation and how upset he seemed as a result of the consultation. Fortunately, my supervisor supported my work, downplayed the complaint, and explained as best he could (without violating my client's confidentiality) to the employer the challenges this person's behavior would present any clinician.

In this instance there may not have been anything I could have done differently. This was a very angry individual in the throws of an active addiction. Also, I needed to be mindful of modeling for his nonviolent spouse that no one is responsible for another person's acts of violence or aggression, or deserving of it, regardless of the circumstances. However, it is clear, in retrospect, that this man felt shamed by my comments, especially delivered in front of his wife. It might have been more prudent for me to have been more transparent with him about the dilemma I faced. I could have offered that I felt in a bind because, although I wanted to be useful, I was concerned that what I needed to say might upset him—or make him feel in a compromised position vis-à-vis his wife—and that backed into such a corner he might feel attacked and unable to participate in the therapy.

These are not uncommon experiences in therapy with men who have a history of violence or verbal abusiveness especially when under the influence of alcohol or other substances. Sometimes men come back after these kind of outbursts and are willing to talk about them. I have also had a great deal of success inviting men to take responsibility for their violence and participate in groups to address their anger in the fashion advocated by White (1989d) and Jenkins (1990). In these sorts of conversations individuals are encouraged to view their violent behavior as a battle between oppressive institutions and problems, on the one hand, and their own subjugated knowledges, on the other. For example, a man's abusive behavior might be described as a struggle of his own values—"I never imagined myself the kind of man who would hit a woman in order to win an argument"—versus the values of patriarchy—women are men's property without rights of their own.

Sometimes I am able to disarm someone who feels so threatened by therapy that they become belligerent. In these interactions I find myself saying something like the following: "I know you want my help, but when you talk to me that way I feel intimidated and bullied by you. And when I feel rattled or attacked in this fashion I'm of no use to anyone. I get defensive and shut down. Could you find a way to help me 'get it' without making me feel that way?"

Occasionally, a well-timed letter can help me negotiate these turbulent waters, as demonstrated in the following therapy with a father and son.

JESSE: AN INVITATION TO COMPASSION

Jesse was an 11-year-old boy who was experiencing family troubles and also participating in a group which I facilitated for children at his school. In one group session, Jesse was having difficulty sitting comfortably in his chair and was in visible pain. At first reluctant to speak to me, with encouragement from other members of the group he told me his father had punched him in his back and thrown him against a wall during an argument at home. Jesse was both relieved and concerned when I explained to him that I was required by law to file a child abuse complaint (and that in this instance I would probably have done so whether I was required to or not).

Jesse was not the only one troubled by this turn of events. Jesse's father was being treated for alcoholism by another therapist at the clinic I worked in at the time. Jesse's father had a reputation for explosive violence and was a prior client of our court-mandated program for wife batterers. I was also seeing Jesse's family, which consisted of two younger sisters, one younger brother, and his mother, at the clinic. Jesse's mother pleaded with me not to file the 51A (a child abuse report). Although her husband had thrown a beer can at her the same evening he struck Jesse, she said she felt that things had been improving.

I had for months tried to get Jesse's father to participate in the family counseling sessions, and reporting him for child abuse was not how I wished to launch our therapeutic relationship. The following letter is how I chose to inform Jesse's father (not required of me by law) of the action I was required to take.

My Correspondence to Jesse's Father

Dear Gere:

I need to set up an appointment for the two of us to meet to talk about your family. In the course of my work with Jesse, it came to my attention that there was an incident that took place at your home on the weekend of the 7th of May that resulted in

Jesse being hit and thrown by you. I know how much you love your children; that is evident even from the brief contact we've had. However, because I am a mandated reporter of child abuse, I have had to file a 51A and make a report with the Department of Social Services. I shared this information in the exact same fashion with your wife and son. I explained to them that I did not think you could live with yourself if any serious physical injury or harm came to any of them. Jesse's recollection of your apology to him also speaks to your consciousness of the emotional and spiritual damage that results when our anger escalates to physical violence and is directed toward others.

Please call me as soon as possible so that we can talk about any options and resources that are available to help that you may not be aware of. I know you have been trying hard to manage your feelings safely. Although over time there has been some improvement, it is my sense recently that things are getting worse instead of better, and desperately need tending to.

Respectfully yours,

Jonathan Diamond

In response to my correspondence, Jesse's father called and requested to meet with me. Following that session, he, Jesse, and I met on three more occasions in what resulted in the most dramatic and sustained improvement in the father's violence and drinking habits in years. The meetings focused on aspects of the relationship the two had inherited from previous father–son experiences within their clan; what aspects of their history they felt good about—were proud of and found useful; what they felt they could do without; and what new stories about fathers and sons they would like to create together.

In these discussions Jesse's father expressed anger and sorrow over the way in which he had bullied and recruited his son into the kind of violent and oppressive relationship that he had been subjected to by his own father while growing up. Jesse's father said that he never felt his own father "ever really gave a damn about me. His only concern was where his next drink was coming from." "That's what happens when you're angry at people," I responded. "You make them part of your life."

For Winnicott (1965), "The word 'concern' is used to cover in a positive way a phenomenon that is covered in a negative way by guilt. . . . Concern refers to the fact that the individual cares, minds, and both feels and accepts responsibility" (p. 8). Consequently, the importance of hope and therapists' belief in their own and their clients' ability to develop this capacity are, for Winnicott, prerequisites for therapeutic success.

I believe my letter to Jesse's father in some small way may have helped transform his anger and guilt into care and concern, mobilizing him to accept responsibility for his behavior and actions. As a result of our conversation together, he began to attend AA again and participated in several family meetings with his wife, Jesse, and the other children.

This "hope" and "belief" in our clients' capacity to develop care and concern for self and others is an essential part of the initial phase of therapy with addicts and alcoholics and their family members. If a therapist starts with a sense of hopelessness about his or her client's drinking problem, it is unlikely that the client will be able to rally the inner resources necessary to take the first steps toward sobriety. That does not mean becoming pollyannaish or protecting people from the reality of their predicament, but it does mean having faith that people can get better, that their situations can improve even in the face of serious challenges and overwhelming odds. Therapists may need to attend some open AA meetings in order to hear, first hand, stories of recovery that have resulted in people overcoming seemingly insurmountable obstacles. Clinicians should listen especially hard for experiences and adversities similar to those their clients faced. These stories of transformation can sustain hope during low points, or stuck places, in the therapy—countering the intense feelings of helplessness and despair addiction creates in clients and therapists alike.

The topic of therapists' self-care and relationship to meetings will be taken up further in Chapter 6 and in more detail in Chapter 11. At this point, I want to discuss the importance of not only inviting clients to deepen the conversation with their addictions and engage in a more honest dialogue about them, but also ways we can expand that dialogue to include others.

MIRANDA, RANDY, AND CRAIG: TRANSITIONAL STORIES

The following set of letters were written by three teenagers in a substance abuse group that I ran as part of a student assistance program in an area school system. Students were referred to the group by school administrators, their peers, teachers, or parents often as the result of disciplinary infractions. As one of the program's objectives was to build bridges between the clinic and the community, parents and children were often in treatment in both settings. Besides making addiction services more available and accessible to the community, an additional effect of this continuum of care was a greater sense of trust and level of intimacy than one would normally expect to find in a school-based group.

The first two letters are by an adolescent girl, Miranda (whom we first met in the Prologue). At age 14 Miranda was suffering physical symptoms from her drinking that are found in alcoholics at least twice her age, and then usually only in the later stages of the disease. Miranda's father was drug addicted and had abandoned Miranda and her mother when Miranda was 4 years old. In a correspondence drafted in the group, Miranda wrote to her father:

Miranda's Letter to Her Father

father,

I know you probably don't remember me as your daughter anymore but I think you should know this. I really resented you for fucking up my life and my mother's. You didn't realize when you did drugs around me I might have picked up some of your bad habits? I just found out you questioned your paternity when I was born, how sleazy can you be. I don't know why my mom married you in the first place, if she even did marry you, I still wonder how many other lies I've been told. I wanted to tell you this for a while but I havn't been able to, but now I can now that I m in a Drug Counsiling group. You treated me and my mother like shit, I sometimes think you would have been closer if i d never been born (i got that impression from some of your letters.) You forgot all about me ten years ago, the last letter! I don't want to hear about you, or hear from you but I wanted to tell you that you left a legacy of hate that i don't think I'll ever forgive you for. I hope your life is terrible and i hope you rot in hell!

Sincerely,

Miranda—"your x daughter."

For the child of an alcoholic the answer to the question "Why did they leave?" always includes, as Hope Edelman (1994) observed in another context, the appendix "me."

Miranda wrote a letter to her own addictions (presented in the Prologue) that expressed many of the same sentiments she expressed in the letter to her father. Here it is again:

Miranda's Good-Bye Letter to Drugs and Alcohol

~~Dear~~ Narcotics, Pot (acid, alcohol) etc.

thanks for all You've done for me. You've helped me forget my problems, You've made me feel good, You've made me see the world in a whole new perspective, You've made me fail out of my freshman year, You've made me Ruin the lining of my esophagus and stomach. You've made the Relationship with my Parents go down hill, You've given me a who gives a shit attitude—i've gotten fucked up Emotionally and Physically. (Relationship wise also) I've gotten used by abusing you: even after all those complaints I don't want to give you up Because i'll be alone.

Miranda

A prior discussion of Miranda's correspondence to drugs and alcohol emphasized how externalizing problems in the form of a letter can create some distance between people and the dilemmas they face, allowing people to feel they are up against a problem, rather than their *being* the problem themselves. In Miranda's case, her letter helped us assess her ability to let go of her addiction. Coupled with her letter to her father, it gave us both a deeper appreciation of how powerful these attachments were in her life.

Miranda's writing further illustrates the difference between constructive anger—an intense emotion in the service of recovery—and destructive anger—the kind of wrath that undermines a person's self-esteem and ability to be present in her life. Miranda's letters contained elements of both, but her ability to express her outrage over the many painful acts of betrayal that had transpired in her life, especially in her relationships with her father and with drugs and alcohol, were mostly positive. Acceptance (i.e., the act of surrender when an alcoholic admits powerlessness over their addiction) does not have to be particularly gratifying to those who witness it in order for it to be transformative for the person experiencing it. People's rage often makes this step more, not less, profound or genuine.

People's anger and denial in therapy often belongs to the moment of hope. When used in the service of their addiction or substance abuse, this anger often precedes a genuine struggle over the decision to change or let go of their habit. In the case of addiction, clients who do not "go quietly into the night" will, once they make up their minds to change, generally seek sobriety with more zeal than those who go quietly into treatment and therapy. The later group often display a lack of investment in the outcome of their care, whereas the former will "rise eagerly from sleep"[4] and use the passion that once fueled their addiction in the service of their healing and recovery. This is especially true for adolescents who have a tendency to behave "as if"—saying what they imagine people want to hear, rather than speaking about what's in their hearts. However, this type of dilemma was not reflected in Miranda's writing. Miranda, as I often found myself saying to her, spoke from the heart because she had no choice in the matter. The hatred and rage expressed in Miranda's letter to her father, who had virtually abandoned his daughter, displayed the depth of her hurt and pain and gave those of us privileged to witness it a glimpse of just how much she lost.

The remaining two letters were written by two older boys to their fathers. In both instances, the boys abused alcohol, cocaine, and marijuana, and came from families with severe legacies of alcoholism and addiction, including both sets of parents. Like Miranda's offerings, these pieces served as (w)rites of passage that saw the boys beginning to come to terms with a significant loss and trauma.

Randy's mother was alcoholic and drug addicted and supplemented her part-time income by dealing drugs. She lived with a man who physically abused her and got into violent fights with Randy. With intervention from social services, Randy (age 17) was able to live on his own in a supervised apartment for emancipated teens. He got himself to school every day, purchased his own groceries and living supplies, held a job, participated in sports, and according to school and police authorities, who referred him to the substance abuse group, smoked too much pot and drank too much alcohol. Randy's father died of AIDS from intravenous (IV) drug use. In group Randy wrote the following letter to his father:

Randy's Letter

Dear Dad,

I wish you wold have came to me instead of just running away from me. I would have loved to have been with you. I just wanted to be your son. When I spent time with you it was great. And now you are gone and I will never see you again: I wish you were here now becuse I could realy use you as my dad. Even though you whernt around when I was yonger I ~~you could use~~ you could make up for it now I miss you so much.

Randy

Craig (age 18) lived with an older brother because his mother was too impaired from her own drinking to care for him. Craig's father died of cirrhosis and other complications from alcoholism. Craig's letter to his father expressed similar themes of love, loss, and abandonment:

Craig's Letter

Dear Dad,

There are a few things I wish you had considered while you were alive. I wish you would have realized that you were an alcoholic. You should have been responsible about your health and you would have still been here today. If you had just remembered my birthday or Christmas once, I would have been so happy. Although I wasn't the greatest of kids, I was there when you needed me, and always loved you more than any person on the face of the earth. But I do thank you for everything you did do.

Love you Dad, Craig

The group and individual sessions in which these pieces were composed and read were followed up by family sessions with their mothers, from whom both boys had been separated from for some time. In Craig's case, that meant becoming angry and staying angry at his "sole"[5] surviving parent. In Randy's therapy, a mending of old wounds and resentments unfolded. Although the former meeting was not as easy to witness as the latter, both experiences helped the participants become unblocked and, for the boys, allowed them to leave home and move on with their lives. At the same time, each young man also made significant strides in addressing his substance abuse problems and either chose to part company with chemicals altogether or at least to begin exploring the issues in more depth.

The letters allowed both boys to recognize and acknowledge their attachments and identification to their fathers via drugs and alcohol. They increased their ability to empathize with both parents, as well as with their own pain and problems—a capacity for caring that friends, lovers, teachers, and future characters in their lives will benefit from as well.

The letters were crafted in the group during one session—refined further at home in some cases—and read the following week. The introduction of writing was not new to the group, as I often brought writing exercises for participants to try in group or at home. In addition, all of the girls and some of the boys chose to keep "recovery journals," where they could keep track of their drug and alcohol use as well as using sobriety days—days that members committed themselves to remaining drug free and tried to "face life on life's terms."

Although encouraged to take risks and experiment with new ways of thinking about themselves and their problems, no one was forced to participate in any activity.* In the same spirit, reading one's work was always optional. However, I found that members—especially boys—who were often not as comfortable sharing their feelings and participating in group discussions seemed more at ease when reading their writing in the group. It provided a way for these young men to take risks, show emotion, and be vulnerable with others in ways to which they were not ordinarily accustomed.

For Randy, this was the first time he had ever discussed the experience of his father's illness with anyone outside his family. He cried when reading his letter, and so did those of us who listened. This led to a profound discussion in the group about members' fears and experiences of losing a parent to alcoholism. Participants talked about the complexities these situations pose when this sadness and grief is colored by a person's anger at one's parents for the emotional and physical absences caused by their addiction and, in many cases, for the atmosphere of violence and abuse it contributed to in their homes.

Randy talked about feeling relieved after sharing his letter, but he was angry at himself for crying. He felt better when the girls and other group members reassured him that they didn't view his tears as a sign of weakness but of strength. Craig was also moved by Randy's piece, as it gave him the courage to read his letter himself, instead of asking someone else to read it for him as he originally planned. Craig was very active in this discussion and said that the most difficult part was knowing, while reading the letter, that the group knew all about his drinking. He said he felt like a hypocrite because he was not having any easier time doing anything about his drinking than his Dad had, and he felt that people would think less of him if they knew his father was a "drunk" (which is how he often felt about his father).

For clients whose addictions are helping them maintain a connection to an addicted parent's life, letter writing can help them to form other, more positive connections. Reading their letters, coupled with the group's compassionate acknowledgment of them, helped Randy and Criag feel less isolated and more connected to others. After this session, everyone in the group reported feeling less isolated and closer to one another. Both boys' correspondence with their fathers helped create a safe space for other group members to talk about their wish for more connection with their own parents and families.

---

*I lent tape recorders to members who were intimidated by writing or whose discomfort with their writing skills kept them from participating. These students would keep audiojournals of their recovery.

The letters appeared to foster a transitional space that helped each teenager recognize his or her own creative intuition as crucial modes of knowledge and experience. Although it was long disregarded as a strictly feminine attribute needed for child rearing, nursing, and other supposed "women's work," developing the capacity for this kind of insight and understanding is highly valued today; we even have a catchy label for it—"emotional intelligence." However, imagination and creativity have always been an essential aspect of therapy and healing as, according to child analyst D. W. Winnicott (1971a), it is creative apperception, more than anything else, that makes us feel that life is worth living. This is particularly the case during adolescence, when creativity, play, and ingenuity are such an important part of a person's growth and development.

NARRATIVE MEANS TO ANALYTIC ENDS

For Winnicott, psychotherapy itself is a form of play that "takes place in the overlap of . . . two areas . . . that of the patient and that of the therapist" (1971a, p. 38). While not the first psychoanalyst to interpret patients' written or artistic communications in psychotherapy, Winnicott pioneered the use of them in a relational context—helping therapists become better acquainted with the nature of their own and their clients' psychic lives and inner worlds. I have in mind his use of the squiggle game. Winnicott developed this type of play which he called "a game with no rules," as a way of "making contact" with his child and adolescent patients: "In this squiggle game I make some kind of impulsive line-drawing and invite the child whom I am working with to turn it into something, and then he makes a squiggle for me to turn it into something, in my turn" (1971a, p. 16).[6]

Winnicott considered these interactions between analyst and patient as sacrosanct, and he was adamant that this was not to be used as some sort of test with rules and techniques and that should the therapist have any sort of agenda of this kind going into the session, "the whole value of the procedure will be lost." He emphasized that this work does not depend upon the cleverness of the consultant's interpretations, whose contributions to the activity are as important as the child's, but relies more on the consultant's ability to be imaginative and spontaneous and learn from his or her patient. He refers to this type of free-flowing human but professional relationship as "a form of 'holding' " (1971a, p. 301).

The squiggle game is not the only aspect of Winnicott's work that I appropriate for narrative designs. Creativity, love, and play are located by Winnicott in the "potential space" between the inner psychic space of "me" and outer social space of "not me." Winnicott coined the term "transitional object" to describe the constructs children create to help them bridge these two worlds. The bridge can be an actual thing (e.g., a baby's blanket or a stuffed animal) or an imaginary toy or companion. An elegant example is the relationship between the boy and his stuffed companion in the story of the Velveteen rabbit. The rabbit was brought to life as a result of the boy's play and love of it; however, because of the way he related to him the rabbit inhabited space betwixt and between our world and the boy's imaginary world. In other words, the rabbit and other chosen objects served as a kind of channel between the two realities. Within this psychic playground children learn to differentiate between themselves and others and generalize from their relationship with their parents to the larger culture.* According to Winnicott, cultural experience itself is located in this "potential space" between the individual and the environment. Thus, Winnicott's is not primarily a theory about certain kinds of objects—teddy bears, blankets, and so forth—but is rather a theory about certain kinds of human experience and ways of being. Winnicott uses a quotation from a work by Margaret Milner to capture the essence and color of what he is trying to say about transitional phenomena and play:

> Moments when the original poet in each of us created the outside world for us, by finding the familiar in the unfamiliar, are perhaps forgotten by most people; or else they are guarded in some secret place of memory because they were too much like visitations of the gods to be mixed with everyday thinking. (Milner, 1957, as quoted in Winnicott, 1971a, p. 39)

Writing can create these sort of sacred moments as well, interactions that allow people to surprise themselves by saying something totally unexpected. As Winnicott (1971b) remarks: "Either the sacred moment is used or it is not. If it is wasted, the child's belief in being understood is shattered. If on the other hand it is used, then the child's belief in being helped is strengthened" (p. 4).

Miranda, Randy, and Craig's letters served as a bridges between the "me" and "not me" and helped give meaning to their experience.

---

*Winnicott discusses the way A. A. Milne immortalized Winnie the Pooh to illustrate the powerful cultural force transitional objects hold for us.

The letters each created a space where their authors could begin to map out their internal struggles with drugs and alcohol and explore what their writing revealed about the nature of their preferences, desires, beliefs, and commitments to others and themselves. Letter writing allows people to externalize the subjective aspects of their experience. Locating the events and feelings that occupy the interior recesses of our minds outside of the self provides us with the opportunity to become more familiar with them and begin tracing their histories. In this realm, stories and events are linked together through time and according to plot, giving people a sense of history and of enduring over time. For all three teens, in the absence of more permanent structures in their lives, the letters provided a kind of makeshift memorial honoring the powerful presence of each teen's connection to a deceased or missing parent.

Winnicott (1971a) contrasts these creative processes with a relationship to the external world that is characterized by compliance, where the world and its details are seen only as something to be fitted or adapted to. For adolescents, these struggles are particularly poignant:

> Compliance carries with it a sense of futility for the individual and is associated with the idea that nothing matters and that life is not worth living. In a tantalizing way many individuals have experienced just enough creative living to recognize that for most of the time they are living uncreatively, as if caught up in the creativity of someone else, or of a machine. (p. 65)

The experience Winnicott is describing is captured in the music of rock groups like Pink Floyd, whose songs, with titles and lyrics such as "Welcome to the Machine" and "The Wall," have served as a rallying cry for generations of alienated youth. Drugs can be the source of these feelings, in and of themselves, or can be used as an escape—a way to soothe and self-medicate painful emotional states. If it is a question of abuse, where problems are encountered in the course of using drugs or alcohol to generate solutions to everyday troubles, common sense and sound hermeneutic practices that restore meaning to people's lives will often help them overcome the adversity posed by chemicals. If it is addiction, these ideas and common-sense solutions will fall short, or result in a period of respite and relief followed by a return to alcohol or drugs that seems to "defy logic" and "boggle the mind."

For example, in the experiences of both Craig and Randy, crafting and sharing their letters with others in the group resulted in renewed and more honest and authentic relationships with their parents (living and dead). In Randy's case, however, the synthetic connections formed by drugs and alcohol were no longer necessary and, like an old tattered comforter, had outlived their usefulness and become obsolete. Craig, on the other hand, found that the role drugs and alcohol played in his life was not only a transitional one and, in a process more akin to Miranda's, he required more time to explore the harsh realities of his addiction.

The next illustration and accompanying correspondence were carried out in my role as a consultant. They represent an effort, on my part, to extend a conversation between myself and a young person about her substance abuse problems to the clinical staff, milieu therapists, and group leaders in her outpatient treatment program. For clients feeling judged and uninvolved in their treatment, writing a letter to them and others involved in their care can avoid the hierarchical one-upmanship that often comes with my role as an outside consultant. The results are always encouraging and often result in clients becoming more involved in their own care.

ANDREA: COPYWRITES

Andrea was a student and patient at a partial hospitalization program for drug-addicted and emotionally troubled adolescents. Andrea's parents were divorced and Andrea lived with her father, an attorney and a recovering alcoholic with several years of sobriety. Andrea's father did not have much patience or tolerance for his daughter's substance abuse problems. He was frustrated and angry with Andrea because she continued to complain about her life but refused to follow his advice and go to AA meetings with him.

Her mother, on the other hand, did not feel that Andrea had a serious problem at all because all she did was smoke pot. Andrea's mother was angry at Andrea's father and the staff at her treatment program for making such a big deal out of Andrea's alcohol and drug use. She wanted Andrea to move back home with her. Because she and her daughter were so much alike, Andrea's mother felt she was the only person who really understood her daughter. She felt that Andrea's abandonment of her to go live with her father was cruel and was the source of Andrea's problems and unhappiness.

Andrea's therapist and the staff that worked with her at the treatment program were frustrated and angry too. They were upset with

Andrea's mother for what they perceived as her lack of support for her daughter's treatment protocol, which stipulated that Andrea attend more AA meetings. However, they were also angry with Andrea for not following her treatment plan more rigorously. They had invested a great deal of energy into Andrea's care and, although they were very fond of her, needed to see more signs of improvement in order to guarantee her continued enrollment in the program. The staff were not in complete agreement about this: her individual therapist and substance abuse group leaders, while concerned, advocated more empathy and acceptance of Andrea's situation; on the other hand, the milieu staff felt that if they did not take a hard line about her pot smoking, Andrea would get the message that they were not serious about her needing to work on her drug problems. After my consultation with Andrea, I sent the following letter to her:

My Letter to Andrea

Dear Andrea:

Thank you for taking the time to meet with me on Friday, March 5. At the time, we talked about the purpose of our interview being more for the two of us to generate some new ideas about your relationship with alcohol and drugs rather than making any decisions about your treatment, as you are already in the CD [chemical dependency] group at Day Treatment and in therapy. When it comes to advice giving, particularly about matters concerning alcohol and drugs, I personally try and avoid it. More often than not, people who come to see me about drinking problems have problems with someone else's drinking and not their own, and if they do see their use as a problem they rarely listen to me (or anyone else for that matter). Alcohol and drugs have a way of taking matters into their own hands, and their voice is a strong one. The word "addict," in Latin, in fact, means "towards (ad) voice (dict)" and people often find themselves, in spite of their best intentions, moving in the direction of the voice of alcohol rather than their own or their therapist's. Even from our brief exchange I can see you're way ahead of the game, as you have clearly put a lot of thought into these concerns. Consequently, part of me feels, as you are already working very hard in group and with Sydney in individual and family therapy on these issues, I should just encourage you to keep at it and trust you'll find your way. However, as so many people believe in you and are eager to find further ways to help you, I have included more ideas here than I might have otherwise or than you may feel is necessary. Also, as you seemed curious yourself about any recommendations I might have, I've included them in this correspondence so you can talk them over (should you choose to) with your family, the staff, and/or your therapist and anyone else on your side and involved in your care.

In addition, I wanted to take this opportunity to ask a few questions that I didn't have the chance to ask on the 5th. Please feel free to discuss them along with any other ideas offered here you find useful, with Sydney or your group leaders, and have them get back to me or pull me aside at Day Treatment if you'd like (I'm almost always there on Fridays). So here goes . . .

Regarding recommendations, I have only two and they're fairly simple. First, try and discover where inside yourself you find the courage to take on these kinds of problems at age 15, and when you find it keep going back to that place to get more.

The second is a bit more complex, so please bear with me. It appears that you have already decided on your own that chemicals (alcohol in particular) are taking up more space in your life than they're paying rent for, and I think the efforts you're making to turn the tables on alcohol, so to speak, so it becomes less in charge of your life and you become more in charge of it are commendable. One of the strategies you mentioned employing is to attempt to let go of alcohol altogether and limit your drug use to marijuana, which hasn't seemed to cause as much trouble in your life, such as sickness, blackouts, or upsetting your friends. My concerns with this approach are twofold. One, I worry that the marijuana will just postpone the inevitable and that you may end up having to deal with your problems with alcohol at the time when more is at stake. I also worry that you may not, at that time, have all the supports and resources that are available to you now. (This point I think you have already heard in different forms from other sources, so I won't belabor it—in AA it's often referred to as "the cannabis maintenance program" or "substitution.") Another thought I had relates to what you said about how the few times you've gone to AA you feel guilty because although you didn't seem to mind the meeting itself, and are invested in doing something about your drinking, in your heart you know you still intend to smoke pot and therefore feel somewhat hypocritical about being there. My suggestion is that you might want to avoid taking on too much all at once and start by trying what people in groups I have run in the past call "sobriety days." Choosing on these days not to use any mood-altering substances (some people include cigarettes, coffee, sugar, etc. as well) whatsoever, and making an effort to go to meetings on these days (that people practice this on the days that they have CD group or therapy is a given). Keeping a journal about your experiences at AA meetings and therapy and your feelings about sobriety is another tool you may want to try.

This will hopefully allow you, at least temporarily, to explore AA more fully without feeling guilty while at the same time not committing yourself to a path you fear you are not yet ready for.

Regarding questions, I have just a few:

1) I was very impressed with the respectful and trusting relationship you have established with your therapist, and I wondered if the uncomfortable feelings you expressed about talking about your marijuana use at AA meetings ever interfere with your ability to raise these issues in therapy? Do you ever feel the need to protect your therapist, or yourself, from your feelings and these troubling dilemmas in the way you did the other participants at the two AA meetings you attended? If you do, what would it be like for you to bring this topic up at an AA meeting, or in a therapy session?

2) If you were to decide that AA was a safe place for you to begin to explore these issues in more depth, what effects would your father's involvement in AA have on your participation? Have you had many conversations with your father about sobriety and recovery? Having just undertaken this journey himself, I imagine he has struggled with many of the same things you're going through. Do you think that makes him more empathetic, or more impatient with your progress thus far? What does your mother have to say about your drug and alcohol abuse? In our meeting you said that sometimes you see her as having been "burnt" from her own drug abuse at different times in her life. How do you think she would feel about your surpassing her own achievements in this area and choosing to explore recovery in more depth? Overall, your predicament with drugs and alcohol strikes me as being similar to the families of the stars who choose to raise children in Hollywood. With so many family members already in "the business," how does a daughter or son find their own path and make a name for themselves that isn't overshadowed by their parents' reputation?

3) Sometimes I see therapists as being a lot like plants: you have to water us or we become droopy and wilt. What signs of progress and change can you offer to keep the people taking care of you healthy and growing? Would you be willing to honor the commitment you said you made to give AA or another 12-step program an honest go of it? If not, what would you be willing to try? Finally, if your therapist started challenging more rigorously the role chemicals play in your life, would that relationship (with your counselor) hold up or would it cause problems?

Thank you again. Should you not choose to talk these issues over with Sydney or in CD group, I hope that at least you mull them over on your own. In addition, should you have any concerns regarding our meeting you wish to discuss with me, please don't hesitate to ask Sydney to set up another appointment.

Respectfully yours,

Jonathan Diamond

cc: Sydney (individual therapist)
Lilly (group therapist)
Tara (group therapist)

Copies of this correspondence were sent to her individual therapist and group leaders, who requested the consultation because they were feeling "stuck," thinking they had exhausted all the possibilities available to them to help Andrea explore her substance abuse problem. I found that colleagues at the hospital where I was employed at the time increasingly preferred this type of approach, as opposed to a more traditional assessment. The custom there would have been for me to do a "substance abuse evaluation" and share it only with other practitioners, or just place it in the patient's "chart."

I always explain my preferred way of working to clients and asked Andrea—well versed in the hospital culture and used to meeting with residents, psychiatrists, and social service workers whom she did not know and never would hear from again—if it was okay with her if I put my ideas in a letter to her and shared them with the team as well. The look of surprise and pleasure on people's faces in response to this question has been one of the most rewarding aspects of this work for me.

Prior to writing my letter, I had informed Andrea's therapist of my intentions and sought his approval as well. Until clinicians are comfortable with my work, I often share drafts of the letter with them to make sure I'm not interfering with some aspect of the therapy. This part of the process—passing drafts back and forth—is also an enjoyable one, as I end up being able to work with others and to teach, not just perform, a different type of therapy practice. When I have time to share sketches of a letter or an intervention with clients as well as therapists, I feel I have been given the opportunity to truly co-construct an intervention with others. Often by the time the final document is completed and received by all of the participants, the problems that led to a person requesting a consultation in the first place are well on their way to being *dis*solved.

Some of what I wrote to Andrea—a 15-year-old teen—was clearly over her head, or included concepts that may have been beyond her grasp. While I was aware of this when I wrote the letter, it did not concern me at the time. On the one hand, the fact that copies of the correspondence were distributed to Andrea's therapist and group leaders meant that she would have plenty of opportunity to look over the material at her own pace, with input from others. Indeed her individual therapist reported that Andrea brought the document to her therapy and talked about it in detail with him. Also, while she expressed some agitation about it's length and recommendations (particularly the idea that she and her therapist have a more mindful discussion about her drug use and its impact on their relationship), she kept it in her back pocket for several weeks—even when attending her day treatment program. On the other hand, the dilemma these other readers faced (her individual therapist and group leaders who requested the consultation) was just as much, if not more, on my mind when drafting the letter.

The letter's primary message was intended for Andrea, her family, the staff, her therapist, and anyone else standing by her side or "involved in her care"—what I like to think of as her and other clients' *community of resistance*. In this situation I was trying to model an overall stance toward addiction that I always strive for as a therapist. This position is one that encourages and supports clients becoming more involved in their recovery through attendance at AA and Al-Anon meetings but is not dependent on them doing so.

Andrea did not become more involved in AA as the result of our consultation, and neither did any other members of her family who were not already attending meetings (i.e., her mother). However, as a result of this intervention, Andrea's individual therapist and one of her group leaders decided to attend some Al-Anon meetings. Both clinicians reported feeling more hopeful about the possibilities for growth and change in their work with Andrea. They attributed this renewed sense of hope to strategies they learned in Al-Anon. They also felt that the rest of the staff was able to benefit from what they had learned.

Another one of my responses documented in my letter to Andrea hints at the next phase of recovery, one which I call "bargaining." It also described a particular type of settlement clients seem willing to negotiate with addiction when they are no longer content with the current arrangement. Recall that in the letter I wrote, "One of the strategies you mentioned employing is to attempt to let go of alcohol altogether and limit your drug use to marijuana, which hasn't seemed to cause as much trouble in your life, such as sickness, blackouts, or upsetting your friends, . . . often referred to as the 'cannabis maintenance program.' "

Driven by the understanding that their drinking and drug use is causing themselves and the people around them untold grief and pain, people are often willing to do anything other than end their relationship with chemicals or other addictions to make the situation right. Remember the description of hitting bottom as the intersection of pain and understanding—if a person's understanding of his or her problem is fundamentally flawed, recovery is unlikely to follow from hitting bottom. Another client made the same point in a "good-bye letter" he'd written to alcohol:

> As far as blackouts go I did what any normal individual would do and say. "Gee, I'll never drink THAT much again!" or better yet, "I got to stop drinking vodka and just stick to beer."

I have come to think of these actions, which AA and some clinicians in the field call "substitution," as a type of joint-custody arrangement whereby drugs and alcohol agree to let people share in the care and guardianship of their lives on a limited basis. Clients aren't the only ones who introduce bargaining into the recovery process. My suggestion to Andrea that she might want to experiment with "sobriety days" as a first step toward separating herself from alcohol was an attempt to appeal to her tendency (shared by many other clients) to want to negotiate a settlement with chemicals that doesn't necessitate dismissing them from their lives completely—an action they may not yet be ready to undertake.

CHAPTER 3

Bargaining

Controlled Drinking and Other Negotiated Settlements

Here are some of the methods we have tried: Drinking beer
only, limiting the number of drinks, never drinking alone,
never drinking in the morning, drinking only at home,
never having it in the house, never drinking during business
hours, drinking only at parties, switching from scotch to
brandy, drinking only natural wines, agreeing to resign if
ever drunk on the job, taking a trip, not taking a trip,
swearing off forever (with and without a solemn oath),
taking more physical exercise, reading inspirational books,
going to health farms and sanitariums, accepting voluntary
commitment to asylums—we could increase the list ad
infinitum.

—ALCOHOLICS ANONYMOUS

Freud's classic paper "Remembering, Repeating and Working-Through"
(1914/1958) remains a template for most Western psychotherapy. In this
treatise he discusses how we remember forgotten traumas not as memories but as actions, actions we repeat and are not conscious of repeating.
Working-through is about making ourselves whole again. It is a process,
as Mark Epstein describes in his *Thoughts without a Thinker*, "of repos-
sessing that from which we have become estranged, of accepting that
which we would rather deny . . . a process of making present that which
was otherwise buried in the past, so that it could, in fact, be experienced
as emanating from ones own present" (1995, p. 204).

Psychotherapy with addicts and alcoholics resembles Freud's psychic passage minus the working through. Like the movie comedy

Groundhog Day, in which Bill Murray's character keeps reliving the same day over and over, addicts and alcoholics seem to repeat self-destructive behavior with a stamina that would wear down the patience of the most seasoned therapist. In postbinge surges of self-revulsion people vow never to drink again only to discover that what Mark Twain said about smoking applies here as well: "It's easy to stop drinking, I've done it hundreds of times."

As this is where the lion's share of people's ambivalence toward both addiction and recovery surfaces, it can be a very frustrating period of therapy for the therapist and client alike. Intense amounts of anxiety rise as people begin to both disclose and become more aware of the severity of their problem. Unfortunately, anxiety is one of the more powerful triggers for drinking. Frequently, these feelings are acted out in a person's therapy with a great deal of oscillating back and forth between use and abstinence, or periods of sobriety followed by periods of abuse. It follows then that one of the most difficult tasks facing therapists treating alcoholism is to lessen a person's denial and encourage increased self-awareness and disclosure while they're trying to keep their client's anxiety to a minimum.

For this reason, John Wallace (1985) cautions, when they are working with addictions therapists are going to have to be content with their clients' gradually deepening self-awareness rather than looking for dramatic breakthroughs.

LARRY: "CANNABIS MAINTENANCE"*

Larry, a full-time social worker and part-time musician, had been feeling good about both his recovery and his therapy. It had been almost 2 years since he'd given up alcohol. Larry went to AA and considered himself a "sober" member of the group. He celebrated the anniversary of his sobriety every year and still remembered the day he decided to stop drinking. His friends had for the most part supported his decision to quit, but when he played gigs he still found it impossible to turn someone down when they offered him marijuana. Larry didn't feel good about the increase in his pot smoking since he'd given up alcohol. Although he no longer found himself embroiled in the drama drinking created in his life—fights with friends, coworkers, and girlfriends; blackouts; hang-

---

*Larry's story has not been altered and this is his real name.

overs; and missed days at work—Larry found the effects of his pot smoking more insidious and his relationship with marijuana more difficult to change. He began feeling a creeping sense of shame and guilt about it. People at the AA meetings he attended were not aware that he used pot. In addition, many of the clients on his caseload had drug problems of their own. At first he considered his clients' problems much worse than his own, but more recently he realized he was giving others advice that he couldn't follow himself.

At my suggestion, Larry wrote a letter to sort out some of his feelings about marijuana and to get a better handle on his relationship with substances.

Larry's Letter to Marijuana

Dear Mr. Marijuana,

It has been 17 years since I first met you. I think my brother introduced us at my request. Emotionally, I don't think I've grown much since I met you. I rely on you now more than I ever have in the past. You've been there for the hard times, the good times and even times that weren't hard or good! You're always there. You've been part of a bond with my closest friends. You were there when I was lonely, when I had time to kill, when I had trouble sleeping and when I was in a pissy mood. You made it right! Or at least you did for the moment. And now my good friend I've leaned on you heavily since I gave up, as the song goes, "Lord Demon Alcohol—sad memories I can't recall." Alcohol was never my drug of choice. It was something I turned to when I wanted to forget about the world, including the pain, and sense of shame I felt about my family—a situation I always blamed myself for. And yes I drank when I was happy or celebrating, but it was you that I turned to when I had to escape *immediately*. No fuckin around with you. Mr consistency—a few tokes of a bong, everything was cool. Yes, I got paranoid occasionally when we met. You let me down a few times— paranoid and self-conscious. But I always looked the other way, choosing to overlook your negative qualities.

Until now. . . . I've got a bone to pick with you. Seventeen years later and you are responsible for:

My weight gain (50 lbs. at least).
My inability to *cope* with the world's curve balls without a toke or seven.
My addiction to you and food.
The cumulative effect of daily pot smoking—never resolving anything.

My alienation from my family, my success, my failures, my
  happiness; and my lousy *concentration* and work habits.
My pathetic financial situation.

Well what have you got to say for yourself? I'm fucked with
you and fucked without you! How am I supposed to get on with
my life and deal with myself and my feelings if I'm messing with
you. When is it going to stop? How is it going to stop? I don't
like you early in the day and if we meet late at night I eat and
put my thoughts on hold. Yeah it's great to be high—to kick
back—think about things like music and my creativity but I can't
control it. I can't stop spinning my wheels. Please, give me a
break-cut me some slack. I'm not through with you yet, but I'm
not pleased with the situation.

Talk to You Soon (Unfortunately), Larry

Many people discover that coming to terms with an addiction is like
peeling the layers of an onion, underneath the skin exist other compulsions
no less compelling, each one closer to the core. As Caroline Knapp says,
"It's a rare addict who hasn't at least danced around another addiction, or
who can't imagine substituting one for another" (1996, p. 134). A lot of
the work at this juncture in treatment necessarily focuses on clients' feelings of guilt about their inability to relinquish their use of drugs or alcohol
on a more permanent basis; or the frustration experienced if, after a great
deal of effort and hard work, they conclude they've merely replaced one
addiction for another. Clients often transfer these feelings of shame and
helplessness onto their therapists—transforming their caregiver's words of
encouragement and AA's principles and guidelines, into voices of authority with set rules and laws to be obeyed.

Larry originally came to see me for an intake to get into a group I
was running for Adult Children of Alcoholics (ACOA). He said he felt
thwarted by his attempts at intimacy in his relationship with his live-in
girlfriend of several years and wanted to strengthen his connection to his
aging alcoholic father before it was too late. When presented with
Larry's own drinking and drug history, I told him I might consider him
for the group in a year if he was able to work on his addiction issues first
and remain sober for a period of time. (Although people often become
aware of their own alcoholism through work on other problems in therapy, I felt Larry's drinking and drug use were too severe for him to participate in a group for nonalcoholic spouses and family members without compromising other group members' feelings of safety.)

Larry took me up on this offer and decided to meet with me on an
individual basis to work on his own addictions. However, during the 2-

year period that Larry struggled with his alcoholism and pot smoking he
often became upset with me when he was not able to meet the goals he
set for himself. Initially his anger might surface in the form of a missed
appointment or his canceling our session at the last minute. If I couldn't
find another time for us to meet, he would become agitated and demanding. When I reminded him that he was the one who had canceled
or missed our meeting, he responded angrily that as he was paying for
my services, including missed appointments and cancellations without
notice (my customary policy), it was up to him how he chose to use our
sessions. Larry's demeanor was humble in our conversations following
these exchanges. Inevitably he would confess that his having "picked
up" (i.e., used drugs or alcohol) was his reason for not wanting to meet
and canceling. During one period of our work together this pattern repeated itself with alarming frequency.

When Larry got high or drank he said he felt that he was letting me
down. These feelings resulted in a conversation taking place between us
in Larry's mind that he described as going something like the following:

> "After drinking, I have these horrendous arguments in my head
> where you get on my case and tell me not to bother coming to
> therapy if I'm not serious about wanting to get sober. Then I get
> mad and say something like I don't need your guilt trip. That if I
> have to put up with this kind of crap, I might as well get stoned or
> drunk so at least I can get something out of it other than aggrava-
> tion. Sometimes, when I'm ranting and raving and carrying on like
> this, even I can see that I am putting all this responsibility for what
> I'm feeling like and what *I* want to do—which is drink—on you.
> Then I decide what you have to say about it and I don't like it one
> bit, and I become full of rage. All this transpires—causing bad
> blood between us—and you're not even in the room! So by the
> time I'm supposed to see you next this huge resentment and anxi-
> ety has built up that I don't know what to do with."

When I asked Larry who or what these dialogues reminded him of, he
responded:

> "My parents. They would argue and carry on like this for days at a
> time. And when my father finally had to stop drinking because of
> his health my mother started focusing her energies on me. I didn't
> disappoint. I guess you could say I simply picked up where my fa-
> ther left off."

I reminded Larry that I was not the voice of his conscience but it appeared that sometimes I stood in for it. When he was having trouble staying sober but didn't want to drink or get high it was not an issue. On those occasions, he experienced my presence in his unconscious life as a welcome ally in harmony with his wants and desires. The problem began when he wanted to drink or get high. In those moments, my voice was transformed from one of a trusted guide into that of a hostile adversary. I also, in an effort to calm his anxiety, shared with him my belief that therapists who take clients' drinking or drugging personally shouldn't work with addicts—that I was there to help, not judge. When not using drugs or alcohol, Larry formed a very positive identification with me; I became the virtuous, sober father figure he longed for. Under their influence, when he identified more with his father's alcoholism, I became the voice of his "overbearing" mother and "critical" wife he resented for denying him his one true pleasure in life.

I didn't mind Larry's forays back to the world of drugs and alcohol when I observed them from the appropriately detached stance of a compassionate therapist well versed in the dynamics of addiction and recovery. However, I found them more than a little disturbing when I felt myself feeling betrayed by Larry's drug use. Sometimes, I was able to offer Larry a gentle hypothesis about what I thought was being enacted between us. Other times, I found myself responding defensively when caught in these binds. Larry would accuse me of behaving just like his mother or girlfriend, the implication being that I was somehow responsible for his drinking or drug use. And the fact is, as a caretaker working with a steady caseload of addictions, it is often difficult for me to see my clients' inability to remain sober as anything other than a reflection of my failure as a therapist.

These dramas are all part of what Michael Balint (1968) describes as the "unharmonious mixup" between client and therapist. My job, as I often had to remind myself, was to help Larry sort out these dramas and manage his anxieties about recovery, not to keep him sober. That was something only Larry could do with the help and support of AA if he chose to avail himself of it. During these periods therapists want to avoid, as best they can, taking responsibility for their clients' helplessness. We need to give people space to experiment with both sober and drinking lifestyles and set limits at the same time. That is, we must somehow resist the temptation to rescue people from the sense of hopelessness and powerlessness they feel, while not allowing them to flounder in that place too long or feel completely abandoned in it either.

Larry moved precipitously between denial and self-awareness, sometimes demonstrating extraordinary commitment to his recovery and at other times showing no signs of investment in his sobriety. Larry, like many addicts, described feeling frustrated at what he perceived as his lack of control over these cycles. I couldn't do much for Larry in these moments except remind him that although it was clear that he didn't have the ability to control his drinking and drug use, he did exercise more influence over his recovery. I noted that, for example, when he took better care of himself by going to meetings, exercising, and tending to his spiritual life through his participation in yoga and meditation (two of his favorite activities) he felt better about himself and his therapy.

When the Past Is Present

One can glean from my conversations with Larry that I find useful the psychoanalytic concept of exploring and listening for both the client's and my own "transference" in the therapy. Transference is not a uniquely analytic or psychotherapeutic phenomenon. It is a human phenomenon, used in a very specific way by analysts and therapists in our work with people. Transference was not invented by Freud; it was taught to him, initially, by his colleague Josef Breuer's patient Bertha Pappenheim (referred to as "Anna O." by Freud). The three, we recall, began thinking about this way of understanding Breuer and Pappenheim's clinical relationship during Freud and Breuer's efforts to help Pappenheim alleviate some very troubling emotional and physical symptoms in her life.[1]

Transference isn't some uncontrollable force that rules our lives. Transferences are simply other storylines in the complex tale of human relations—narratives we can use to explore unexamined aspects of our relationships with our clients and of our clients with us. Listening for these voices in the therapy conversation requires a kind of suspended disbelief on the part of the therapist, an attitude akin to Anderson and Goolishian's (1992) "not-knowing" stance. Countertransference produces what Bollas describes as an "inevitable, ever-present, and necessary uncertainty about why we feel as we do" that gives our work a certain humility and responsibility (1983, p. 4).

Stiver (1992) reminds us that transference is very much a relational phenomenon. There is nothing mystical or obtuse about such experiences; they are feelings with historical resonances created in the context of relationships among people. In other words, like the analytic concepts of repetition, compulsion, and reenactment, transference is another way of remembering. This can be as simple as asking how clients' experiences of their relationships with us remind them of past relationships, or it can be more complicated and involved, such as when a therapy relationship reenacts some unconscious, or unspoken, fantasy or story of pleasure and pain in the client's or (in the case of countertransference) the therapist's life. Analyst Glen Gabbard (1996) writes, "To get to the most primitive transference issues, one often has to go to the brink of despair with the patient, where one questions whether or not he can continue and whether or not he is being an effective analyst" (p. 202). Therapists who work with addictions will find themselves walking this knife-edge of faith and despair with alarming frequency. Sitting with the paradox of having to embrace one's powerlessness over drugs and alcohol before discovering the strength needed to combat them is a prerequisite to recovery. If therapists can't tolerate the feelings of failure and despair that come with recovery—to accept it as part of the journey—clients are not going to learn how to do so either. Therapists are most likely to experience this sort of discouragement when they haven't personally experienced powerlessness as a prelude to liberation in their own lives.

The goal of therapy in this phase of care is to allow clients to hit bottom and focus on taking responsibility for themselves rather than trying to change them. Many people become terrified at the prospect of coping with life on its own terms—without chemicals—and seek to run away from it. It is important for therapists to name this experience for clients. Therapists should make clear that to get through it clients will have to experience emptiness and despair, but it is also essential to remind them they don't have to do it alone—they have therapy and AA to serve as guides and companions.

Next to the existential angst that arises when one is hitting bottom, anger, more than any other emotion, undermines recovery and attempts at sobriety. Freud was the first to point out that the opposite of love is not hate but indifference. In therapy, clients often find themselves using aggression in the service of love. Bollas (1992) uses the term *loving hate* as an example of how some people bind others to them with intensely hateful feelings. The expression "loving hate" also describes many addicts' ties to alcohol and drugs, and the way that intensely hateful feelings toward significant others in their lives can be remembered and preserved in the form of an addiction. This was certainly true of Gere (in Chapter 2), who held onto, drank at, and reenacted his resentment and traumatic memories of his alcoholic father in the relationship with his own son, Jesse. And although Karen (in Chapter 1) took a different tack than Gere did, choosing, as many women do, to "act in" rather than "act out" her pain, Karen's drinking also helped her ward off past hurts and traumas.

Before moving on to a description of the next phase of care, I want to offer a few other thoughts about sitting with clients who are bargaining with an addiction and present some additional strategies that therapists can use to help them.

Once Larry decided that he no longer wanted to get high, he went through the same dance of intimacy, anger, and deception with marijuana that he had with alcohol. At this juncture, I found myself asking Larry if he might consider entering into a bargain with me. But this time, I warned, my proposition might seem a bit unorthodox. A little curious and more than a little desperate, Larry agreed. I asked him to promise that he would go to an AA or NA (Narcotics Anonymous) meeting that week, but only on condition that he would also promise to smoke some pot the following morning.

More than a bit surprised, Larry said he would keep his pledge but wanted to know more about the unusual nature of my request. I explained that it appeared that Larry had gotten himself into a bind where he felt that in order to go to AA or NA meetings he had to have come to a decision to stop drinking or using drugs *forever*. This left him paralyzed. No longer wanting to continue using substances but unable to stop, he was framing his dilemma in such a way that he was unable to draw on valuable supports at the time he needed them most. My agreement with him was intended to free him from this impasse and invite him to explore what resources AA or NA had to offer without having to commit himself to a course of action for which he wasn't ready.

Andrea (in Chapter 2) and Karen faced the same dilemma as Larry did; they all quit drinking for a period of time before they were willing or able to let go of marijuana or other drugs for good. Each felt that if they chose AA it had to be "all or nothing," that there was no room for doubt or struggle. It's helpful to remind clients who find themselves in this situation that not drinking is an accomplishment in and of itself, and that the success they met with there can be applied to other habits as well. In fact, AA's response to people who turn back to the bottle or to another drug is always more compassionate than judging. The use of sobriety days (a concept discussed in my letter to Andrea) can also be helpful during these times. This exercise helps individuals discriminate between sober versus alcoholic behavior. Keeping a behavioral inventory of their drinking and drug use allows people to view their histories of chemical dependency as a whole rather than in fragmented episodes.

For many people, this period comes with a painful realization that abstinence is only the beginning of their journey, not the end. Imagining themselves in pain without alcohol or something else to numb their feelings (pot, prescription medication, sex, food, etc.), is terrifying to most addicts. This fear is what drives most clients' desire to negotiate a kinder and gentler resolution to their quandary regarding the issue of abstinence versus controlled use. Larry turned to pot and food. After Larry formed a stronger bond with AA he expressed renewed enthusiasm for taking on all his compulsions, including compulsive overeating, at once. We discussed the destructive role that food played in Larry's life but agreed that dismissing pot from his life for good was a "huge next step" for him. While doing so would inevitably help with his weight gain, I didn't want to see Larry give up all his crutches, so to speak, at the same time. The "all or nothing" thinking that is such a signature trait of addiction can pose similar problems for people in recovery. Instead, I suggested that Larry use the opportunity of being completely drug free to gather data about his relationship with food, to really notice his eating habits and become more mindful of how, when sober, his emotions impacted on them.

Larry explained that in sobriety he felt emotions but had no logical explanation for them, and would often want to respond to them by drinking. AA's firm guidance and slogans, such as "Don't get too hungry, angry, lonely, or tired" (H.A.L.T.), are often enough to get people through the initial stages of sobriety but will start to feel empty in later recovery. As Whitfield (1987) observed, the newly recovering person can easily take this maxim to mean "hold in your feelings" rather than the intended message, "take better care of yourself so you don't become overwhelmed by these emotions." However, AA's slogans and supports do give people something to do, an action to take, that impacts on their mood and feeling state. As one recovering alcoholic remarked, "When I can not understand or explain what I'm feeling, I call someone or go to a meeting. The awareness will come, and the action reduces my fear" (Brown, 1985, p. 218). Again, in later recovery, taking these steps will work to prevent the act of drinking but will not address the emptiness and depression that contributed to the onset of such feelings in the first place.

Lockard (personal communication, 1992) refers to this depression as the "18-month crisis." It is a crisis of self-comprehension that following nearly 2 years of successful sobriety and loyal attendance at AA meetings leaves the person wondering, "Who am I?" The introduction used at meetings by most recovering people—"Hi, my name is Bill, and I'm an alcoholic"—experienced as freeing and liberating when they first become sober, is no longer an adequate identity in and of itself.

Once Larry had given up drinking, whenever these feelings surfaced he turned to pot and overeating to help him manage them. The same recovering person quoted above concludes: "Beneath the fear is the trust that comes from the knowledge that if I work the program and rely on my higher power for guidance, I do not need to repeat these old self-destructive patterns. I am really amazed at the idea that I can trust myself. I think the big surprise in my life is finding I'm okay and not a failure" (Brown, 1985, p. 219). No matter how much a person receives this message—about needing to put trust in themselves and their recovery—from their therapist or others, often they will not be able to hear it until it's delivered by fellow sufferers in AA. A quick explanation for AA's success in restoring people's faith in themselves may be drawn from pop culture. In interview after interview John Lennon was asked to speak to what was so special about the Beatles. Usually interviewers were looking for him to reveal something hidden in the music or some untold story about the band's strained backstage relations. On one occasion, however, Lennon responded differently. Accent in Britain, he said, is like race here in North America. It really marks you, and the prejudice about it is hard to overcome. Before the Beatles, British pop music stars who made it big cultivated accents from nowhere, what in North America we call "mid-Atlantic." Raised in the industrial city of Liverpool in Northern England, the Beatles kept their own accents. Similarly, AA has no pretensions. The people in these rooms speak in the addict's own language.

As Stephanie Brown (1985) observed, returning to an alcohol focus in therapy and recovery not only offers the refueling people need to proceed back "out" and continue enjoying life's rewards and facing its challenges, it also provides a secure territory and safe environment for a "timeout." These themes will be discussed further later in this book. However, as the next chapter suggests, therapy can help people manage the tension of not being in control by gradually becoming more confident and familiar with the experience of being out of control that not drinking creates. As Brown writes, "The primary focus of advanced alcoholism is on alcohol. Most of the individual's energy and attention go into the maintenance of denial in order to preserve the two basic beliefs: *'I am not alcoholic'* and *'I can control my drinking'* " (1985, p. 220; emphasis added).

Drinking and getting high provide people with the illusion that they are involved with the world and others but they're out of touch. The connection and love they desire is, ironically, most inaccessible when they are under the influence of addictive chemicals. The moment at which a person's life is no longer being used in the service of these deceptions—or compromised by them—and their energies are transformed into a genuine acceptance of their dilemma is when true healing and sobriety can begin.

CHAPTER 4

Telegrams from God

Reauthoring Spirituality

Praise me, says God, and I will know that you love Me.
Curse Me, says God, and I will know that you love Me.
Praise Me or Curse Me,
And I will know that you love Me.

Sing out My graces, says God.
Raise your fist against Me and revile, says God.
Sing out graces or revile,
Reviling is also a kind of praise, says God.

But if you sit fenced off in your apathy, says God,
If you sit entrenched in "I don't give a hang," says God,
If you look at the stars and yawn,
If you see suffering and don't cry out,
If you praise and you don't revile,
Then I created you in vain, says God.
            —IF YOU LOOK AT THE STARS (Prayer from
            the Jewish New Year, *Amherst Prayer Book*)

More perhaps than any other human activity, psychotherapy provides a model for what Søren Kierkegaard called the "passionate inwardness" involved in making existential decisions. What we do is at the interface of the spiritual and the therapeutic. Discussions of people's faith and spiritual values in this book are intentionally more tacit than explicit. Spirituality is talked about in the context of my work with clients rather than being presented as a separate lens through which to view therapy. This reflects my preferred way of addressing people's spiritual needs in therapy as well as my overall philosophy and approach to the subject. However, these are paths that clients and therapists can't ignore when faced with problems of addiction and trauma.

Many clients are uncomfortable with the spiritual aspects of recovery, what many in AA call the "God stuff." And, if they're able to overcome these feelings and embrace the need for a spiritual component in their treatment, the whole concept of prayer raises their insecurities. These concerns used to bring up my own feelings of inadequacy until a colleague told me about one of his clients, a recovering alcoholic, who came to see him because of the trouble he was having with the "God stuff." He was especially unnerved by what AA had to say about prayer and meditation. He said he didn't know how to pray, that he'd never done it. Then one time he came late for an appointment very upset with himself. He said he was ashamed of his behavior. He'd really "hit bottom" with his addiction—all his problems seemed to be crashing in on him. He was desperate to see his counselor and got stuck in traffic. Instead of using what he'd learned in AA about taking things "one day at a time" and "easy does it," he became furious. He started hammering his steering wheel with his fist, cursing God and shouting at the car in front of him "Jesus Christ Almighty" and a litany of other epithets. My colleague interrupted him, "I thought you said you didn't know how to pray?" he asked. The point is that our prayers needn't read like scripture or sound like poetry in order to reach a compassionate or understanding "other," including the being or presence we call God. The prayer this chapter opened with "If You Look at the Stars" makes the same point. It's okay to cry out in protest.

This chapter explores the less-traveled road of spiritual growth and healing overlooked by or omitted from most psychotherapies. It asks if we are finally ready, as Hans Loewald said, to explore how psychotherapy and psychoanalysis "might begin to contribute in their own way to the understanding of religious experience, instead of ignoring or rejecting its genuine validity or treating it as a mark of immaturity" (1980, p. 73).

Clinicians often wrongly interpret people's reliance on an external source of help, or "Higher Power," as a failure of the will. However, when it comes to treating addiction, psychotherapy's emphasis on independence and self-reliance can get in the way. Recovery is based on the continuing acceptance of loss of control and the need to continue to ask for help. It requires giving up one's belief in the power of self and the recognition of an ongoing need for support.

AA has long recognized that it takes both tough-mindedness and faith to get by in this world. This willingness of AA to remain open minded when investigating spiritual experience, and its encouraging its membership to do the same, is what distinguishes AA's voice from most other theories and methods. It also counters what Erik H. Erikson referred to in his epilogue to *Childhood and Society* (1950) as the "talmudic orthodoxy" he felt had descended on the psychotherapy community.

A CORRESPONDENCE BETWEEN
AN ANALYST AND A DRUNK

> A man stands alone and cannot sing. Another man stands
> with him and the first man can also sing.
> —MARTIN BUBER

In a correspondence between Bill Wilson, cofounder of AA, and Carl Jung, Wilson traces the origins of AA back to the analyst's consulting room and the "hitting bottom" experience of one of Jung's patients. Roland H., an individual whom Jung had been treating for a severe drinking problem, had shown improvement and terminated therapy feeling much better about himself. After approximately a year of sobriety he started drinking again and, in worse shape than ever, returned seeking additional help from his former analyst. Wilson described what happened next in a letter that he wrote to Jung 30 years later:

> First of all, you frankly told him of his hopelessness so far as any further medical or psychiatric treatments might be concerned. This candid and humble statement of yours was beyond a doubt the first foundation upon which our society has since been built.
>
> Coming from you, one he so trusted and admired, the impact upon him was immense.
>
> When he then asked you if there was any other hope, you told him that there might be, provided he could become the subject of a spiritual or religious experience. In short, a genuine conversion. (*Best of the Grapevine*, 1985, p. 164)

Jung's patient subsequently joined the Oxford Group, an evangelical movement popular in the 1930s, and did indeed have a spiritual experience and was able to stop drinking. Jung's patient then worked with an old drinking buddy of Bill Wilson's named Ebby, who in turn became sober and showed up at Bill's house proclaiming that "I got religion" (Berenson, 1987).

More is written about these events in *Alcoholics Anonymous* (1939/1976; what's often referred to as the "Big Book") and other biographies of AA. It suffices to say that Ebby's sobriety had a profound impact on

Bill—a "release" or serenity that Bill felt wasn't accounted for by Ebby's brief association with a religious group. One aspect of the experience that Bill could identify as crucial for him, even in his intoxicated state of mind, was the relief that hearing those words from a "kindred spirit" brought him at the time. Ebby's visit led to Bill's own "spiritual awakening" and his eventual recovery.

A closer examination of these events will also help readers understand the traces of traditional Christian vernacular still found in AA and other 12-step programs today. Sometimes providing portions of this history to clients can put some people—those whose reactions to the word "God" and its use in meetings interferes with their participation—more at ease.

Jung enthusiastically responded to Bill's letter, as he had always wondered what had become of Roland H.:

> His craving for alcohol was the equivalent, on a low level, of the thirst of our being for wholeness, expressed in medieval language: the union with God.[1]
>
> How could one formulate such an insight in a language that is understood in our days?
>
> The only right and legitimate way to such an experience is that it happens to you in reality, and it can only happen to you when you walk on a path which leads you to higher understanding. You might be led to that goal by an act of grace or through personal and honest contact with friends, or through a higher education of the mind beyond the confines of mere rationalism. I see from your letter that Roland H. has chosen the second way, which was, under the circumstances, obviously the best one. . . .
>
> You see "alcohol" in Latin is *spiritus*, and you use the same word for the highest religious experience as well as for the most depraving poison. The helpful formula therefore is: *spiritus contra spiritum*. (*Best of the Grapevine*, 1985, pp. 167–168)

Following Jung, clinicians and researchers need to recognize the strength and hope of AA and other 12-step programs as legitimate sources of knowledge and scholarship.

PAIN AND PARADOX

Bill Wilson's own experience of "hitting bottom" and the spiritual awakening he experienced following his visit from his friend Ebby is a powerful illustration of our reliance upon, and faith in, the power of story, as well as its prominent role in the growth and development of Alcoholics Anonymous. A vision that came to him during his final stay and detox at Towns Hospital (in New York) is, in the folklore of AA, commonly referred to as Bill's "white light" experience:

> My depression deepened unbearably, and finally it seemed to me as though I were at the very bottom of the pit. For the moment, the last vestige of my proud obstinacy was crushed. All at once I found myself crying out, "If there is a God, let him show himself! I am ready to do anything!"
>
> Suddenly the room lit up with a great white light. It seemed to me, in the mind's eye, that I was on a mountain and that a wind not of air but of spirit was blowing. And then it burst upon me that I was a free man. Slowly the ecstasy subsided. I lay on the bed, but now for the first time I was in another world, a new world of consciousness. All about me and through me there was a wonderful feeling of presence, and I thought to myself, "So this is the God of the preachers!" A great peace stole over me and I thought, "No matter how wrong things seem to be, they are all right. Things are all right with God and his world."[2] (*AA Comes of Age*, 1985, p. 63)

When Bill returned to his ordinary state of consciousness, he began to panic, thinking that maybe he was hallucinating, or worse, that he might be going crazy. He immediately sent for his physician to ask if he was still sane. After hearing Bill's story, his doctor said, "Something has happened to you that I don't understand. But you had better hang on to it. Anything is better than the way you were." Bill never drank again.[3]

According to cultural anthropologist and family therapist Joan Laird (1989), storytelling and mythmaking are themselves definitional. We come to know the world through our own storying or mythologizing of it. Only when events have been languaged—put into words—do our experiences become endowed with cognitive, moral, or aesthetic meaning. Bill Wilson, reflecting on his experience some years later (which, incidentally, he felt a certain embarrassment about as a reserved New Englander and often called his "hot flash"), showed a deep appreciation for the power of myth and story to define our lived experience:

> Perhaps you raise the question of hallucination versus the divine imagery of a genuine spiritual experience. I doubt if anyone has authoritatively defined what an hallucination really is. . . .
>
> Some might think me presumptuous when I say that my own experience is real. Nevertheless, I can surely report that in my own life and in the lives of countless others, *the fruits of that experience have been real, and the benefactions beyond reckoning.* (*As Bill Sees It,*

1967, p. 182 [formally *The AA Way of Life*], from a talk delivered in 1960; emphasis added)

The point Wilson is trying to make is that regardless of the veracity of his spiritual encounter, the story about it has had an effect on the people whose lives have been touched by it and its impact has, for the most part, been a positive one.

Pragmatics aside, one cannot underestimate the importance of tending to a person's sense of spirituality and faith when that individual is developing ideas about addiction or recovering from it. Psychotherapy generally remains obsessed with uncovering the underlying structure or causes of a person's problems—systemic, psychic, biological, cybernetic, or otherwise. AA, on the other hand, emphasizes acceptance over understanding and places the mystery of the human spirit much closer to the recovering person's center of gravity.

As David Berenson explains, the resistance most therapists have to the spiritual message of AA is isomorphic to the paradox most alcoholics find themselves in when they hear the same message. A person admits that she has a drinking problem but is sure she can control it without declaring herself an alcoholic. A therapist admits that AA produces positive results but is sure it can be explained by group hypnosis, a person receiving a "corrective emotional experience," or the substitution of an addiction to AA for her alcoholism. "In both cases," Berenson concludes, "there is an attempt to maintain a mindset that offers logic, predictability, and the illusion of control and an avoidance of a way of being that offers serenity, peace, and self-acceptance" (1985, p. xi).

On a personal note, one of the most spiritually affirming experiences in my professional life took place at one of Berenson's workshops (1986) more than 10 years ago. I can't describe what an epiphany it was for me to see a Harvard-educated MD stand in front of a room full of educated professionals—who were expecting to grapple with issues of "wet" and "dry" phases of family interaction, "high" versus "low" bottom recovery, and the effects of problem drinking in couple treatment—and say, "Folks if you want to know what gets alcoholics better: *It's the God stuff.*"

The terms "spiritual experience" and spiritual awakenings are used many times in AA's Big Book and other literature, which, according to the former:

> Upon careful reading shows that the personality change sufficient to bring about recovery from alcoholism has manifested itself among us in many different forms.
>
> Yet it is true that our first printing gave many readers the impres-

> sion that these personality changes, or religious experiences must be in
> the nature of sudden and spectacular upheavals. Happily for everyone
> this conclusion is erroneous. (*Alcoholics Anonymous*, 1939/1976,
> p. 569).

Without dismissing this kind of transformation out of hand, the authors
go on to explain that the majority of these experiences are what psychologist William James called the "educational variety," because they develop slowly over a period of time. This is what is referred to, in the family therapy speak of Bateson and his colleagues at the Mental Health
Research Institute, as "second order change." Through the accumulation of healthy loving interactions with other alcoholics, the person finds
herself having undergone a profound alteration that could not have been
brought about on their own. It is suggested that the newly discovered inner strength needed to accomplish this shift is what the majority of AA
members identify as their concept of a power greater than themselves:
"Most of us think this awareness of a Power Greater than ourselves is
the essence of spiritual experience. Our more religious members call it
'God-consciousness' " (*Alcoholics Anonymous*, 1939/1976, p. 570).[4]

PARADOX WITHOUT ANGUISH

AA makes it clear that the concept of a Higher Power is for each individual to define for her- or himself. In order to flesh out these concepts further and provide the reader with a better sense of how they effect the
way I think about my practice, I find myself turning to traditions from
my own religious and cultural heritage. I have already made reference to
Martin Buber's philosophy. Further mention of his ideas warrants more
background.

Buber's thinking about spirituality appeals to me because it keeps
me from treating people and their addictions generically. In Buber's vision, "Every person born into the world represents something new,
something that never existed before, something original and unique. . . .
If there had been someone like her in the world, there would have been
no need for her to be born." Buber's poetic use of language, florid and
obscure as it often is, resonates. It offers therapists a way of helping clients rid themselves of problems without losing sight of the person. Buber
was once asked, "If you had to characterize God in one word, what
would it be?" He replied, "If I had to use one word only it would be
presence."[5] It is a good word because it indicates that where we human

beings are sometimes present God is always present and accessible to all human beings at once. Buber's concept of I–Thou can be best summarized as a mandate to relate to all beings with respect for their otherness—to view every moment of engagement with another person as an act of faith conjuring up the presence of God. It's about being touched by and touching others. This is no less true of our relationship with God. According to Buber, we do not worship God, we relate to God; or, more accurately, worship is just another way of relating—it's a particular kind of conversation within the human dialogue.

In contrast, "I–It" relations are about interactions that do not require reciprocity. They are more about events that involve detachment, such as when we interface with technology. I–It interactions are not inherently exploitative or evil; in fact, just the opposite, they are indispensable for life. They're the floor, the basis of all routine experience. They become corrupted only when they presume to have the I–Thou quality. If someone tries to palm the floor off as the ceiling, then it becomes evil in that context. For example, often in political and economic spheres, we are told that thermonuclear, chemical, and biological weapons are essential for keeping the peace; or computers are depicted as saviors, rather than instruments, of modern civilization; or the care of our sick and elderly citizens is described as something that needs to be "managed" (i.e., reduced).

According to Buber there are not two kinds of people—the pure I–It types and the pure I–Thou types—but two poles of humanity, and we all relate to one another in both ways at different times. Similarly, I find there are not different kinds of addicts but people afflicted by varying poles of addiction. Buber calls these two poles "ego" and "person." No one is a pure ego (I–It) or pure person (I–Thou); rather, the words represent tendencies. Recovery is about helping someone become less ego and more person.

Note that Buber is not talking about achieving higher levels of consciousness or transcending the material world. When he refers to I–Thou relations he is talking about ordinary human experience. We can have such I–Thou encounters in nature, too—with a bird, a rock, or a tree. A biologist, a botanist, a chemist, and a physicist all approach the tree in terms of their own preoccupations. The result is I–It. We have our own version of this in our professional communities. Just as the painter is inherently not in an I–Thou relationship with the world, neither is any particular branch of the mental health professions or any school of therapy more in touch with people's needs than any other; each illuminates a different aspect of experience. The artist who simply sees the tree as an instrument of her art is no better than the paper manufacturer who sees it as potential wood pulp. So, too, is the novelist who only sees the tree as a symbol or as the subject of a story. It is a matter of approach not occupation. At our best we treat all aspects of nature—all rocks, trees, birds, and human beings—as though they had a spark of the divine in them. (Agnostics might well opt to use a more Einsteinian vocabulary and perhaps call that spark "energy.") We do not look at them with an eye to their utility or how neatly they fit into our theories.

While a tree or a rock may not be able to reciprocate (i.e., we cannot be certain that there is an awareness or consciousness of the interaction on its part), we can approach it as if it has. We approach these sorts of interaction with what Buber calls an "uncertain certainty." If I have both the will *and* the grace to consider the tree as a manifestation of the divine, then I become bound up in an I–Thou relation with it and the tree is no longer an "it."

You cannot force an I–Thou relation; it must be spontaneous. It cannot be controlled. That is why we speak of falling in love rather than planning our way into love. But there has to be a willingness—it is both passivity and activity at the same time. It is difficult, Buber notes, to bear the episodic and ephemeral character of the I–Thou relation with God. In fact, any I–Thou relation is threatening because it is not subject to control, which is one explanation of why spirituality, in general, and AA's spiritual concepts and practices, in particular, are often so intimidating to the active or newly sober addict.

Buber always deals with relations—what transpires between people. His concepts are moving pictures of relationships, never still photographs. The word of God is like a meteor flashing across the sky, it is I–Thou; but our relationship with the Bible, or another holy book is like that with the stone-cold meteorite in the ground, it is I–It. The meteorite must light up again for us in order for us to encounter the eternal I–Thou in an I–Thou relation. It is like when you taped a great concert at which you had an I–Thou experience. When you brought it home and played it, it felt like an I–It, just sound. To become a vehicle for another I–Thou encounter, the experience of listening to the tape must be as spontaneous as was the original concert. But the harder you try to force it and rekindle the original I–Thou experience, the less likely it is to happen. Similarly, for example, we are unlikely to succeed when we find ourselves using a technique in therapy with a client to try and invoke an I–Thou moment because it had that effect on a different person some days earlier.

The I–Thou relation converts sounds into music, color splotches into paintings, touch into affection. And most important it is not a rare occurrence. It is the joy of interacting with a pet that takes us out of ourselves. It transformed Miranda's words into poetry and her letters (in the Prologue and Chapter 2) into a form of prayer and meditation—what AA's 11th-step would call "conscious contact" with a power greater than herself.

I am not trying to provide answers here. Rather, I am just offering one of the many ways (out of an endless array of possibilities) that I try to think about or conceptualize a sense of the sacred in my work—how I personally try to hold onto a concept of a higher power when I practice therapy. This is not a map for infusing spirituality into the therapy process. It is simply an example of how I try to stay connected to myself and to the Divine—to what we call God—in my life and remain open and willing to show up for these moments when they present themselves in my consultations with my clients. It is an attempt to make a connection between AA's emphasis on "the God stuff" and all clients', not just addicts' and recovering persons', need for more I–Thou encounters in their therapy and healing.[6]

These dialogic approaches to spirituality and psychotherapy also provide a way of responding to the egocentric stance of Descartes's *cogito, ergo sum* ("I think, therefore I am") presented in the Introduction and its pernicious effect on modern culture, in general, as well as the culture of therapy and recovery, in particular. In this worldview all beliefs must appear before the omnipotent "I" and stand up to cross-examination. The point is captured in a saying that was popular when my parents were kids: "I am from Missouri; you have to show me." I need proof.

Buber's answer, similar to AA's response to the addict, is that beginning with the isolated ego you cannot get to a genuine involvement with the world and with other selves. It's like the traveler in the Irish village who asked a resident how to get to Dublin. And the villager answered, "If I was wanting to get to Dublin, I wouldn't be starting from here." So AA, in effect, says to the alcoholic what Buber says to Descartes and to the many modern philosophers who have followed him: "If you want to get to a life that resonates with meaning, then don't begin with the isolated ego." What Buber does is start with the self interacting with other beings—just as AA situates alcoholics within a protective wall of humanity—for Buber there is no self apart from other beings. We are constituted by our relations to others.

ANALYTIC MEANS TO SPIRITUAL ENDS

Author Leon Wieseltier in his book *Kaddish*—a moving memoir of his father's death and his search for the origin and meaning of the Jewish mourners' prayer—says "Jews who open their books do so for one of two reasons: to make themselves more like the tradition or to make the tradition more like themselves" (1998, p. 76). My own father used to say, "There are two types: those who divide the world into two types and those who don't." Nevertheless, if one were to apply Wieseltier's axiom to the secular world of psychoanalysis, object relations theorist and child analyst D. W. Winnicott would fit into the latter category. Winnicott once remarked that it was difficult for him to read other people's work, as by the time he got to the bottom of the page he had already made the words his own, transforming them into something completely different than the author intended. Winnicott appreciated that true creativity—coming to know and share our authentic self—is itself an act of faith.

Winnicott's work focuses on the magical and sacred aspects of everyday life. Winnicott, like Buber, is interested in exploring the connections between the routine and the extraordinary, between the everyday and the more intense. For both men, philosopher and therapist, ordinary events are the miracles of people's lives. "Play," says Buber, "is the exultation of the possible." Winnicott uses the concept of "good-enough" parenting to make this same point. It is for parents (and therapists) the daily routine of showing up (i.e., being there) for the child, day in and day out, as well as their willingness to play and be played with in the potential space that exists between the two that transforms ordinary experience into a magical event. Winnicott's celebration of and straightforward language about naturally occurring events invites us to examine the complexity and multiple meaning of our everyday lives. He seems to be reminding us—in the words of the popular Bonnie Raitt song—"just how good 'good enough' can be."

Winnicott's thoughts about the joy that can be found in everyday experience or derived from the simplest pleasures would bring little comfort to most addicts. T. S. Eliot wrote in "Burnt Norton," the first of the *Four Quartets* (1943/1962a), "human kind cannot bear very much reality" (p. 118). This might serve as a text of what happens with regard to the progression of addiction in people's lives as well as Buber's analysis of people's alternation of "it" and "thou." People shy away from the uncertainty and insecurity of the thou, which involves spontaneity. They run away from the I–Thou relations, into I–It experiences that can be controlled. Buber (1958) claims that we "flee from the unreliable, unsolid, unlasting, unpredictable, dangerous world of relation into the having of things" (p. 126). Addicts turn to substances in an effort to guarantee pleasurable experience in the same way people brandish religious symbols in an effort to guarantee spiritual experiences. In both instances they make God into an object and try to drag the divine into the It-world.

"BY THE GRACE OF GOD":
PSYCHOTHERAPY, SPIRITUALITY, AND RECOVERY

> It requires moral courage to grieve; it requires religious
> courage to rejoice.
>
> —SØREN KIERKEGAARD

Similar to Buber's I–Thou dialogic, concepts of spirituality in AA are viewed as forms of social activity cast in the context of human relationships. As Buber puts it, "Meeting with God does not come to man in order that he may concern himself with God, but in order that he may confirm that there is meaning in the world" (1958, p. 115). Addiction is what some people turn to in order both to avoid painful feelings *and to provide meaning.*

From the standpoint of recovery, acceptance is about having faith in someone or something greater than oneself. It can be something in nature—a tree, a tranquil spot by a riverbank, or the cosmos itself—or it can be faith in other human beings, which often takes the form of a person's 12-step support group. It makes no difference, as AA members like to remind one another, whether your Higher Power is God-G-O-D—or God—G.O.D. (group of drunks)—"The only thing you need to know for certain is you ain't it!"

What all these various descriptions of a higher power have in common is the manner in which people infuse their relationships to these experiences or phenomena with a sense of the sacred. We use many words to describe this feeling and our relationship to it: God, Higher Power, Majesty, Infinite, Eternal, Divine, Truth. These words, said a well-known rabbi, are all metaphors for a mystery whose nature eludes us but whose presence sometimes makes itself known in our lives, seeking a relationship with us.

The relative silence, until recently, in the psychotherapy community regarding people's spiritual and religious concerns has many origins, not the least of which is the great many clients in recovery who have experienced religious abuses of one kind or another. Most of these incidents are not the headline-grabbing sort that involve parish priests or other religious leaders committing acts of sexual abuse. They are much more mundane but no less damaging. A devout Catholic who has taken communion is told she is sinful and risks excommunication because she wants to make a home with the woman she loves. A son and daughter whose parents are practicing Jews who keep a kosher home and attend temple reject their religion because they cannot reconcile their father's spiritual practices with his violent behavior at home toward his wife and children.

These experiences are not unique to alcoholic families but, because of the increased risk of violence and erratic behavior in homes with high incidents of substance abuse and addiction, show up in larger numbers within them. "Religion is for those of us afraid of going to hell; spirituality is for those of us who have already been there" is how one client explained his understanding of the difference between spirituality and religion to me and the important role that faith played in his recovery.

For another client, the way God is talked about at meetings was painful for other reasons. A deeply religious person, he felt that AA treated God too lightly. The second of the 12 steps declares: "We came to believe a Power greater than ourselves could restore us to sanity." The third testifies to having "made a decision to turn our will and our lives over to the care of God as we understood him." Members are encouraged to develop their own views. What results is often what we might call, Higher Power as "celestial valet." One AA member extols her Higher Power for providing a parking space when she was hassled and short on time; another, for supplying someone to help her fix a flat tire. Yet, many of these statements represent a failure of articulation rather than a failure of faith. What underlines these testimonies is the sense that an individual is related to a power that is always there, a power not one's own.

The concept of acceptance or surrender in AA does not advocate people becoming accepting or tolerant of abuse, injustice, or other degrading situations in their lives. On the contrary, people who are no longer willing to put up with self-abuse are less likely to submit to it in other contexts or to accept it from others. It means accepting the fact of a situation and then deciding what we will do about it. In AA, Al-Anon, and other 12-step programs, learning to accept the things we can't change and to change the things we can means knowing what it is to have power *in relation to,* rather than power *over,* someone.[7]

Thomas Moore, in *Care of the Soul* (1992), also worries about our tendency in the modern world to separate psychology from religion. He says that we like to think that emotional problems have to do with the family, childhood, and trauma—but not with spirituality. However, for the person subjected to them, trauma and abuse are spiritual crises. These problems are also symptomatic of a spiritual breakdown in the values and psyche of the perpetrator of the violence and, when it reaches epidemic proportions, the culture in which it takes place.

As a consequence, for many people only the concept of a being or presence as omnipotent as God may be large enough to heal the scars of violence and abuse and the shame that can stem from addiction, or fulfill an undying need for a parent or unconditional love. To paraphrase poet Louise Gluck, what has driven many of these clients' letters and stories—as well as my own—from the first is terror and the need for an understandable other: "When the terror becomes unbearable, the other becomes God" (1994, p. 22).

My introduction to this process—my "white light" experience, so to speak—took place in my own therapy and through my participation in Al-Anon. My own mother continues to suffer from alcoholism, as she did throughout much of my childhood and adult life. When I decided to marry Dana, my partner of many years, my mother's drinking became the source of much stress and anxiety for me, as it had on numerous other occasions. Unsure how to handle the presence of alcohol at my wedding and concerned about her alcoholism, I sought a personal consultation with my colleague, Roget. After listening patiently to my dilemma, Roget asked me to entertain the following scenario:

> "Imagine, Jon, if tomorrow morning you went out to your mail box and discovered a telegram, and when you opened it read:
>
> Dear Jonathan,
> > I am sorry, it is not in the stars for your mother to get better.
> > Love,
> > > God."

I fought back tears when I heard these words. Their message led to a profound shift in my relationship with my mother from one of grieving for the past to living for the present. And although it is far from ideal and can at times still be quite painful, it remains a growing relationship. My mother's alcoholism, while still active, is in the midst of a process that I have come to describe as "bottoming up." With so much love, care, and change in her own life and the people around her, the alcoholic can't help but feel better about herself and her circumstances.

This imaginary telegram had a greater impact on my life story than any real correspondence I've ever received. I have since passed this intervention on to numerous clients. I have also not missed the irony or, in literary terms, "poetic justice" in discovering that my own Higher Power often channels such communiqués through my most challenging and difficult relationships.

If There Has to Be a God, Can She Be a Committee of Women Dedicated to Wiping Out Earthly Oppression?

For Karen (in Chapter 1) and Angela (in Chapter 2), locating their spirituality in the context of relationships with others resulted in their feeling less isolated and more willing to reach out to others. This process unfolded in therapy, with other members of AA and Al-Anon, with others at church, and most importantly for each woman, with herself—or, as expressed in one of Karen's letters, "by the Grace of God, being in AA and becoming my real self."

Karen's spiritual beliefs and commitments have undergone many transformations as a result of her participation in AA:

> "I used to see things that happened to me as lessons God wanted me to learn. I've since gotten rid of that idea. I used to prefer judgmental religion. I was a 'good catch,' a 'big prize' for the fundamentalist church I joined when I got married the first time [to a physically abusive man whose father was the minister of the church she attended]. I hated it, it was always, 'Look at all those things Karen did.' It makes me want to get up on a podium in the park or town commons and shout, 'This is what happened to Karen!' God is no longer a judge. I feel that kind of thinking does more harm than good. I can no longer think of myself as acceptable and think of God as condemning."

After an extensive search Karen joined a Unitarian church in her community from which she derives a great deal of support. She was particularly drawn to its nonhierarchical structure and the strong and spirited presence of its woman minister, with whom Karen felt an immediate connection. Karen also helped found and co-led a weekly support group for troubled teenagers, sponsored by the church.

Angela, too, viewed her letter to her "fear of loneliness" as an opportunity to dialogue with her Higher Power—in my metaphoric shorthand, her version of a telegram from God or Western (Com)Union:

> You were the reason I turned to God for strength. You were the reason I found the church full of Christian friends who care for me. . . .
> However many of the painful relationships I jumped into

were your handiwork also. I looked for anything to fill the gap in my life. I would take any abuse because of you.

For both women, a reauthoring of their spirituality resulted in their loosening the grip that fear had on their lives and relationships, a renewed commitment to fighting forces of terror and oppression in their homes and communities, and an unwillingness to organize their lives around and tolerate abuse. Overall, their writing and the conversations it generated had the effect of transforming their faith into what bell hooks and Cornell West (hooks & West, 1991) call a "combative spirituality."

For Karen and Angela there was a gentler more personal side to this journey as well. For them, and for many of the other contributors to this book, reclaiming their sense of spirituality—their faith and belief in others—helped them discover a greater sense of acceptance, love and compassion for themselves. When people come to trust in this aspect of their spirit through AA, psychotherapy, or writing, not only does it help them to connect with the larger culture and external world in ways they did not think possible, but it also helps them to create a sense of interior space they may not have known they had. Spirituality—the power of love and faith—strengthens our connection with ourselves, others, and the world around us. It allows us to inhabit parts of ourselves we had long since abandoned.

CHAPTER 5

Epilogues

Letting Go

It always comes back to the same necessity: go deep enough
and there is a bedrock of truth, however hard.
—MAY SARTON

A common thread running through all the stories and letters collected in
this volume is the sadness and grief expressed over lost years and opportunities. This is an experience shared by addicts, alcoholics, and their
family members from all walks of life. David Treadway once described
AA as an ongoing funeral (i.e., it's difficult to sit in these meeting rooms
without having some kind of pain or grief from your own past come up).
Al-Anon is another space where people can mourn the loss of friends
and family to addiction. Judaism has a saying that "the mourning of one
human being cannot be separated from the mourning of a people." AA
seems to embody this principle. Many gatherings offer a moment of silence "for the sick and suffering alcoholics who are still out there" prior
to the start of the meeting. This ritual and others like it help people let
go of their pain and suffering. Grief experienced by oneself opens
wounds while grief experienced in the company of others heals them.
The goal of therapy in the final stage of recovery is to move people from
a position of saving to that of grieving.

JEFF AND SYLVIA: "STORIES WITHOUT ENDINGS"

Jeff and Sylvia were a couple with whom I met for therapy in a New
England Hospital. After a year of working together, I had to leave the

hospital and their story had "to be continued" with another therapist. I wrote the following letter in response to the couple's request that I give their new therapist an "extensive summary" of our work together. (The gift I thank them for at the beginning of the correspondence refers to a book of quotations entitled *Great Thoughts* that they gave me in our last meeting together.)

My Correspondence to Jeff and Sylvia

Dear Sylvia & Jeff,

I want to thank you again for both your presents and your presence in the therapy. I am having a hard time putting the book down, but have managed to pull myself away to send this note off to you.

You had asked me to provide a summary of our work together for Margaret. I have decided to include it in this letter instead so that you can share parts or all of it as you deem appropriate with her whenever you decide to continue your therapy. So here goes.

I remember when you first came to my office in January you were trying to heal from a very traumatic incident in your marriage. At that time, Jeff had just disclosed his involvement with another woman whom he had met through his work. You both were in agreement, a unique and unusual occurrence at the time, that had this event not happened it would still have been extremely important for the two of you to seek some kind of counseling or help with your marriage. When reflecting back on that painful period in your lives, several thoughts and ideas come to mind as having been particularly helpful. Our collective decision to view the affair as a serious violation of Sylvia's trust on Jeff's part and as a wrong and hurtful action and behavior rather than just a symptom of a "bad marriage" was one turning point in your relationship that transformed this crisis into an opportunity for growth and change. Sylvia needed this to feel understood in order to even begin contemplating any attempts at mending the relationship. Jeff, feeling more remorseful and angry at himself than any therapist could imagine, would not, I feel, have been able to undertake any meaningful therapy process if his guilt and other emotions were not validated and taken seriously. This unwelcome and intrusive sense of shame about the state of your relationship, coupled with a shared undying love for your daughter, Rose, is what I believe kept the two of you together and committed to coming to therapy at the time. The other turning point was Sylvia's decision to seek individual counseling for herself. It was clear that while the events and problems that threatened your marriage were scary and upsetting for both of you, it was disorienting for Sylvia to such an extent that it had her questioning not only the future of the marriage but her very own existence as well. Acknowledging that she would carry on alone for Rose if she had to, the possibility of her marriage ending felt like a schism that cut all the way to the core of her being and personhood. This we understood as having something to do with the differences in the way that men and women are raised to see themselves in the world. Women's sense of self stems so strongly from connection to others, while men are raised to be much more independent and reliant on themselves alone. Although the thought of dissolving the marriage felt devastating to you both, Sylvia had few, if any, descriptions of herself without the relationship.

Through her work with Leslie, Sylvia became much more confident of her own abilities and in turn empowered in the relationship. Sylvia discovering her power and Jeff (with Jack's help) learning to accept responsibility for his actions, while also accepting that his needs and feelings are worthy of love and nothing to be ashamed of, are, in my view, important and irreversible strides you both have made together. As two equal partners (in and outside the room), you then began the difficult and complex process of exploring your feelings about your marriage and determining your respective needs in the relationship. I feel strongly that your decision to separate during this time is what allowed you both the time and space you needed to accomplish all this, while providing the most loving and nurturing environment possible for Rose. In our meetings, the dialogue moved sensitively and sensibly between support for your daughter's needs (and your shared concerns about parenting) and your sense of how events in your lives had unfolded so that you had "grown so far apart."

I was in awe of the determination with which you pursued this task, leaving no stone unturned. The myriad of themes that emerged are too numerous to mention, so I will highlight what I feel were some of the more important ones. You both looked honestly and openly at your families of origin. Sylvia decided that sacrificing herself unconditionally without regard for her own needs was an heirloom handed down from generation to generation by women in her family that she did not want to pass on to her own daughter. Protecting others from her anger and then directing it inward or having it surface in the form of stomach pains and other physical discomfort is another unwanted side effect of this legacy. Jeff's willingness to look at the role that alcohol and pot in particular may play in buffering him from intimacy and/or unwanted feelings of dependence in relationships

was another very important development. Just as Sylvia had
trouble coming up with descriptions of herself without a marriage
or relationship, Jeff, in turn, had similar difficulties developing a
strong sense of self within a marriage. Having met at a very
young age, what you both discovered, or one idea we discussed,
was that you often felt more married to roles that ended up
feeling like obligations rather than choices and/or compromises.
Together, on paper, these thoughts are more like a collage of our
relationship and your work. No one idea stands out more
significantly than the other, and I haven't put them in any order
of importance. I'll leave that job for you.

What I do want to emphasize is that much of what you
discovered about yourselves on this journey was extremely
positive—not the least of which has been the care and support of
both of your families for each of you as individuals and as a
couple.

I realize that as our work is coming to an end, many of the
feelings that surfaced recently have been extremely painful ones.
At this point, your decision to move back in and make a go of it,
in addition to bringing a sense of relief and joy, must be
extremely scary and anxiety provoking. Returning to the
marriage with so much more mindfulness and awareness of who
you are and your strengths and limitations must bring a certain
finality with it. If it doesn't work, you won't be able to blame
youth, inexperience, or one another. It will mean having to
accept that you've done the best you can, celebrating and
embracing your successes and grieving the loss of some of the
dreams you shared together as you let go and move on.

I am not surprised that sex came up in our last session as
the forum for our discussion of these fears. It embodies most, if
not all, of the topics explored in our work and in this
correspondence. It requires a great deal of trust for it to feel safe,
and the intimacy and feelings of dependency generated can be
frightening. For these reasons, many couples have, at one time or
another, felt overwhelmed and constricted by the expectations,
stereotypes, and gender roles associated with the acts of
performance themselves. Consequently, I think there is a wisdom
in your moving slowly and not rushing into things. I realize this
feels like a giant step backward for you, Jeff, and you worry that
you're right back to where you started 3–4 years ago. I assure
you you're not, and continuing in a dialogue with a third person
will help keep things moving forward. (*Choosing* not to be sexual
for a time with one another to help facilitate other kinds of
intimacy and ways of communicating with one another is *not* the
same as not having sex because you're not communicating!) I
hope you continue to explore these feelings with one another and

in the therapy so that neither of you experiences this development as a punishment but instead as an important and acceptable part of reestablishing a successful partnership.

Finally, I believe it is *very* important for you both to think about what your *assumptions* and *expectations* are regarding your decision to move back in with one another. A quote from *Great Thoughts* may shed some light on this point: "The definition of insanity is doing the same thing over and over again and expecting different results!" What are the guidelines each of you has established for your *own* behavior? What signs of change will you look for? What would you need more of to keep enabling these changes to happen? How did you know you were ready to take this step? I hope these are useful ideas and questions for you both and Margaret.

Again, thank you for both the gift and your trust. Please don't hesitate to call me if I can be of any further assistance.

Fondly yours,

Jonathan Diamond

Therapy with Jeff and Sylvia reminds me of Peter Drucker's words that there are risks you cannot afford to take and there are risks you cannot not afford to take.

I sent my correspondence to the couple, leaving it up to them as to what information to share with their new therapist. All of what was highlighted in the letter was shared first with the couple over the course of our relationship, meeting every other week, and is a poignant example of what analyst Christopher Bollas (1983) refers to as "working in the subjective." Interpretations are shared tentatively and cautiously, and in fact any decision about the entire value of the therapy is left in the clients' hands, with them having the final interpretation. In this sense, the letter reflected an effort on my part to make the work more accessible and transparent to my clients as well as any colleagues planning on continuing the therapy with them.

The themes addressed in my letter to Jeff and Sylvia, and our work together in general, illustrate many of the clinical questions found throughout this book—particularly those related to issues of power, gender, and addiction—and will be explored further in subsequent chapters.

However, what I especially appreciate about Jeff and Sylvia's story, along with Karen's (in Chapter 1), Larry's (in Chapter 3), and so many others stories included here, is that it counters prevailing thought in both the psychotherapy and the 12-step recovery communities that therapy with people who are struggling with alcohol and drug problems is never effective or warranted unless their addiction issues are resolved first. While this may be the ideal, it is often an unrealistic objective and, as witnessed in much of the work presented thus far, not always preferable. In some instances a great deal of productive dialogue can take place before people are ready to tackle their troubles with drugs and alcohol.

This couple's experience also helps dispel the myth that people who suffer from an addiction do not have other problems to contend with, or that everything in their lives is put on hold in the service of drinking or drug use. While this is one possible scenario, it is one of many. It is important to remember that people suffering from an addiction are often capable of functioning well, or at least adequately, and tending to other aspects of their lives while in the throws of a severe problem.

"MAKING A CUP OF GREEN TEA, I STOP THE WAR"

In his book *Healing into Life and Death* (1987), author Stephen Levine tells the story of how during the Korean War Paul Reps, a long-time meditator and writer, gained entrance into Japan so that he might spend some time studying and practicing at a Zen monastery in Kyoto. At the time Japan was being used as a military staging area for UN air and troop movements to Korea. As a result, nonmilitary Westerners were not being given visas. Levine continues:

> Filing the necessary documents with the Asian immigration officer, [Reps] was told it would not be possible for him to visit Japan as he was not "militarily allied." Sitting opposite the immigration officer, he turned his visa request over and on the back wrote, "Making a cup of green tea, I stop the war," and handed it back to the official across the desk. The immigration officer took a long look at the poem, reading it silently to himself, "Making a cup of green tea, I stop the war." Turning the paper over he initialed approval for Reps' entry into Japan. Looking up he said, "We need more people like you in our country right now." (1987, p. 284)

What does it mean to make a cup of green tea that stops the war? Reps wasn't being clever, explains Levine, he was being real:

> He was speaking of the incessant struggle for control, our long conditioned inner conflicts, with something other than the mind's old ways of violence and "victory," of mercilessness and inner strife. To make a

> cup of tea that doesn't continue the war, that doesn't deepen the con-
> flict, the impatience, the waiting, the desire for things to be otherwise,
> one simply lets the water boil. (pp. 284–285)

Have you ever boiled a cup of water without goals, asks Levine, without
needing the water to be different? "Without waiting? Waiting is war.
Impatience is war. The moment is unsatisfactory and there is no peace to
be found" (p. 285).

Not taking a drink, I stop the war. Holding onto anger and resentment causes harm to ourselves and others. It dominates our lives and
consumes us. By realizing and accepting our inability to control everything in our lives, and by transforming fear into trust and self-pity into
gratitude, we learn to let go of our resentments and stop the war within
ourselves. More than anything, recovery involves showing up. Frequently, we need others to help us accept realities we do not want to face
or simply don't like. My letter to Jeff and Sylvia describes such a moment:

> Returning to the marriage with so much more mindfulness and
> awareness of who you are and your strengths and limitations
> must bring a certain finality with it. If it doesn't work, you won't
> be able to blame youth, inexperience, or one another. It will
> mean having to accept that you've done the best you can,
> celebrating and embracing your successes and grieving the loss of
> some of the dreams you shared together as you let go and move
> on.

There are many ways that writing this type of correspondence affects me personally. From the standpoint of literary theory, I find it encourages me to "personify" rather than "thingify" people's problems
and leads to my developing a sense of "alterity" (or otherness). This is
how novelists, by putting themselves in the place of their characters, develop attachments to them; they identify with them. They can then return to their own position, one of alterity, of difference, where this exchange transforms their experience and gives rise to new voices.

As in good story writing, the personification of people's problems in
the form of such letters leads to the creation of a dialogue between clients and the characters and objects in their lives. Today, for example,
when I ask people to write good-bye letters to alcohol and drugs I encourage them to include what they are angry about, what they are sad
about, and what part of their relationship with alcohol and drugs they
are grateful for. I find this type of narration and dialogue increases cli-

ents'—and my own—capacity to experience compassion and empathy in therapy toward their own and other people's addictions and problems.

The letters I write to clients and the liminal inner space I access when writing them feels like my own version of Winnicott's "healing dreams." Oftentimes I complete them in the early hours of the morning or late at night. At these moments, it can feel like, in Winnicott's words, "my arrival at a new stage in emotional development" (1949, p. 71)— that is, a reworking of my own relationship to the themes and experiences addressed in the letters.

Finally, these correspondences, along with the other letters presented in this book, remind us that some stories don't fit inside our theories. Some stories have to tell themselves.

HEALING STORIES, NOT CLIFF NOTES

None of my own or my clients' letters are intended to serve as a recipe or "quick fix" for problems or as "gimmicks" that replace sound clinical practice. In some instances the therapy took place over a period of several months; in others, several years (or longer). If some of these techniques result in people resolving their troubles and alleviating their suffering in a more timely fashion I am all for it, but none of the work presented here was "time driven." Overall, I prefer to think of letter writing and narrative approaches to people's care as simply another way to share our experiences and adventures with clients and colleagues in this odd business we call "therapy."

Letters create a place where I can offer my own thoughts on clients' addictions—and other dilemmas—to be tossed about, digested, or discarded, away from direct exchange and the need for normal personal defenses. In this sense the letters, and the fate they meet, are a bit like the paper toys Winnicott made for children when they left his consulting room. Like these parting gifts, Winnicott viewed all his thoughts and interpretations as subjective objects that were meant to be played with— "kicked around, mulled over, torn to pieces." He would give them to his clients as objects between the client and therapist, as one possible version of their story, "rather than as official psychoanalytic decodings of the person's unconscious life" (Bollas, 1983, p. 7).

Neither do I intend, by organizing and sharing my thoughts this way, to give the impression that people move through these "stages of recovery" in an epigenetic fashion or that one stage is more important than another. We therapists get into trouble when we privilege one aspect of recovery over another. For example, the challenging and often frustrating stages of "anger" and "denial" are just as crucial as the more transformative processes of "acceptance" and "letting go." As Stephanie Brown points out, clinicians need to exercise great tolerance for a client's shifting back and forth between drinking and abstinence, "always providing a safe climate for both risk and retreat." A therapist who does not understand the ebbs and flow of these cycles may, as Brown concludes, "put undo pressure on the patient or become hopeless when abstinence is not maintained" (1985, p. 274).

In my metaphoric shorthand it is helpful for me to think about these stages of a person's healing and recovery as phases of the moon: while each one is connected to the other and are all part of the same satellite or whole, anyone of them can be observed and appreciated independently. Additionally, no astronomer would bother to argue as to which lunar phase is more important or came first; ideas that would be considered of greater relevance are what that particular lunar phase tells us about the gravitational relationship between the moon and the sun, earth, and stars at any given time and the impact of this relationship on the tides. In the same way that Martin Buber invites us to look for the word of God wherever it is manifested, we need to be open to finding traces of the divine in the most hardened and unyielding places of a client's story—even within the thickest denial.

Furthermore, anger and denial is as relevant to the alcoholic after 10 years of sobriety as it is to the "newcomer." AA has a saying that the further you are from your last drink the closer you are to your next, or (as a popular rock lyric puts it), "The nearer you are to your destination the more you keep slip slidin' away." Alcoholics who have good sobriety and years of abstinence frequently find themselves in reckless states of denial that have them willing to risk everything for a brief period of "normal" or "controlled" drinking—only to discover that their alcoholism picks up where it left off. Additionally, most discover the bottom falls out much quicker this time out. I can't count the number of clients and recovering alcoholics at AA meetings I've heard describe their disappointment and dismay at how many, and how fast, problems associated with drinking return when they've relapsed, and how the pleasurable feelings associated with drinking and drug use don't.

Relapse is also about fighting hopelessness and despair. As one client described it

"The first time I went into treatment I was all polished and smooth—like a shiny new penny—with hopes and expectations that I would never pick up again. The second time I went to detox I felt jaded and scuffed up, but I said to myself, 'Well I screwed things up pretty good, but I've been given a second chance and I am going to make the most of it this time.' The third time it was like 'What's it matter.' I started to recognize people's faces and just knew my situation was hopeless."

Ironically, this is where real change or transformation begins, and it often takes people at least several attempts before they are ready for it. I once heard an administrator from the Hazelden Institute being interviewed on the radio. He was talking about prevalent attitudes about relapse, spurred on by "managed care," which limit people's access to treatment. He made the point that when a person has advanced heart disease and is lying on the surgeon's table for the second bypass operation in a year (a much more costly procedure than a 30-day stay in a rehab center), the doctor doesn't tell the patient, "I'm not fixing your heart again; you've already been in one time this year for this procedure." Nor does the surgeon punish him and refuse care because the patient hasn't been disciplined about changing his diet and exercise habits. That is why AA builds Step 10 into its practices: *"Continued to take a personal inventory and when we were wrong promptly admitted it."* It is a way to prevent addicts from getting complacent. Called the "maintenance step," it reminds alcoholics that sobriety isn't an event, it's a lifestyle, and developing the art of self-reflection comes with the discipline of daily practice.

There is at the heart of many of the letters in this book a profound sense of loss and sadness. Clients expressed grief over time not spent with a parent—whose life was ravaged by drinking and drug use—as in Craig's and Randy's experiences, or the sense of loneliness and emptiness created by just imagining the absence of a drink or drug, as expressed by Miranda. In all of these stories the letters expressed a deep sense of sorrow and anguish.

For Angela and Karen, their grief stemmed more from the loss of self. Fragmented and discordant storylines were a predominant theme in these clients' care. Each woman's use of letter writing in therapy helped her reauthor her life story and reestablish a sense of personal agency.[1] Becoming the author of her own actions, and recapturing the sense of a nonfragmented physical self, as well as reclaiming her past, her self-history, were key elements in each woman's recovery.

Recounting past experiences in the form of a letter, for all clients, resulted in their discovering and making available a myriad of "lost or forgotten knowledges" of themselves in the fashion Michael White describes in his article "Saying Hello Again" (1989a). Certainly Angela and many of the other women whose narratives are presented in this book have had the experience of having their grief labeled as "pathological mourning." The letters and the ideas they generated about their own relationships to substances (or a family member's addiction) allowed them to incorporate different and less pathological views of their grief and sadness. Also, circulating these newly discovered and "preferred" stories of themselves in AA (and other such groups) with people up against similar troubles has been a crucial aspect of their recovery.

Loss of fulfillment, or loss of the possibility of fulfillment, due to alcoholism, drug addiction, or other self-defeating habits, was a significant theme in every client's story as revealed in their writing. Each author experienced intense feelings of abandonment and grief when letting go of or imagining letting go of his or her relationships to substances. These moments in therapy and writing when people feel truly alone with the addiction remind me of Audre Lorde's words, "for the embattled there is no place that cannot be home nor is" (1978, p. 55).

My own experience and relationship to the letters and their authors are also an integral part of this process. Writing this chapter has made me aware of how deeply mutual the shared grief-work of patients' relinquishing their addiction—or any other part of their identity—truly is. Healing is a process of learning to live with the loss, not under it—to, as Edelman (1994) says, let it become our companion rather than our guide.

In the end, all of us have something broken, some aspect of our lives that can't be mended or put back together: for Jeff and Sylvia it was the marriage they had; for Angela, the marriages she lost; for Miranda, Randy, and Craig their connection to their fathers; for Karen her connection to her body; for Jesse and his father the years of growing up in alcoholic homes marred by violence; for Larry and the others, the lost years. On some people it doesn't show. In today's times the less broken have to take care of the more broken. I learned that from my clients.

PART II

Detoxing the Theory

i like, in the early morning, to dig in my garden:
chard, lettuce, radishes, tomatoes;
with slow bucketfuls, i water the short furrows.
i pull up weeds.

today the newspaper said men had landed on the moon;
bent over the furrow, i turned up to look at it,
i couldn't see a thing and went back to work.
                              —VICENT ANDRÉS ESTELLÉS

CHAPTER 6

Becoming 12-Step Literate

The spiritual life is not a theory. *We have to live it . . .*

If we are painstaking about this phase of our development, we will be amazed before we are half way through. We are going to know a new freedom and a new happiness. We will not regret the past nor wish to shut the door on it. We will comprehend the word serenity and we will know peace. No matter how far down the scale we have gone, we will see how our experience can benefit others. That feeling of uselessness and self-pity will disappear. We will lose interest in selfish things and gain interest in our fellows. Self seeking will slip away. Our whole attitude and outlook upon life will change. Fear of people and of economic insecurity will leave us. We will intuitively know how to handle situations which used to baffle us. We will suddenly realize that God is doing for us what we could not do for ourselves.

Are these extravagant promises? We think not. They are being fulfilled among us—sometimes quickly, sometimes slowly. They will always materialize if we work for them.

—"THE PROMISES" (From *Alcoholics Anonymous*)

These words are found on pages 83 and 84 of *Alcoholics Anonymous* ([1939/1976]; more commonly referred to in AA as the "Big Book"). Known in the program as "the promises," they are meant to offer comfort and hope to the newly sober alcoholic. The message being that if you stick with it good things will happen. For Freud the goal of psychoanalysis, as he once put it, "is to convert hysterical misery into common unhappiness." A more feelingful and inspiring treatment plan than

Freud's, the goals of family therapy—"differentiating from one's family ego mass," "dissolving problems," "providing solutions," or "reauthoring stories"—also pale in comparison to AA's message of strength, hope, and recovery. As David Berenson writes, "People find in AA a new vision, a sense that there is more to life 'than business as usual,' that beyond the desperate chaos that drinking creates and/or is an escape from, there is hope and a future" (1987, p. 30). This may explain, in part, why alcoholics and addicts flock to AA in such great numbers, as well as accounting for so many peoples' desire and willingness to remain there and continue investing energy in their recovery once they're sober. However, after the slogans and clichés are stripped away the two processes—psychotherapy and AA—have more in common than one might think.

A parable (of whose origins I'm unclear), tells of a father who while at his workbench was being badgered by his 8-year-old child to come and play with him. Working under a stressful deadline on a difficult project and not wanting to be disturbed, he set upon the idea of giving his child a jigsaw puzzle of a map of the world. The child took the puzzle and went out to start working on it. The father felt he was safe from interruption because the child did not yet know what the world looked like, making it next to impossible for him to put the puzzle together. Remarkably, within the hour the child was back with the puzzle completed. The father asked, "How could you do that so quickly? You don't even know what the world looks like." And the child replied, "That was only one side of the puzzle. The other side of the puzzle was a picture of a man. I know what a man looks like, and when I put the man together, the world fell into place."

If one had to describe a philosophy or ontology that captures AA's approach to living, this parable would pretty much sum it up. Get your own house in order and the rest of life's problems will take care of themselves. It is very similar to the concept in Zen and in other forms of Buddhism that emphasizes approaching all tasks—both simple and worldly—with a clear head and an intimate knowledge of what's in one's heart.[1] This is what is meant by Step 4 of AA—"made a searching and fearless moral inventory of ourselves"—in which participants are asked to make a list of all their "character defects" and "personal shortcomings." While the language and context of this step is outside the realm of experience of most psychotherapists, the process is not.

"What," asks Stephanie Brown, "do people talk about in psychotherapy?" The answer: we discuss our fears, needs, anger, and resentments. Through the process of exploring and revealing these feelings we come to an understanding of how our attitudes and beliefs structure our view of the world and often get in our way. Extending the analogy further, having character defects does not mean that we are defective individuals; perhaps, in the words of one recovering person, it would be better to think of them as "character defenses." Furthermore, failing to take stock of one's strengths and the more radiant aspects of one's personality qualifies as a personal shortcoming as well, and belongs at the top of many people's 4th Step inventories.

A STORIED PROGRAM

> "Our stories disclose in a general way what we used to be like, what happened and what we are like now." So long as they do, Alcoholics Anonymous lives. For AA's story is one of those stories that will never end so long as there are human beings who discover, however painfully, having tried to play God, that they are not-God, that they can be *both* "sober" and "alcoholic," both whole and flawed.
> —ERNEST KURTZ

AA is rich in tradition and ritual. However, as Leon Wieseltier (1998) says, a ritual life is not an unexamined life. From the standpoint of literature and sociology, the Big Book is, in a manner of speaking, AA's Rosetta stone. Colorfully and inspirationally written, it tells of the program's origins, serves as a handbook for individual groups and members, and provides clues and insight into the program's local customs and idiosyncrasies. More than anything, the Big Book is a collection of people's stories that infuse the text with human spirit. Its pages teem with signs of life.

Experience taught that the telling of their stories by now-sober alcoholics is what made the program work. Better than half the Big Book's text consists of individual accounts of people's experiences of what it was like for them to give up drinking and how their lives have changed as a result. As Kurtz (1979, 1988) describes, from the program's earliest moments, "the telling and re-telling of 'stories' began unselfconsciously to develop into the practice that best embraced the core therapeutic process of what would soon become Alcoholics Anonymous" (p. 68). The Big Book suggests that people's stories ought to "disclose in a general way what we used to be like, what happened and what we are like now." The purpose of telling one's story in the company of fellow sufferers is to find wholeness in limitation. It is about sharing for witness, not confession. It has proven an effective method of keeping alcoholics sober and reaching out to others less fortunate. It's simple and it works.

However, while the Big Book is an important text that contains sound advice for psychotherapists and recovering persons alike, much of the language and cultural references found in it are dated and sexist. Consequently, I find it helpful to remind clients that the Big Book ought to be taken seriously, not literally. A rabbi finds his disciples playing checkers when they should be studying Torah. The students stop abruptly, but it's too late to hide the board and the pieces. The rabbi picks up the pieces and the board, looks them over, and proceeds to tell his young followers the rules: (1) you can't make two moves at once; (2) you can only move forward or backward; and (3) when you reach the last row, you can move wherever you like. The point is that you can learn from anything if you approach it in the right way. This is another good analogy for AA's pragmatic philosophy and approach to recovery, and I encourage clients to take this same attitude into meetings with them, as well as applying it to any literature they read.

Drawing on the stories presented in Part I, I am going to review some critical issues that clients and therapists face in addictions treatment and demonstrate how a closer reading of AA's steps and traditions and the spiritual narratives found in its rooms can guide therapists' work with active alcoholics and people in recovery. The steps refer to AA's well-known collection of spiritual practices and guidelines—12 in all—members can use in service of their recovery. While the steps form the core of AA, there are no doubt as many ways of *working* them as there are people in AA. Some are only aware of them in a general way, whereas others make them an intricate part of their recovery and apply them systematically to every facet of their lives. The traditions, which also number 12, refer to a less widely encountered set of principles intended to help groups govern themselves and resolve problems and conflicts among individuals and within the program at large. I will try to weave both processes—the steps and the traditions—into a narrative that breaks down some of the borders between psychotherapy and recovery. My hope is to provide a bridge that will allow therapists, clients, and the reader to travel more freely between the two worlds. It is for therapists a journey that begins with a concept I call *12-step literacy*.

Re-visioning the Disease Model

In his beautiful book *The Songlines*, Bruce Chatwin tells the story of an aboriginal creation myth in which "legendary totemic beings wandered over the continent in the Dreamtime, singing out the name of everything that crossed their path—birds, animals, plants, rocks, waterholes—and so singing the world into existence" (1987, p. 2). Over the course of time, these songlines became a sort of musical road map tracing the territorial spaces and paths that people inhabited and shared with the spirits of their ancestors. Individuals would be born into one of the songlines but would only know a section of it. The way the Australian Aborigines extended their knowledge of a particular songline was to go on periodic "walkabouts" that led to encounters with others living far away who knew of other melodies and stanzas, so to speak. Called "the dreaming," exchanging songlines was a means of sharing wisdom—an important way for people to learn more about themselves, their past, and the world around them.

Many therapists (Hoffman, 1993; Bollas, 1992) use this story as a metaphor to illustrate the mix of psychic, spiritual, and relational aspects of the self—an elegant example of the social construction of the self as well as our movement through the object world and the self states it invokes in each of us; "walkabouts" are also a good analogy for the 12-step self-help community as a whole.

In fact, one of the traditions in AA and other 12-step recovery groups are "commitments," where several members of an AA group or one representative go to another meeting in another part of the district or region to share their history and stories. The emphasis, similar to that at all speaker meetings, is on messages of hope, strength, and recovery. This tradition is used to keep groups from becoming isolated from one another, to assist new groups that are just beginning, or to reinvigorate old groups when members feel meetings are becoming stale or stuck. Also, in a process similar to the one described by O'Neil and Stockwell (1991) in their piece "Worthy of Discussion" (an article that explores the authors' application of narrative ideas to group work with schizophrenia), groups often take on names that portray the predicaments participants face, such as "Freedom from Fear," "Here, Because We're Not All Here," "Saturday Night Live" or "The Loony Nooner."

"Commitments" are a form of "service," referred to in AA as "12-step work." Step 12—"having had a spiritual awakening as a result of these steps, we tried to carry this message to others, and to practice these principles in all our affairs"—is what makes and keeps AA a living, breathing organism. It is how new ideas, blood, and nutrients are infused into the system. This is how new members access strength and hope and give back energy and wisdom to "old-timers" by helping them maintain a healthy amount of fear and humility through memories of what life was once like.

At the conclusion of our work together my client Larry (see Chapter 3) offered, in the form of a letter, a narrative version of this step. Larry invited me to share this correspondence with others who found themselves struggling to overcome an addiction or experiencing problems similar to the ones he encountered in recovery.

Larry's "12-Step" Letter

To Whom It May Concern

So you want to get sober. In two weeks I will have been sober for one year. Although I have made a lot of progress I am still in the woods as far as sobriety is concerned. Here are some thoughts that may/will help you on your road to sobriety. I don't expect you will follow all or even some of these "suggestions" at this time. Like myself you may have to bang your head against the wall before you walk around it.

Don't get too bogged down with the God stuff. If you stay sober for any length of time, you are not doing it, some Higher Power is. Now don't get me wrong, you are being responsible. Just because you are "powerless" over alcohol, doesn't mean you aren't responsible. Just because you give up "control," doesn't mean your not responsible for your own actions. GOD can be Group Of Drunks, or GOD can be whatever you want it to be. No one in AA needs to Know. Anyway, keep your mind OPEN.

Also treat AA like a new job. This thought came to me at the Laundromat today. I wondered why I wasn't gongs to meetings regularly. Was I afraid? Did I feel vulnerable? Did I not feel worthy of receiving the gift of sobriety? Yes, yes, and maybe. Then it came to me. I was thinking that I was supposed to know the answers to these questions. I was supposed to understand what was happening to me. I was thinking I'm eleven months sober and I should be OK with this stuff. But I wasn't. I am confused and I don't know why. Then I thought of my new job. How did I acquire the skills I have and the confidence to stand behind my work. I did it the AA way. I opened my mind, I was humble, I was like a sponge, I took all suggestions (not all at once mind you, just like AA), I made mistakes and got up and kept going, I did not get defensive. I did get frustrated, I did get angry, I did get scared, I did get confused. And I got good at what I do, I got confident. The problem is I became a workaholic. Better that than drinking. I feel good about myself, or at least better about myself. I can hang with adults without feeling ashamed and guilty about being an addict. If I don't know what's up, I know there are others with the same questions at AA. But I can't answer or even ask the questions from home . . . I have to go to meetings. So I went to a meeting tonight and got this off my shoulders and feel better about my confusion.

Make friends, AA friends. Stay clear of friends that will influence your old ways. Take responsibility for your life. You're going to have to change your life. But it will come naturally, if and it's a big if. . . . You go to meetings. You have to open your mouth and get your feelings out. You have got to shut up at times and listen. You will identify with other alcoholics. You will feel their pain as they will feel yours. You will get HOPE. . . . This has been one of the most precious gifts I have received to date. I never felt I would ever find my way out of this madness "without getting killed or caught" (as Jerry Jeff Walker once sang).

And it does work. You will see that as you grow. You will see that you let things go that you used to obsess about for days. You will feel a peace of mind that you never knew existed before. You will be able to look at yourself, really look at yourself without feeling ashamed. But you've got to go to meetings. Without that relationship you will never have an honest relationship with anyone, including yourself. Read the books, join a group, do the steps, and get a sponsor. I feel a little bit of a hypocrite as I have not joined a group or asked someone to be my sponsor. But look at me, eleven months sober and I'm barely out of the starting gate.

Oh yes, one more thing. If you can afford it, get a therapist My therapist has stuck it out with me and has helped me grow into AA. I sometimes wonder if I would still be in AA without his assistance. I know I am doing this for myself but sometimes I wonder if I am using our sessions as check-ins, to make sure I am doing the right thing, staying on track. It's like I have training wheels and I wonder if I can ride the bike without them. I have started to feel trust for the first time in my life. I feel that it's okay to share my feelings with not only my therapist but with others at meetings.

So get out there and just do it. And by the way, if you need someone to talk to, call me day or night.

Good luck,

Larry

Sponsorship

One theme raised in Larry's letter that I have made little mention of thus far is the importance of people obtaining an AA sponsor and how these relationships affect therapy. Sponsorship offers newcomers to AA a sort of mentor relationship to help them get acclimated to the program while they begin the difficult task of getting sober. But sponsorship is not limited to new members. Many participants with years of sobriety continue to use sponsors well into the middle and late stages of recovery. Some stay with their original sponsor while others find that, like therapists, different people meet different needs at different times in their lives. And, similar to many models of clinical supervision psychotherapists are familiar with, sponsorship provides people who spend most of their time working in groups an opportunity to receive one-on-one support in the context of an intimate caring relationship. Sponsorship differs from therapy, however, in that it is not a professional relationship. There is, for example, much more mutuality and genuine give-and-take between people in AA sponsor relationships than occurs in most therapies, even those therapies that are informed by relational theories and pride themselves on being more egalitarian in their approach. While each sponsor relationship is different and negotiated by the two parties involved, it is not unusual for sponsors and sponsees to become friends and socialize with one another outside the context of meetings. Also, sponsors often make themselves available 24 hours a day, 7 days a week, especially when a sponsee is newly sober, but again these boundaries are established by individuals, not the group.

Perhaps the biggest difference between psychotherapy and sponsorship is that AA is very clear that sponsorship is as much for the person providing the service as it is for the person receiving it. Members are encouraged to take this kind of service on for their own benefit, not just for the good of the person they're helping. It is not unusual for people who have been in an AA program for 2 years or more and are struggling with sobriety to find their own sponsor recommending that they volunteer their time to work with others who are just starting out in AA or fresh out of treatment. In addition to this being a way to give back strength and hope to others and take their mind off their own problems, for those considering a return to drinking or who have started to romanticize the experience, it helps them remember what life used to be like before they got sober.

What Larry didn't mention in his letter is that one explanation for the difficulty he was having in this area may have come from some advice his therapist gave him. I suggested to Larry that he *not* go about pursuing a sponsor the way he pursued his addiction. Instead, I asked that he think of the process as having more in common with finding a mate: "Don't just walk up and propose to someone that he be your sponsor. Get to know him first. Go out for coffee or tea—and use a temporary sponsor in the interim."* Of course for people whose track record with marriages and relationships more closely resembles their history with drugs and alcohol, this analogy will need more fleshing out.

The shared intimacy of recovery work can pose a challenge to therapists who are used to people's healing unfolding within the context of the kind of intimate dyadic relationships generated in psychotherapy. Clients' relationships to the 12 steps, literature, or sponsors can serve as transitional objects, in the Winicottian sense of the word, ushering people into a world of less destructive and more loving attachments and connection to others. It is difficult for all clients, but recovering persons in particular, to allow themselves to share inadequacies when they do not know that the therapist is also imperfect. The sharing of drunkalogues and other experiences in AA highlights people's similarities with others. As Stephanie Brown (1985) observes, no matter what awful things the alcoholic has done, someone else at some time has done the same things. Discussing the events with a sponsor or another person from the program is often less threatening to people because they know the person is, or was at one time, in the same boat.

Clients in recovery will occasionally express a desire to do some form of step work with their therapist. This may include reading and discussing books together, working on their "personal inventory," or creating an "8th step list" of people they need to make amends to for their behavior when drinking. Usually done under the guidance of a sponsor, this often represents clients' efforts to transfer their attachments from AA objects (literature, books, sponsor, etc.) to their therapy or to include their therapist in this menagerie of significant others. This provides clients an excellent opportunity to integrate these two worlds and develop trusting relationships outside of AA. Therapists just need to be careful that clients do not use therapy as an excuse to avoid meetings. It is important to encourage clients not to limit their step work to therapy for another reason. Step 5 of AA—"admitted to God, to ourselves and to another human being the exact nature of our wrongs"—is about breaking silence and removing feelings of secrecy, isolation, and shame.

The key words in this step are "to another human being." Because

---

*A temporary sponsor is just that—someone who agrees to serve in this capacity for a while, until a sponsee can find someone willing to participate in an ongoing relationship. People willing to be temporary sponsors are usually asked to identify themselves at the beginning of meetings.

of the strict confidentiality surrounding the process of psychotherapy and it being a paid professional relationship, sharing a 4th or 5th Step with one's therapist can be important meaningful work but is not completely in keeping with the spirit of the program. When sober individuals share their story in a meeting or tell others in the program what they did when under the influence of alcohol or drugs, they step out of the secrecy and isolation necessary to maintain any feelings of shame they may feel about themselves.

The desire to do step work in therapy can, in some instances, be driven by clients' fear of intimacy and their need to buffer themselves from feelings of closeness and dependency upon their therapist. Therapists just have to trust their own instincts and intuition and be willing to talk to clients about their concerns when it comes to determining what these kinds of requests mean to people. However, clinicians should tread lightly in these places. Even in situations where it feels as though clients are using their recovery issues to block intimacy, in my experience this is almost always an effort by people to strengthen their connection to me and increase the level of safety they experience in therapy. Transforming their therapist into a sponsor or placing him or her in this role (if it feels as though that is happening) is often an attempt to make an extremely threatening and confusing relationship into something more familiar and comforting—or, even more importantly, a way of modulating intense feelings that in the past would often lead to drinking.

Cara*

Cara had 7 years of sobriety. I had been meeting with her weekly (sometimes more) for 6 of those years. Cara expressed a desire to tell me her story in therapy or for me to hear her tell her story at an AA meeting. In AA this refers to a very specific event, discussed earlier, where a person talks about what life used to be like and what it's like now. Cara's request puzzled me, because although I had not been to a meeting where she had spoken I felt like I knew her story as well as anyone in her life (with the possible exception of her sponsor). When I asked her to say more about the feelings surrounding her request, Cara said that although we had done a lot of talking in therapy, because I had not heard her story the way she told it in AA, she felt that I didn't really know her.

---

*More of Cara's story and experience in recovery is shared in Chapter 8 and briefly at the start of Chapter 7.

This sense of distance she experienced between us bothered her. While she felt that we had accomplished many good things in our work together, she found herself questioning whether I was the right therapist for her.

I was surprised by Cara's remarks and felt pushed away by them. I knew that at meetings people rarely speak for more than 30 minutes at a time. Furthermore, many of our sessions focused on experiences that were very personal and difficult for her to talk about. Because of the emotions these conversations stirred up for her, Cara frequently sought my input about how much of this material I thought she should include or not include in her AA story. Consequently, not only did I feel that I had heard her story before, I felt that I was privy to the unedited version of it. Upon further exploration, Cara brought up her concern that my not being an alcoholic was still disconcerting for her.

This concern was one that Cara had expressed at the beginning of our work together, but it hadn't surfaced in some time. At the start of our relationship the issue for her was my not knowing recovery from "the inside out." Her assumption was that if I wasn't a recovering alcoholic myself I could never fully understand her experience or be trusted with her problems. After a while she came to feel that I did have an intimate enough knowledge of addiction even if I wasn't a "drunk" myself. At the time, Cara felt badly about challenging my credentials for working with her in this fashion. While she recognized that this was her way of being a smart consumer, she also needed my reassurance that her wanting us to be able to identify with one another in this way was not bad. She needed to know that what she was asking of me was not unreasonable, even if it was not possible.

Early on in our relationship she needed to keep me at a safe distance, especially if our differences prevented her from knowing what I might be thinking or feeling. Later the issue was about her feeling threatened or ambivalent at having allowed me and others, such as her sponsor, to get close to her. For Cara sponsorship and therapy were the first relationships in which she'd formed a genuine dependence on another human being that was not clouded or buffered by alcohol. At this juncture, Cara and I agreed that her dilemma was about *both* her need to push me away *and* her desire for us to be closer, and that this unfamiliar territory we were entering was unsettling to her. We saw it as a positive development that our relationship did not fit neatly into the models of intimacy which Cara had created when drinking or in recovery. It was a sign that she was broadening her horizons.

This exchange with Cara is a good example of clients' need, discussed earlier, to return to a "recovery focus" in therapy. It is a way of providing a firewall, as it were, between an individual's sobriety and the intense feelings of anger, intimacy, and loss that often surface in therapy. Following this particular discussion, which took up several meetings, I can't remember whether Cara and I did or did not return to a more immediate focus on recovery issues in our sessions. My guess is that we continued, as we always had, talking about them as they came up in the context of our relationship and as Cara's experiences in AA and other relationships dictated. However, not long after this conversation, at her AA anniversary, Cara asked that I help her celebrate her sobriety by presenting her with her "8th-year" medallion in front of her home group. In addition to its providing Cara the opportunity to honor how much our relationship meant to her, we both saw this ritual as a powerful acknowledgment of the significant role therapy and recovery working conjointly can play in people's lives— one I felt privileged to witness and be part of.

People's need to attend meetings, a theme Larry was emphatic about in his correspondence, will be taken up shortly. However, his letter, along with Cara's story, brought to the fore two other issues critical to psychotherapy and recovery: (1) the acquisition of independence through intense dependence on others and (2) taking responsibility for one's actions in the context of extreme powerlessness and helplessness.

12-Step Epistemology

The AA program, as Berenson (1987) describes in his article "Alcoholics Anonymous: From Surrender to Transformation," is based on paradox. Trying to unpack its mysteries reminds me of a cartoon by Gary Larson. A scientist is standing in front of a blackboard filled with calculations. At the head of a long string of formulas are the simple words, "Then a miracle occurs!" In the foreground are three colleagues and one of them whispers to the presenter, "I think they're going to want you to be a bit more specific than that."

The Twelve and Twelve*—a book that helps guide members through AA's steps and traditions—says, "Step One showed us an amazing paradox: We found that we were totally unable to be rid of the alcohol obsession until we first admitted we were powerless over it." Berenson (1987) describes numerous other paradoxes built into the program:

The Twelve Steps and Twelve Traditions of Alcoholics Anonymous.

One has to put one's sobriety ahead of everything else, yet to maintain sobriety one has to care for others. One has to do it totally for oneself, to stop being dependent on the bottle or addictive relationships, and at the same time to stop trying to do it by oneself, to accept the help of the group and/or one's personal higher power. One comes to see Higher Power or God as existing both within and outside of oneself, not adopting a psychological view of God as only identical with the self or a conventionally religious view of God as existing only outside the self. Alcoholism is seen as a disease beyond one's control and not a moral failing, yet much of the process of recovery is about taking a moral inventory, healing character defects, and making amends for the damage that one's behavior has caused. (p. 30)

That AA puts so much stock in paradox is not surprising, because, as Lockard observed, the lives of alcoholics and addicts are, in a very real sense, a study in tortuous paradox that embodies thinking like this: "In order to survive, I must persist in behaviors which are killing me" (personal communication, 1999).

Paradoxes, a core aspect of addiction, carry many different meanings in our culture and are incorporated into our thinking about a range of human and nonhuman experience. A concept first applied to psychotherapy by Watzlawick, Weakland, and Fisch (1974) of the Mental Health Research Institute in Palo Alto, California, and taken up later by the founders of the Milan school (Selvini-Palazzoli, Boscolo, Cecchin, & Prata, 1978; Boscolo, Cecchin, Hoffman, & Penn, 1987; see also McKinnon & Miller, 1987), paradoxes are not applied the same way in AA as they are in family therapy. In strategic family therapies, paradoxes (packaged as "invariant prescriptions," "therapeutic double binds," "prescribing the symptom," etc.) form the building blocks of "therapeutic" interventions meant to induce change in individuals and their families. In recovery and other spiritual endeavors, these mysteries are respectfully acknowledged but are not used to solve anything or change anyone. In this scenario, the absence of paradox in a person's recovery becomes a warning sign that alerts him or her to the presence of potentially dangerous behavior and thinking—"people, places, and things"— that threaten sobriety and increase the risk of relapse. When, for example, individuals spend more time trying to figure out how to *fix* or *manage* the uncontrollable forces and *insane* relationships in their lives, rather than learning how to *accept* and *let go* of them.

Many therapists have difficulty embracing this stance toward paradox, especially when it comes to the kind of spiritual narratives found in AA. As Brown (1985) suggests, summarizing Bean's (1975a, 1975b) work, educated individuals have trouble accepting the inspirational focus and message of AA. Yet, as we have observed, and as many of the people's stories gathered herein will further demonstrate, the suspension of intellectual explanation is essential at certain phases of recovery. In these moments, it is precisely the intellectual wish to explain what is happening, to attribute cause in a way that will make some sense of prolonged irrational acts of drinking or drug use that impedes a person's movement into recovery. A believer remarks, "An honest person is the noblest work of God," to which the atheist replies, "An honest God is the noblest work of people." Reading these statements, adherents of the AA approach might respond, "An honest program is the noblest work of both."

AA can't be understood using an analytic positivist model or framework. A phenomenological, subjective perspective is required to understand the meaning of addiction, the self, and the world. According to Berenson (1991), as soon as therapists fall into believing in cause-and-effect explanations for alcoholism, they are incapable of effectively treating alcohol problems. At the same time they must be willing to allow clients to accept cause-and-effect thinking, such as the disease model of alcoholism, if that will assist them in helping to resolve their drinking or drug problem. In other words, Berenson concludes, therapists must not commit themselves to any causative notion of alcoholism but act as if they had one.

My way of adapting Berenson's directive in my own work is to be as transparent as possible with my clients about my views. I do not argue with people who embrace the disease concept. I am comfortable "languaging" about addiction in that way—even to the point of offering interpretations and ideas in that idiom. However, I often simply share my own version of Berenson's remarks with them as representing my position or "opinion" about these matters. I find that for people who are having trouble making a connection with AA, an exchange like this is very freeing. It allows them to "act as if" the notions AA has about the "disease" of addiction were true and apply them to their lives without compromising their own ideas or beliefs. They are thus able to invest in their recovery in a fashion consistent with AA's approach while maintaining a healthy skepticism toward any dogma or ideology that does not resonate with them. I also point out that this is consistent with AA's philosophy, which is always to "take what you need and leave the rest."

Many people take issue with AA's unique spiritual slant. They fear it absolves individuals of personal responsibility for their actions. Within both Christianity (the religious tradition that informed most of AA's early writings and work) and Judaism, confession and repentance atones only for transgressions between human beings and God. For transgressions between one individual and another, atonement is achieved by reconciling with the person who has been offended. However, in psychotherapy these issues are more complicated because, as therapist and philosophy of religion professor Malcolm Diamond points out, "in our culture the debate over the power of the will has shifted from the religious battleground of sin to the secular one of addiction" (1994b, p. 9).

The issue of responsibility versus willpower is the primary paradox each therapist must resolve for him or herself before providing care to people suffering from addictions. As AA has demonstrated, willpower is almost useless in stopping alcoholic drinking. Step 1, "We admitted we were powerless over alcohol and our lives had become unmanageable," is AA's most important step. At the same time, AA and other successful therapeutic approaches emphasize the importance of taking responsibility for one's actions.

AA appears to have anticipated these struggles and tried to formulate its own response:

> Some strongly object to the AA position that alcoholism is an illness. This concept, they feel, removes moral responsibility from alcoholics. As any AA [member] knows, this is far from true. We do not use the concept of sickness to absolve our members from responsibility. On the contrary, we use the fact of fatal illness to clamp the heaviest kind of moral obligation onto the sufferer, the obligation to use AA's twelve steps to get well. (*As Bill Sees It*, 1967, p. 32)

WHAT DOES IT MEAN TO BECOME 12-STEP LITERATE?

> A discovery is said to be an accident meeting a prepared mind.
> —ALBERT SZENT-GYÖRGYI

When I think about what it takes to "get well," what it means for a person "to use AA" to overcome an addiction, I no longer find myself thinking of AA as a culture per se but as an ecosystem (Lockard, 1985b). In other words, what's toxic to one organism can be pure sustenance for others. Or, as my colleague Roget is fond of saying, "Some meetings are to my spirit as breath is to my body—others would drive me to drink if I went to three in a row."

A deeper appreciation of this point might result in therapists showing more compassion, empathy, and patience for clients trying to estab-

lish a working relationship with AA and other 12-step recovery programs. More importantly, therapists might come to view this process as
a *collaboration* between clients and themselves, and a crucial aspect of
their work with people in recovery.

Larry's 12-step letter to other alcoholics (above) hit hard on the
need to attend meetings, but clearly one approach is not going to work
for all people. Similar to the myriad of therapy mediums and choices
available to clients, AA and other 12-step groups are not necessarily beneficial for everyone who is chemically dependent or affected by alcoholism, but 12-step programs and their body of knowledge can inform our
work with all clients who face these challenges in their lives. AA, Al-
Anon, and ACOA (Adult Children of Alcoholics) are all prominent
"songlines" that I have encountered on my own professional "walk-
about." The ideas found in these programs, while extremely useful to my
professional and personal growth and development, have a unique no-
menclature of their own. Clinicians should not let the terminology distract them from some of the more substantial issues raised in these gatherings.

A Selfish Program

An oft-used expression by recovering alcoholics is that AA is a "selfish
program." It means that members have to put their sobriety above everything else. Without it they are useless to themselves and others. It requires a narcissistic investment in the self but, in another of AA's endless
series of paradoxes, the alcoholic must rely upon and keep the focus on
him- or herself by helping others. This paradox, already touched upon in
our discussion of AA's 12th-step, is one of the most misunderstood concepts in AA. The slogan "It's a Selfish Program," is often interpreted as
one of two extremes—either people needing to nurture a heartless ego-
ism or people abandoning themselves in cult-like fashion to the needs of
the group. Many, unfortunately, have misconstrued AA's concept of a
therapeutic community. Individuality, what makes people unique, need
not be sacrificed so that a sense of community can be achieved. John
Wallace (1985), a pioneer in alcoholism treatment, observed that identifying and connecting with others does not require one to give up the precious aspect of self not shared with others: "true therapeutic community
does not stamp out individuality but encourages it and enhances it" by
providing the necessary spiritual and emotional supports for its growth
(p. 48).

This tension surfaced in my discussion of Karen's story (see Chapter

1) and her struggle to remain sober. In Karen's case taking the necessary steps to improve her life out of a sense of loyalty to herself ran counter to the cultural messages she had received about her duty as a woman to remain selflessly available for others. Each individual needs to resolve this tension in her or his own way, discovering over time how to strike the right balance. Some of us are very good at caring for ourselves but may look after our own interests to a fault, whereas others are geared too much toward meeting other people's needs sometimes to the point of obsession. In addition, as we discussed in Chapter 5, people's needs change over time and often the best assistance a therapist can offer is to try and help clients remain flexible and be compassionate with themselves when wrestling with this emotional rubric.

Wallace uses an analogy from ancient times to highlight the need to balance ones obligation to self and others when treating addictions: "The Ancients recognized that life is often a matter of choosing a safe course between two equally hazardous alternatives. Navigators operating off the coast of Italy were cautioned to find the narrow passage between Scylla, the rock, and Charybdis, the whirlpool, since sailing too close to either meant certain disaster" (1985, p. 37). However, in psychotherapy and recovery, finding a safe passage between the Scylla of narcissistic investment in the self at the expense of others and the Charybdis of obsession with others at the expense of self requires a rereading of ancient myths and aspects of the psychological theories based on them.[2]

"A Selfish Psychology"

There are many different versions of the myth of Narcissus. The most common interpretation is the idea that Narcissus was tricked into looking into a pool of water, whereupon seeing his own reflection he fell in love with himself, as punishment for his self-centeredness and self aggrandizement. Narcissus's kismet was, the story goes, the result of a curse put on him by the goddess Nemesis, whose fury over Narcissus's cruel treatment of Echo, a beautiful wood nymph who had pledged her love to him, sealed his fate. A version I prefer is that Narcissus had a twin sister who died in utero. Narcissus's mother was told by the oracle not to let him see his reflection, for the pain and memory of his dead and forgotten sister would destroy him. While each reading (and there are many others) emphasizes different aspects of the story, what they all share in common is an appreciation of the relational context in which the events took place.

Plight or curse, no rendition implies that Narcissus's troubles were the result of an inborn personality trait. Similarly, the idea that an alcoholic's cruel or neglectful treatment of others is driven by malice or sadism, or the result of a flawed character structure is one of the more unfortunate legacies of psychoanalytic grappling with addiction.

However, not all analytic and depth psychologies are alike. Heinz Kohut's (1971, 1977, 1984) self psychology sees narcissism as part of the human condition and locates it on a positive and necessary developmental path or continuum, rather than seeing it through the lens of psychopathology, as Freud did. For Freud the goal was to move from self-love to *object* love (Freud's term for our ability to empathize and care for others).[3] Failure to do so was viewed as a sign of immaturity and delayed intellectual and emotional growth. Kohut rejected Freud's ideas about narcissistic pathology because he felt it encouraged moralizing and the denigration of patients on the part of the analyst. Kohut managed to accomplish this without giving up psychoanalysis's sensitive and complex insight into the harsh and often painful experiences people struggle with when tying to create an authentic sense of self.

An appreciation of the significance and meaning of these crises of identity and narcissistic injuries is particularly relevant to work with persons and families struggling with addiction. For alcoholics, messages of shame and worthlessness they receive about themselves are two of the biggest deceptions addiction plays on them: the first lie is that "I need my drugs and alcohol in order to feel like a valuable and lovable human being"; the second, "I'm not a valuable and loving human being in the first place."

Rather than focusing on the structures of the mind—id, ego, and superego—Kohut sees the self as the centerpiece of the analytic theory and human behavior. According to Kohut, we develop the capacity to grow and love through our interaction as young children with what he calls "selfobjects." Through gratifying responses, small frustrations ("empathic failures") of parents and other caretakers, children gradually internalize the protective presence of these adult figures and learn to negotiate their own way in the world. When this process is impinged upon or breaks down under the stress of too much trauma, other significant problems can occur. Selfobjects are defined as objects experienced as part of the self or in the service of it, which is why the theory offers such an elegant way of understanding the intensity of people's experience and identification with alcohol and how they can come to believe that their very existence depends on it.

Borrowing the triadic structure of Freud's theory, Kohut's self is made up of three major selfobject states inherent in human development.

Kohut's trinity consists of the need to experience affirmation and acceptance (mirroring); the need to merge with the calm, strength, and wisdom of others (idealization); and the need to feel that one is like the other (twinship).[4] Again the parallels with the unfolding of recovery and development of a sober identity and sense of self in AA are also strong. In my shorthand, it helps me to break down Kohut's ideas into people's basic need to be *accepted*, *embraced*, and *celebrated*. The primary need is to be accepted and affirmed for who we are. A child who isn't accepted by others will have great difficulty feeling like a whole person. Being embraced (i.e., showered with love) and given a sense of pride and competency about what they bring to the world is what makes children resilient and joyful. For people in recovery who were deprived of these experiences in childhood, AA is often the first place they've been embraced and celebrated just for being who they are.

The difference between Kohut's and Freud's approach is captured in their understanding of transference. In classical theory transference represents the projection of past conflict onto the blank screen of the analyst. In the transference the patient is viewed by Freud as reexperiencing these significant object relationships or as resisting remembering those experiences by acting them out. In contrast, transference in self psychology is about the actual transfer of selfobject needs.[5] In other words, clients bring to therapy an expectation for the kind of care, love, and responsiveness that's been missing from their lives and relationships. The role of the therapist is to provide the missing link. In the case of addiction, a person turns to alcohol and/or drugs, rather than people, to mend a rupture in a selfobject relationship or to fill the void or emptiness created in its absence.

Put another way, chemicals often fill a gap in a person's life that otherwise would have exposed an intolerable emptiness. Had the person not soothed these feelings at the time with drugs and alcohol, he or she might have felt compelled to turn to even more extreme measures to relieve the pain. Clients' writings often reveal these powerful attachments and fulfilling aspects of their addiction. Holly wrote, "You put me in a different world when I really needed it." Miranda's letter uncovered similar feelings of despair, abandonment, and relief: "i've gotten fucked up Emotionally and Physically. (Relationship wise also) I've gotten used by abusing you: even after all those complaints I don't want to give you up Because i'll be alone." And Karen, summing up her experience of her relationship with alcohol, wrote, "I always came back to you—you of course always being faithfully available." *

Many argue that once the cycle of abuse or addiction is set in motion, the question of "why" a person drinks becomes less important than "how" to stop it. Nevertheless, it's crucial to remember the primary role alcohol played in organizing that person's life and sense of self. Furthermore, although the predisposition to alcoholism is random (i.e., no one asks to be born into an alcoholic family or with a physiology predisposing him or her to addiction), the timing of a person's bout with substances is usually less accidental. This accounts for the great number of men and women speakers in AA who, after identifying as a "gratefully recovering alcoholic," share through their stories how alcohol or drugs saved their lives—since the alternative may have been insanity or death.

1-800-Denial Busting

Therapists and anyone else who is living on a steady diet of addiction or substance abuse in their caseload need a working knowledge of 12-step recovery programs, preferably through a relationship to meetings. This is particularly important if the therapist's own story, or his or her family's, is colored by substance abuse or addiction.[6] When therapists become 12-step literate, they are more likely to appreciate that the two main ingredients of any successful intervention are love and respect. Confrontations need not be aggressive to be effective.

Clinicians, in other words, should try to avoid what I call "1-800-Denial Busting." I think there is a growing impression in the mental health and addiction fields that there is a different set of rules that applies to addicts; in regards to alcoholism, the common practice of "meeting clients where they're at" is no longer fashionable.

The emphasis in the addiction field on earlier and more aggressive treatment approaches has created a therapy climate that views these attitudes as acceptable. This, I believe, is one of the few negative side effects of what has otherwise been a positive move away from treatment of addicts and alcoholics to early intervention and placement of the family at the center of treatment efforts.

The challenge, it seems to me, when inviting family members, friends, and employers to take a more active role in therapy with addicts and alcoholics (or any other person) is how do we talk about the toxic effects of blame without blaming? The answer is similar to the one given

---

(footnote from p. 119) Holly's letter can be found in Chapter 2; Miranda's letter is in the Prologue and Chapter 2; and Karen's letter is in Chapter 1.

to the tourist in New York inquiring of a passerby, "Could you tell me, Sir, how to get to Carnegie Hall?" The New Yorker's answer: "Practice, practice, practice!"

Michael White's ideas about externalizing conversation helps me to identify, but not attribute negativity to a person's relationship with drugs or alcohol—to acknowledge the presence of this relationship in a person's life, but not its ownership of that life. Externalizing problems in the form of a letter offers clients the opportunity to feel more compassion for themselves and enhances their ability to let go of their addictions—or their therapists' ability to assist them in accomplishing this daunting task. It allows both parties to get more distance from the "problem," and to keep their feelings about the therapy relationship separate from their feelings about drugs and alcohol.

Anytime an addict behaves in ways she is ashamed of, she is at risk of drinking or relapsing. When such a client engages in some act of dishonesty or deceit (or acts out destructively toward herself or someone else), the therapist's job is not to support her unconditionally but to name and confront any reprehensible or harmful behaviors. This does not need to be done heavy-handedly—such harshness merely adds to the shame and humiliation the person already feels. A gentle hypothesis is all that's required: "Of course you feel bad about yourself. How could you feel otherwise given your present behavior?" Steps 8 and 9 of AA— "made a list of all persons we had harmed, and became willing to make amends to them all" and "made direct amends to such people wherever possible, except when to do so would injure them or others"—can be useful here. Suggesting clients drop the "a" in "amends" and simply think about doing what they need to "mend" any given situation can make both these steps feel more manageable while still capturing their essence. In addition, I often have to remind people that failure to make amends to oneself is the most common oversight on an alcoholic's 8th-step list.

Therapists who become 12-step literate are also in a better position to help clients find and choose meetings that are a better fit with their experience and outlook on life. Or, conversely, therapists may suggest a meeting that challenges a person's outlook in a particular way. (Although AA meetings, and sobriety in general, pose so many "new ways of knowing" for people, most clients will find AA stretching their thinking on just about every topic imaginable.) Clients who are well versed in the practices and principles of AA but find the process of therapy unfamiliar and foreign—if not frightening—often have an easier time making the transition to therapy if a therapist is grounded in the workings of these recovery programs. That is, clients are likely to enjoy better communication with a therapist who is willing to make the effort to speak their own language. All of these strategies require therapists to become familiar with the culture of recovery in their own communities (at a minimum, the types and kinds of meetings offered) and to explore, in depth, their clients' experiences of them.

My conversation with Karen following her request for help coping with her anger was illustrative of this process (her story can be found in Chapter 1). Karen's anger was laced with a spiritual quandary: "I'm angry at God." During that exchange, I suggested that she "view her rage and despair as a form of prayer and 'conscious contact' with her higher power—'owned and accepted, it's your friend and ally; denied, it undermines your sobriety.' " My reference to the 11th step of AA—"sought through prayer and meditation to improve our conscious contact with God as we understood him/her, praying only for the knowledge of his/her will and the power to carry that out"—was a conscious effort on my part to describe Karen's dilemma using the language of AA. One AA text offers the following explanation of how prayer and meditation work: "*Perhaps one of the greatest rewards of meditation and prayer is the sense of belonging that comes to us. We no longer live in a completely hostile world. We are no longer lost frightened and purposeless*" (*The Twelve and Twelve*, p. 105).

After years of feeling like an outcast, Karen was trying to make a positive connection to AA. My ability to explain my interpretations and ideas in these terms strengthened that alliance and supported her newly discovered view of AA as a resource that could help her with the problems she faced. My using AA's spiritual language to frame her dilemma allowed Karen to see her anger and her courage to express those feelings in our relationship as an important part of her recovery. Bringing her anger to therapy and expressing her rage at God was therapeutic for Karen and an important part of her healing journey. As one AA speaker at an 11th-step meeting* put it, "Prayer is just a crying out for the power to make our lives count. It is a petition." The 11th step is the spiritual heart of the program. AA and Al-Anon meetings that focus on this step, and the reflections heard at them, often feel like poetry readings to me. This, in my view, is where the song of the program is created.

---

*An AA meeting where the topic is the 11th step.

Identity Stories: Creating a Sober Sense of Self

When clients comes to therapy excited about meetings or their discovery of the benefits of a sober lifestyle, I genuinely share in their joy and delight. I find that this enthusiasm over their new-found ability to stay sober, and the renewed sense of self they feel as a result, is contagious. When they report specific decisions reached or situations handled sober, I ask them to consider how they might have handled them while drinking. I then ask them to consider what these sober experiences tell them about themselves and what they want out of life. In sum, any interactions during this period are seen as opportunities to support the person's growing self-identity as a competent, responsible, and sober person.

What about clients who are grateful for the discovery of new behaviors and for a source of support that provides an alternative to drinking but are ambivalent about identifying as an alcoholic at AA meetings or embracing an alcoholic identity? Can they benefit from AA without taking this step? And how do you respond to those people who see AA as a good solution to their immediate problems but look forward to the time when they can return to "controlled" or "social" drinking?

Wallace (1985) has a way of situating himself in these sorts of conversations which guides my responses to my own clients' struggles with this issue. In the beginning of therapy I support any self-categorizations by clients that realistically appraise their problems with alcohol: "problem drinker," "in trouble with alcohol," "potential alcoholic" and "possible alcoholic," are common labels that people apply to themselves and their addiction narratives. I invite people to explore these self-categorizations in more depth and to examine the implications of each. In many situations they do eventually arrive at the self-categorization of "alcoholic"—though clearly not always.

Some therapists regard this labeling process as unimportant, and others find that it gets in the way. While I agree that this issue isn't what makes or breaks clients' chances for recovery—it is, for example, much more important that they accept their powerlessness over alcohol than their labeling themselves as "alcoholic"—I, along with Wallace (1985), do not feel that a person's struggles with identifying or labeling themselves alcoholic are unimportant or countertherapeutic.

Construing the self as "alcoholic" is an important new identity. For some clients, sobriety and their identity as a "recovering alcoholic" is, writes Wallace, "all that they have to cling to in lives beset by unbelievable complexity, devoid of opportunity, and surrounded on all sides by the wreckage of the past" (1985, p. 117). For many people it is, in fact, the only thing that gives meaning to the past, makes the present bearable, and promises hope for the future.

After people are over the stigma associated with admitting their problem and going to meetings, the process of identification can help alleviate any shame they may experience as a result of their circumstances. While AA's first step, admitting powerlessness over alcohol, is clearly the most important move toward health an alcoholic can make, identifying with others and shaping an identity to go with this new understanding of their problem is a close second.

NOT GOD

The sun will set without thine assistance.
—THE TALMUD

Regardless of how a person resolves the question of whether to identify in therapy or at meetings as "alcoholic," AA's point is that it's the willingness to actively engage and struggle with this issue that counts. The words, "First of all we had to stop playing God," found on page 62 of the Big Book, refer to a kind of selfishness and grandiose thinking—*alcoholic pride*—many believe accounts for the lion's share of trouble alcoholics face when trying to become and remain sober. Alcoholism, says the Big Book, is an extreme example of "self-will run riot," which, according to AA, is the driving force behind people's efforts to control their drinking and all other aspects of their experience. The solution requires a shift in attitude. AA's first step calls for humility. Ultimately, what alcoholics and their caregivers are grappling with here are questions of faith not pride.

A story recounted in Buber's *Tales of the Hasidim* illustrates this point:

> A Hasid of the Rabbi of Lubin once fasted from one Sabbath to the next. On Friday afternoon he began to suffer such a cruel thirst that he thought he would die. He saw a well, went up to it, and prepared to drink. But instantly he realized that because of one brief hour he had still to endure, he was about to destroy the work of the entire week. He did not drink and went away from the well.
>
> Then he was touched by a feeling of pride for having passed this difficult test. When he became aware of it, he said to himself: "Better I go and drink than let my heart fall prey to pride." He went back to the

well, but just as he was going to bend down to draw water, he noticed that his thirst had disappeared. (1955, p. 316)

The message for alcoholics to be gleaned from Buber's story is that faith is vital to sobriety because without it there is only willpower upon which to rely. Those of us who work with people in recovery can fall prey to our own version of this sort of willful pride. A clinician who has devoted his or her career to working with addicts and alcoholics, or any other group, may feel that he or she has heard every addict's story imaginable. The therapist may begin to feel as if he or she knows exactly what every alcoholic needs to do to get sober. Clients are seen as challenges rather than individuals, and every session becomes a test of our skills and commitment to help others. Therapy, the process of discovering what changes people want to make in their lives and readying people for them, becomes more about what changes the therapist thinks the client should make. Every clinician is susceptible to such lofty moments. In these instances, the first thing we have to do in order to put things in their proper perspective, is, to borrow AA's expression, "Stop playing God."

Recovery Is a Time-Dependent Process

When we say recovery is a time-dependent process, what we are really talking about is *not* time but timing. Ideas on the creative use of time in the therapy hour can be found in a section on brief therapy in Chapter 12. However, recent preoccupations with time and the effective management of it in therapy, more often than not, contribute to therapists feeling more harried and pressured in the already difficult and stressful climate that exists in addiction treatment. In fact, many times the internally or externally driven panic a therapist feels to hurry up and get this person "better" or sober is isomorphic with the alcoholic's experience of his or her crisis. For the alcoholic these time pressures often lead to thoughts like "I don't have time for this now, I have to 'take care of business' and then I'll deal with my drinking problem," or "I've already put my family through so much I can't make them go through a costly and lengthy treatment ordeal." As a result, many alcoholics may end up taking shortcuts and trying strategies to control or manage their situation and their drinking that lead to ineffective solutions.

In the world of addiction, possessing a good sense of timing means appreciating the varying kinds of emotional and mental spaces people occupy during their recovery. Clients face distinct problems and dilemmas at each stage of recovery, and clinicians need to encourage people to draw on different aspects of AA's steps and other rituals to meet these changing needs. In the early stages of therapy and recovery, I often find people more willing to attend meetings if I make it clear to them that their participation is as much for me as it is for them. "I will be of no use to you," I'll comment, "if I burn out trying to respond to your needs without enough help and support for our work. Without AA or some other kind of group we risk becoming too isolated and self-sufficient, two things you said contributed to your feeling so overwhelmed in the first place."

This can also be a useful way of pulling off what has to be one of the most difficult and challenging balancing acts a client can ask a therapist to perform—"I want to deal with my drinking problem but I want to work on 'other' things as well." A person's willingness to go to at least a few meetings can, I explain, prevent us from using up all our time tending to the drinking issues, thus freeing us up to discuss other topics: "This way I can be a resource for you—a sounding board for your experiences in AA—but I won't have primary responsibility for tending to your recovery issues." If a person declines all of these offers, just raising these ideas is important role modeling on my part and can become grist for future conversations. If, for example, a client opts to go it on her own without using AA or other supports, I can, should she later get stuck or find herself in one crisis after another, suggest that she really ought to avail herself of these resources rather than relying exclusively on therapy to provide all the support she needs.

Finally, what of the question about clients who see AA as a way station on their voyage back to controlled drinking? AA allows for people going in and out of sobriety. People are encouraged to try AA's methods with the understanding that they may discover it's not for them. Therapists, too, can remind clients that they've had a lifetime of drinking and learning about life from the inside of a bottle. Why not try recovery for a while? They can always go back to their old lifestyle—they're not going to forget how to drink or use drugs. Remember my letter to Andrea (in Chapter 2) and my discussions with Larry and Karen (in Chapters 1 and 3)? All three needed reassurance that making the decision to go to meetings did not mean having to commit to never picking up a drug or a drink again. It is imperative that clients not be pressured into making these kinds of choices before they're ready and that they see them as two separate decisions.

Relaxation, breathing exercises, and other forms of meditation can be very useful during what many clients find is an extremely anxiety-ridden time for them. AA's slogans and self-commands, such as "easy does it," "one day at a time," "this too shall pass," "keep it simple," "turn it over," and the serenity prayer can help people stay more grounded in the present and feel less tyrannized by the future. As Wallace (1985) says, just as some of us allow ourselves to become victims of our biographies, others "become victims of biographies yet to be written" (p. 123). The emphasis in AA on taking life 24 hours at a time is intended to help people quiet this kind of obsessive thinking.

The Disease Model Revisited

A *New Yorker* cartoon carries a message we could apply to the importance of keeping a variety of perspectives when trying to grasp the larger picture of psychotherapy, addiction, and recovery. An old farmer is standing in the middle of his field speaking with two aliens, wearing long white coats and stethoscopes, their spaceship—just landed—in the background. The farmer is scratching his head and saying, "Orbistic medicine? You treat whole planets? I never heard of such a thing."

I like this picture because it reminds me that the healing of our human hearts is inseparable from the healing of the planet as a whole. Unfortunately, progress in developing integrative approaches to alcoholism and addiction treatment have been slow to catch on in the mental health community. One explanation for this is the history of mistrust between AA, recognized by many as the treatment of choice for addiction and alcoholism, and the field of psychotherapy as a whole. I had a colleague at a local substance abuse clinic who told me that when she began working in the field—some 30 years ago—alcoholism counselors had to pass notes to their patients, on tiny slips of paper, with directions to AA meetings, as hospital policy prohibited them from discussing AA's possible benefits.

While we've come a long way since that time, one of the reasons for the continuing schism between the two groups is the tendency of contemporary theories of psychology to tell AA what it is all about. With the exception of the psychoanalyst Carl Jung, psychiatrists, psychologists, and social workers have ignored the potential for rich dialogue with AA.* Instead, the majority of the studies of these "fellowships" have been conducted by "professionals" who have used these "nonprofessional" lay support groups to test their own or others' theories. This too is unfortunate, as it robs the remainder of us in the intellectual and

---

*A description of the unique part Jung played in the history of AA—and the correspondence between Jung and AA's cofounder Bill Wilson—can be found on pp. 74–75.

clinical communities of the opportunity to have our lives and work enriched by the practices and wisdom of these traditions.

AA's significance, from the standpoint of narrative therapy and postmodernism is due in large part to its ability to provide healing without healers (i.e., professionals), spirituality (i.e., faith and hope) without religion (religious institutions in particular), and solidarity and community without organization and bureaucracy. As one colleague put it, "AA is more like an 'un-organization.'" It does not seek approval, legitimacy, or money and does not adhere to a dominant political ideology. Its *raison d'être* could be summed up as helping its members, whose ranks include all kinds of people, face their feelings with more courage, think more clearly, and experience life with more reckless abandon (and less alcohol).[7]

Also, while an interest in narrative and storytelling has been experiencing a renaissance in the psychotherapy community and so many other disciplines, AA has lived in story and lived by story since its inception in 1935. Today the telling of stories remains the heart of the AA program.

Most criticism of AA from narrative and other postmodern perspectives actually targets other addictive phenomena and compulsive behavior (e.g., "codependency"). These perspectives hold that the proliferation of 12-step culture has resulted in the "diseasing of America," a view in which women are seen as helpless victims and no groups or individuals are held accountable for their actions. These concerns constitute a harsh and more deserving critique of the billion-dollar self-help publication and workshop industry, rather than being grounded in any serious empirical study or experience of 12-step meetings, literature, or traditions. It is important when raising these concerns to specify whether one is talking about the recovery movement or the recovery marketplace, as each phenomenon has had quite a different history and story to tell.

As David Treadway (1990) points out, the self-help recovery movement is, regardless of its successes or failures, driven by people's attempts to regain the "lost spirit of community." It is an example of what Buber calls an "I–Thou" relationship, whereas the recovery marketplace best describes what he refers to as an "I–It" stance. The latter's story is more closely aligned with the history of consumer capitalism and the commodification of people's intimate connections and personal relationships.

However, as feminist author bell hooks (1993) observes, self-help books can serve as important guides for many who cannot afford therapy or have had endless hours of it without results. In addition, many women and men find it safer to take risks in their lives and embrace change when ideas are presented in writing. The main problem with this literature is its failure to suggest that people need to organize politically to change society in conjunction with our efforts to transform ourselves.

STORIES OF GENDER AND JUSTICE: THE CULTURE AND POLITICS OF RECOVERY

> The struggle to end domination, the individual struggle to resist colonization, to move from object to subject, is expressed in the effort to establish the liberatory voice— that way of speaking that is no longer determined by one's status as object—as oppressed being. That way of speaking is characterized by opposition, by resistance. It demands that paradigms shift—that we learn to talk—to listen—to hear in a new way.
>
> —BELL HOOKS

We are trained to think of our work in clinical terms, not political ones. The two processes—politics and therapy—are treated as separate worlds. Frantz Fanon's *The Wretched of the Earth* (1961/1978) revealed the intense personal revulsion and self-hatred that can be manifested when people try to embrace a sense of self and family in an atmosphere colored by oppression and fear. Addiction can fuel these psychic dramas or unfold as a consequence of them. In sum, both phenomena, internalized racism and the intense feelings of shame and worthlessness addiction generates, are intimate forms of violence that can feed off each other or be experienced independently of one another.

Ervin: Race Matters

Ervin, a 22-year-old biracial man, was 2 years sober when he started experiencing anxiety attacks. Ervin was attending an elite private college on an athletic scholarship for basketball. He said his anxiety was effecting his play on the court, which naturally increased his worry. Ervin was 2 years old when his mother left the tough inner-city neighborhood where he was born and returned to the much wealthier white suburb where she was raised. Ervin's mother was very concerned about her son becoming alienated from his African-American heritage. She tried to stay in contact with some of Ervin's relatives from his father's side of the family, but this was difficult because of his father's alcoholism and violence. Eventually she and Ervin stopped having any contact with them at all.

Ervin always experienced a certain amount of unease about his racial and cultural heritage, particularly his blackness. On the one hand, Ervin expressed a kind of survivor's guilt about his privileged education and upbringing. On the other, he constantly found himself calling into question his own self-worth and competence. He worried, for example, whether he was simply an "affirmative action entrant" at the college he attended. He also wondered if he would have been accepted in the white community he grew up in had he not excelled in sports or had he looked more "African." This was a particularly intense source of pain for him. Because of his light complexion many of his black friends resented him—a dilemma that confronts many people of color in a society where the media-promoted standards of beauty and attractiveness are still based primarily on European features and characteristics.

Ervin loved playing basketball and possessed a real talent for the game. He knew he'd been given a gift, but often thought about whether he played basketball because it was what he wanted for himself or to please others. He wondered if people would have been as encouraging and supportive had he chosen to develop his talents in math, his best subject in school, but one that doesn't conform to people's racial stereotypes or culturally based role expectations.

Most of all, Ervin wondered where he belonged. Like many people of color he possessed a double consciousness of sorts. When hanging out with his black friends at school he felt pressure to talk and think black: "If the school recognized Ebonics as a legitimate dialect, I'd have met my foreign language requirement before I started college," he joked. However, when surrounded by his white classmates or visiting his mother's parents, he found himself changing his mannerisms and language so he would fit in better with upper class white culture and customs. Ervin said this experience more than any other fueled his drinking. He described feeling split at times and said that alcohol was the only thing that quieted the feelings of shame and self-doubt he experienced. Since getting sober, Ervin said he no longer felt ashamed of being black but said he felt just as confused about his identity. He talked about how these feelings were getting in the way of his ability to compete with his teammates and his enjoyment of his sport:

> "So many black kids I faced on the court growing up were playing to get out of the ghetto. My mother made it clear to me that if I didn't get to college playing basketball the money was there. I was going to get an education. She said it to take the pressure off me. But all these other guys who came from nothing, basketball is all

they got. They play the game angry. They have the eye of the tiger, there's an edge to them. They're playing for a shot at a better life. What am I playing for?"

Complicating matters further, many of Ervin's relatives (black and white) drank heavily. This made it difficult for Ervin to spend time with them. They didn't understand his recovery: "You have a job, you're going to school, how can you be alcoholic?" Some of his black relatives used to invite Ervin to take a walk with them around his old neighborhood so they could show him some "real drunks." Some said they felt that Ervin had been "brainwashed" by the white people in the AA program. Ervin explained that many of his family members were suspicious of "outsiders" and felt threatened by his decision to get sober: "Most of them have never missed a game, but couldn't make it up to see me during all the months I spent in treatment." However, these objections to Ervin's recovery, voiced by his black relatives, were about more than just their denial of their own problems; they were a reflection of a general mistrust of the treatment establishment and other white-run institutions common within black communities. This sort of minimization of the alcoholic's problem and mistrust of the medical profession are obstacles many recovering people from alcoholic families face, but they may be especially difficult for members of black and other marginalized communities to overcome.

Ervin and I discussed the importance of his being as honest about his feelings about his racial identity as he had been about his drinking. This meant being frank about his feelings about our relationship as well. Having grown up in a predominantly white community Ervin was accustomed to seeing white professionals, which only contributed to the problems he was having developing a stronger sense of a black identity. Ervin came to see me because I had seen his mother and him in family therapy when he was a child and met with him on his own when he was an adolescent. He said he was torn between his desire to find a black male therapist (not an easy task in either the community where he lived or went to school) and not wanting to start over again with someone new.

Consequently, Ervin and I talked about his needing to seek out successful recovering black men as role models. This was an especially sensitive topic for Ervin because it brought him face to face with his father's absence in his life. Ervin had never met his father. This fact, coupled with his desire to better understand himself and where he came from—"my roots"—haunted Ervin. Up to this point, Ervin depended on everyone's voice but his own for what little insight he had into his past. We talked about his need to begin forming his own relationship to these events. I suggested he start this quest by reading a letter he'd written to his father when he was a teenager and last in therapy with me.

Excerpts from Ervin's Letter to His Father

Dear Dad,

You know who this is right? Yeah it's me. YOUR SON! The child you had with that white woman. My name is Ervin Munroe. I am your son. I'm 6'2". Only about an inch or two shorter than you. I'm 16. DO you remember me? I got this picture of you holding me. You're looking at me, you seem proud. But I am looking somewhere else, far off into the distance. I knew I wasn't going to stay.

Why have you never tried to reach us? Do you even care? I don't know I'm part black. Really, I can't believe it. I play basketball, Dad I listen to rap music, I watched Belly, but that's about as black as I can make myself feel. Where were you to tell me I was black? I think you should come see me play basketball. I'm good, really good. Sometimes I get afraid on the court, but that's about all that can stop me. You stop me. I do something great on the court, and I look in the stands and see all these fathers cheering for me. But you're not there so it doesn't mater.

Mom says you're a nobody a failure, that you can't hold down a job, that you pee on yourself, that you hit her, that you threatened to kill her, that you hold a bible in one hand and a baseball bat in the other. C'mon I say. It can't be like that. Look at me! I play the saxophone like Coltrane, I play basketball like Jordan, I write like Jesse Jackson, I make music better than anything you've ever heard in your life. But you have never heard it. You haven't even heard me talk. I am your goddamn son, and you haven't even heard me talk yet. You should see me. I'm distinguished, I'm handsome. Mom tells me everyday. I've got straight teeth. My calf muscles are huge, which helps me jump high. I get good grades too. There is no possible way that I am not going to succeed in life. But you're not there. Oh what you are missing out on! You should hear what people say about me. Glowing comments, wonderful attitude, great effort, charisma, creativity. I'm not a robot Dad. I'm not going to fall off like everyone tells me you did. I have never taken a drink in my life and I never will. I swear I never will. Never drugs never. Cuz I am not going to miss out on all the greatness my kids are going to have because I can't stop pissing on myself. No Dad, not like you.

Mom sometimes complains that when I do certain things,

like yell at her when we get into fights, that I remind her of you. That scares me more than it scares her. I don't want to be you. I am the last hope for this family, both sides, white and black, when it comes to men. You have failed. Mom says you tried but you just couldn't do it. Good try. I will not be like you. I work hard at school, hard at basketball, hard at loving, hard at life. I just wrote a letter to a girl that I was going with back in school. I mistreated her, and I am apologizing. That is what you need to do, Dad, apologize. To me and to mom. I don't think you can ever apologize enough, but it would be a start. I know mom fears and hates you. She hates you with good reason, Dad. You didn't treat her well. Me, I don't hate you. I have nothing to hate about you. You cannot hate someone you do not know. You have given me nothing to hate and nothing to love except this tint in my skin and some large calf muscles.

Mom said that you are really into Jesus and Christianity. You're not going to find God through Jesus, I'm sorry Dad. No religion can find God for you. You've got to put down that bible and pick up your baby.

Mom and I are Buddhists. I read in religion class at school that Buddhism and Christianity are now considered to not be that far apart. You should try it, it improves the condition of your life. I chanted for you tonight. It's hard to think about you, Dad. I get all queasy and nervous. You have always been this figment of my imagination. This small myth of "Dad" that lies in the back of my mind as part of my story. You're like the white whale in *Moby Dick*! You hear that. I've been searching for you in all these places. In my musical creations, in my sporting endeavors, in my schoolwork, in my writing, but I never found you.

Dad. Daddy. Pops. Poppa. Father. All these words are foreign to me. I've waited so long for you Dad. I have waited so long to love you. Every man I see. Every male relationship I have is based on finding a replacement for you. I want your guidance, I want your knowledge, I want you to tell me how the world works, how I fit in, and how I will become great. I want to hug you so badly. I want to hug you and have your big body engulf me. I want to cry on your chest and feel safe, and know that nothing is going to touch me, absolutely nothing. I want you to say, "I love you son," and push me hard to excel in future endeavors. I want you to see me do something really mediocre and then praise me as if I just recreated the world. I want that. All this I want, all this I will never have. It is too late to tuck me in bed at night. It is too late for me to come screaming into your room at two in the morning, positively sure that there are robbers outside my window. I was always terrified in the dark.

Mom would be home, but mom is constantly marveling at my paltry physical strength, so how could she possibly defend me. Where were you to defend us? When I find you, Dad, I will take you in my arms and cry on you. Whether you like it or not. I am going to lift weights, get strong, and grow three more inches so that when I take you in my arms and cry on you, you won't be able to get away.

Just asking myself who you are is really affecting me. For the first time in a long time, I have been able to breath and see some things as they really are. I feel like an adult almost, if feeling like an adult is being aware of oneself. You have taught me so much. You don't know it but you have taught me so much about how to be a man. You taught me with what you haven't done. You must have found Buddhism in a previous lifetime.

Dad, I am smart and I am going to do something other than basketball with my life. But, I would like to master basketball. I have worked a long time at it and I think I can do it. There's one thing about basketball, Dad. Everyone wants to sky above the rim and dunk the basketball. They get off on it. I am the same way. But one thing I have noticed is that those guys that recognize that basketball is played on the floor and not in the air have a much easier time with themselves. It doesn't matter how tall you are, how big you are, or how good you are. Everyone's feet come back on the floor. That's all I want to do, Dad. Keep my feet on the floor and my mind in my head. Every coach I've ever had has told me how I should reach you. Work harder on Defense, Hustle, Get Rebounds, Be a Leader. They call it winning. In order to reach you, I've got to win and play well. That's what they tell me. I believed them for so long, Dad. All the black people told me if I could dunk the ball I could reach you. If I could jump and touch the top of the basket, the top of the world, that I could reach you. Now I know. You are on the floor, just like me.

I've got to go now, but I'll write to you again. Please help me keep my feet on the ground. Let me remember you.

For Ervin, this correspondence represented the culmination of years of struggle, first as a child and then as an adolescent, trying to come to terms with his father's abandonment of him and his identity as a young black man. Ervin said that reading it again made him feel like Ebenezer Scrooge, the character in the Dickens novel who receives a visit from the ghost of Christmas past and begins his life anew.

Especially disturbing to Ervin was reading about his commitment not to ever use drugs and alcohol as his father had. He said that whenever he found himself on the verge of picking up a drink or a drug again, usually the thought of ruining any chance he had at a career in professional basketball was enough to stop him from acting on these cravings. He felt sad that so many of his issues from childhood about where he belonged or fit in were still with him. However, reading his own words as a 16-year-old youth ready and willing to take on these concerns inspired him: "If he had the courage to handle all that, to overcome all that adversity so I could have this opportunity, the least I can do is take advantage of it and not throw it away just so I can get a buzz on. I think I owe us both that much."

Ervin accomplished a lot in recovery, but because he did not adequately deal with his racial pain and father loss during his chemical dependency treatment his healing felt incomplete. The concept of 12-step literacy advocates that therapists need to assist clients in overcoming cultural obstacles and barriers—including issues of race, gender, sexual orientation, and class—that keep people from making healthy connections to AA and recovery. Clients who do not receive help understanding and coping with these societal problems in treatment are at much greater risk for relapse. It is too often wasted work when we address clients' emotional, mental, and spiritual needs and fail to identify and assist them with the sociopolitical and economic challenges they face.

Although we continued meeting for several months, after a few sessions Ervin reported that his play on the court had settled down and he was no longer as anxious about his performance. He said that reading the letter had reminded him that there were more things he wanted to do with his life than play basketball. I, in turn, no longer worried about Ervin's sobriety. Ervin had his feet on the ground.

Gender, Culture, and Power

The couples therapy with Sylvia and Jeff (presented in Chapter 5) is a good illustration of the constricting impact that gender stereotypes and roles imposed by the larger culture can have on relationships. In this instance it would have been too convenient, as well as simplistic, to label Sylvia "codependent" and her relationship with Jeff as "dysfunctional."

This stance, in addition to being demeaning, ignores the complex lacework of cultural, familial, and psychic factors that influence people's choices in life and relationships. It also, as the feminist critique of codependency protests, pathologizes women's innate talent for caring for others, taking something good and turning it against them. As Bepko and Krestan (1991) caution, these terms—initially meant to help people identify behaviors that were interfering with their enjoyment and ability to take responsibility for their lives—can become just another oppressive discourse that places the blame for what's wrong in families at the feet of women.

Similarly, my efforts on behalf of Jesse's family (in Chapter 2), while appearing to have improved the possibilities of their lives, could have had alarming results. The incident that eventually led to his father becoming more involved in Jesse's therapy (punching his son in the back and throwing him across the room) made this clearer. My initial determination to engage Jesse's father in family therapy placed too much emphasis on a point of view that sees families without an active and involved father as incomplete and more difficult to change. Jesse and his mother obviously needed help managing their relationship with Jesse's father. However, the essential point here was that these relations were still characterized primarily by the "abuse" of power—*not* the "absence" of it.

As Schafer (1992) points out, from the standpoint of writing—for Karen and many others whose stories are collected in this book—women are the pages on which men write their stories of power. Karen's experience of oppression as a woman colored her experience of addiction and recovery, as well as her participation in AA. It impeded her ability to make a meaningful connection to AA—a "fellowship" whose assistance we both felt she needed. For Karen, recognizing and understanding her need to connect with other women (not just other alcoholics) was an integral part of her therapy. Put another way, Karen needed a safe haven from the effects of *both* sexism *and* alcoholism.

For Karen, therapy and recovery challenged some of her most deeply held beliefs about herself. Exploring what mattered to her in life, what was possible, and how it all came together (i.e., her reality, values, and systems of meaning) were questions she had never been invited to ask herself. Every therapy asks these questions of clients. However, narrative and other feminist-minded therapies recognize that any inquiry into how people use stories to make meaning out of their lives and give voice to their experience is an inherently political one.

AA, on the other hand, emphasizes the importance of its groups staying focused on helping people's personal recovery, encouraging each person's responsibility for him- or herself and other alcoholics over social responsibility or involvement in politics and public policy issues. To ensure this, AA's fifth tradition (adopted along with its steps by all the other 12-step programs) says, "Each group has but one primary purpose—to carry its message to the alcoholic who still suffers," while tradition 10 states "Alcoholics Anonymous has no opinion on outside issues; hence the AA name ought never be drawn into public controversy."

While AA chooses not to get involved in politics for purposes of group cohesion, it is nevertheless political and has an impact on our culture and the contemporary postmodern landscape. AA and other 12-step programs offer an alternative to the growing sense of randomness and disconnection people experience in their lives today. These groups not only buffer people from the chaos of their alcoholic pasts, but for many they also provide protection from the random violence and disconnection they experience in the present.

From the standpoint of gender, while the Big Book did not speak to women's experience when outlining its fundamental premises about addiction and recovery, the ideals expressed in the text clearly meant to include women's voices even though the prevailing social arrangements of the time did not make space for or value them. Today, women are represented at meetings in the same numbers as men, and alcoholism is no longer seen as a man's problem. Beginning with the second edition published in 1955, many women's narratives were included in the collection of stories that make up the book's second part.[8]

Although AA literature is one of the worst offenders when it comes to perpetuating sex role stereotypes, often portraying men and women as caricatures of 1950s American life, members' attitudes and sharings at meetings are more in sync with prevailing cultural moods and sentiments. Also, while much of AA's written material is dated, there is a plethora of more recent literary productions in AA written specifically for people of color, gays, lesbians, and women. This literature addresses contemporary problems particular to the era we're living in now (such as AIDS, single parent families, and blended families). Furthermore, many of AA's efforts to reach out to marginalized groups and populations were way ahead of their time when compared with other institutions in both the private and public sector. Much of the debate about changing or rewriting AA's major texts concerns members' fears about losing their connection to the program's past with its rich sense of tradition and history.[9]

However, therapists need to continue to help clients interpret AA and Al-Anon's spiritual narratives and principles in ways that will both fit with and challenge people's world outlook. This has to include challenging and scrutinizing the political messages found in AA and other 12-step programs when necessary, or their practices will lose any relevance they have to people's everyday lives.

Hermeneutics, Story, and Voice

All people, including alcoholics and other recovering persons, who lack the ability to confront the sheer absurdity of the human condition, what Cornel West (1996) calls the "tragicomic" sense of life, propel themselves toward suicide, madness, or addiction unless they are, as West admonishes, buffered by ritual, cushioned by community, or sustained by art. What sociologists call the interpretive turn in psychology and the human sciences was, in part, a response to people's experience of the absence of community and meaningful ritual in their lives. The rise of narrative in other disciplines ushered in a number of new metaphors for psychotherapy, including hermeneutics, story, and voice.

A great deal of literature is dedicated to exploring the differences and interplay of hermeneutics, story, and voice as they apply to the process of psychotherapy. There is a great deal of overlap and cross-pollination among the three concepts. However, as I understand the term, hermeneutics is more concerned with systems of meaning and matters of epistemology (how we know what we know). Descended from the study and interpretation of the Bible and religious texts, the word *hermeneutics* is derived from the Greek. It means interpretation, and I prefer this more familiar expression. However, in the past decade a new psychology has cropped up that shares this name with a radical philosophy linked to the work of Martin Heidegger and of Hans-Georg Gadamer (1960/1975), so it is worth it for therapists to become familiar with the ideas associated with the term.

Hermeneutics, as applied by the authors and therapists whose work is presented in this book, is "based on the premise that human beings, both individually and in concert with one another, actively construct and co-construct meaning out of their experiences as opposed to receiving knowledge in pure form directly from the external world" (Rosen, personal communication, 1994). According to this perspective, psychotherapy is conducted as a clinical dialogue that alters in crucial ways our consciously narrated presentations of the self and its history by destabilizing, deconstructing and defamiliarizing our life stories. Clinicians whose work is informed by this tradition (e.g., the conversational approach of family therapists Harlene Anderson & Harold A. Goolishian, 1988, 1992, or the work of analyst Roy Schafer, 1976a, 1992) locate therapy in the domain of language and meaning.

On the other hand, *story*, while sharing a meaning-making approach, emphasizes the role that myth, ritual, tradition, creativity, and imagination play in people's lives. However, the use of "story" as a metaphor for psychotherapy and recovery has political implications as well. Stories and rituals can help us make connections between oppressive cultural narratives (e.g., racism, sexism, and homophobia) and the intimately personal ways these negative messages shape our experience of our spiritual practices, sexual relations, parenting, work, and other human relationships. Examples of this perspective in the family therapy community include what I call the "narritual" approach of Evan Imber-Black and Janine Roberts (Roberts, 1994; see also Imber-Black, Roberts, & Whiting, 1988), "the letters to ourselves" which Peggy Penn and Marcia Scheinberg (1991) encourage us to write, as well as the narrative work of White and Epston (1990, 1991; see also White, 1989g).

Finally, *voice,* is about agency, identity, and self-determination. Its domain includes relations of power; people's resistance to domination, exploitation, and abuse; and other acts of courage. In the face of increasing attacks on many people's personal and cultural identities, breaking silence and speaking out sustains us and offers hope. Many therapists (Hoffman, 1993; S. Levin, 1988; M. Olson, 1995) are adding this metaphor to those associated with hermeneutics and other literary forms (such as story and narrative) adopted by psychotherapy. Drawing on Ong's (1982) work, they examine how women have historically been excluded from male preserves of knowledge, which since Plato have been based on literacy, oratory, and rhetoric. These authors see women's identity as having closer ties to an oral tradition, less rhetorical and more conversational in nature—practices that contributed to the rise of the novel and the growing presence of women's voices in literature and the humanities. They join the call by Gilligan (1982), Belenky, Clinchy, Goldberger, and Tarule (1986), and J. B. Miller (1976) for research and therapy "in a different voice," based upon an "ethic of care," empathy, and concern.

Collectively, these new ways of thinking about human experience are changing our understanding of how therapy helps people heal. They also help bridge the gap between the 12-step recovery and psychotherapy communities, linking AA's storied past to psychotherapy's narrative future.

Hermeneutist or Heretic?

Aspects of the concept of 12-step literacy outlined in this chapter are my own testimonial, of sorts, to the knowledge and wonders of AA. This is cause for concern as it counters AA's own credo of "membership by attraction, not promotion." I do not mean to give the impression that I believe AA or 12-step groups are meant for every client struggling with an addiction. They're not. Recovery is a fluid process, and clinicians must give clients the space they need to define it for themselves. This requires therapists to remain flexible in their application of AA's concepts to people's stories while steadfastly refusing to join clients in their denial. It also requires that clinicians consider working with people who choose not to make AA or another 12-step group part of their healing. The enthusiasm displayed in this book for 12-step customs and practices represents an effort to close the gap between the AA and psychotherapy communities. As I said earlier, historically, scholars, physicians, and therapists, when writing about alcoholism, have marginalized AA's contribution to the growing body of knowledge about addiction.

I've intended in this chapter to enhance the reader's understanding of the story behind my own efforts at narrating clients' stories of addiction and recovery, and to show how AA and Al-Anon help me access this world. Such an understanding might, for instance, explain why I was not more confrontative when dealing with a client's denial of a problem with alcohol or drugs, or why I chose to work with someone in therapy for as long as I did while he or she was actively abusing substances. These insights may explain why, for example, I did not stamp Holly's letter (presented at the beginning of Chapter 2)—or anyone else's—"return to sender," choosing instead to accept her understanding of her problem and then trying to focus on issues that were of concern to her.

A note of caution: therapists who collaborate with people utilizing AA and other 12-step programs in treatment must be capable of resting on the perimeter of the important action, allowing the therapy arena to play a secondary role in a person's recovery. This is especially true during early recovery (the first 1 to 2 years of sobriety). During this period, stripped of their chemicals, people often find themselves extremely vulnerable and raw. They may become more dependent on AA, and they have little tolerance for the kind of strong affect and feeling that tends to surface in therapy.

Suffice it to say, after much hard work fielding angry transferences and crises calls; receiving blame for the alcoholic's problem ("kill the messenger"); providing extra sessions; arranging detox, hospitalization, family meetings, and aftercare planning; attending AA and Al-Anon meetings to learn more about the process of recovery and the disease concept of alcoholism—therapists must be prepared for a client to come into the session one afternoon and credit her sponsor, AA, and her

Higher Power for saving her life and making it all possible! Step 1: humility.

From Recovery to Discovery

In sum, in a narrative approach to drug and alcohol abuse, the process of healing may be viewed as one of *discovery* rather than *recovery*. As a result, therapists who work with people suffering from addiction should think of themselves as possessing a sort of clinical poaching license— raiding other psychological theories and intellectual disciplines for whatever treasures they hold or insight they can afford. Roland Barthes, discussing the increasingly popular topic of interdisciplinary work, observed that such study is not about confronting already constituted disciplines: "To do something interdisciplinary it's not enough to choose a 'subject' (a theme) and gather around it two or three sciences. Interdisciplinarity consists in creating a new object that belongs to no one" (Barthes, as quoted in Clifford & Marcus, 1986, p. 1).

PART III

Stories for Our Time

Thirty years ago my older brother, who was ten years old at the time, was trying to get a report on birds written that he'd had three months to write. It was due the next day . . . . he was at the kitchen table in tears . . . . Then my father sat down beside him, and put his arm around my brother's shoulders, and said, "Bird by bird, buddy. Just take it bird by bird."

—ANNE LAMOTT

CHAPTER 7

Trauma and Recovery

Wherever the bird with no feet flew
she found trees with no limbs.
—AUDRE LORDE

In the beginning of her book *Women Who Hurt Themselves* (1994), Dusty Miller invites us to imagine a memorial wall inscribed with the names of women who have died by their own hand through some kind of self-inflicted abuse. Alcoholism, drug addiction, anorexia, bulimia, excessive dieting, self-inflicted burns and cuts—the monument or fabric, says Miller, would cover acres and acres of land and the names would stretch for hundreds of miles:

> These women are not remembered as brave victims of a war or epidemic illness, but they should be. Instead they are often blamed for their deaths because the fatal wounds were inflicted by their own hand. These wounds, however, were a direct consequence of earlier injuries inflicted by parents, grandparents, and other primary caretakers, injuries that never healed or proved deadly. (1994, p. 3)[1]

There are still no permanent monuments to these survivors, however the Clothesline Project is one of a growing number of national and local grassroots campaigns that has tried to fill this void. Women survivors of rape, incest, and other sexual trauma are invited to tell their stories on a T-shirt (similar to a "loved one's patch" on the AIDS quilt), and thousands of such T-shirts are displayed on clotheslines hung in large public spaces. The exhibit is open to everyone and is a powerful and moving sight. One of my clients, Cara (introduced in Chapter 6), saw the exhibit when it came to a nearby college. Inspired by what she saw, Cara came to her next session with a letter describing what she would say if she had contributed an article of her clothing to such a project.

Cara's Letter

This is what I would put on a T-shirt.

Sometime between the ages of 6 yrs to 8 yrs old I was traumatized by the man next door. As a result of this now until age 44 I have lived with a distrust. While in therapy at the age of 42 (while working on my addiction) the nightmares all fell in place. His name was Billy M.—his crime would only be listed as: sexual assault of a minor, but it was much more. It's lasting effects have stripped me of many things. My child's mind remembers this HUGE penis with milk—that tasted awful— dripping from it and 2 faceless little girls. One was Billy's daughter the other was me. My mother had always told me not to be alone with men but never told me why. Mom I wasn't alone. I had a friend whose name today I don't remember. The other part of this nightmare that still hasn't come full circle is a large knife. I remember nothing at all of my childhood until my parents moved out of Missouri to Indiana when I was 12½.

Then at the age of 14 I was molested by a neighbor George R. and I knew I couldn't tell. I used to baby-sit his kids. He was a doctor and he was sexy and handsome. He called me "elephant" and made fun of the fact that I was fat for my age— but I hated my body—thanks to Billy and the nightmares. He would tell me that no boy would want me but he would show me sex—teach me more than science which he was tutoring me in. I let him molest me and felt his penis but we never had sex (until I was 19 years old and went to him to live out what I couldn't between ages 14–17). While he was molesting me between 14–17 he gave me medicine that would help me lose weight so men would want to be with me and I could have a boyfriend. He promised me antibiotics if I caught any STDs [sexually transmitted diseases] and condoms so I wouldn't get knocked up.

From the age of 23–40 or 41 I was (still am) married to and allowed Marty, my husband, to be emotionally abusive because he did want to have sex with me. Through these years came heavy drinking and drugging to attempt to cover the pain that started between 6–8 and has lasted through today. He blamed me for Sam (my second child) even though he told me he wanted 2 kids. He blamed me for our financial ruin—even though I worked 2 jobs and went with only the new clothes I got at

X-mas. He would spend $100 to $200 a month on clothes and shoes for himself. Clothing money for me went to the kids. He gave me money to drink because I left him alone (and the world) when I drank. He blamed me for his being unfaithful because I wasn't a good enough lover to satisfy his needs. He blamed me for my son's violent temper when actually he copied his father. He treated me like I didn't have the right to stand up for myself and my child's mind knew nobody would listen any how. At least I knew he had no right to beat me and I stood up to that.

Jim—he was a professional who treated my body, his hurt was also of an emotional nature. He would accidentally slip and feel my breast sexually. He also again accidentally would slip into my groin when working on my thigh, gluts or abdomen. Because I trusted you [Jim] I knew you would remain professional—after all you were the one person I had told all about Billy, George, and Marty. I then thought I felt your hard penis rub on me, but again I knew it was just in my mind—after all I trusted you completely. I thought I heard you unzip your pants. Again it was OK because you had gained weight and your pants were too tight. You had helped me get sober and had fully won my trust by telling me to stand up for myself—all the time you were taking sexual liberties you should not have been. I know now you were touching me with your unprotected penis— you were stroking yourself with your pants unzipped and your penis out while working on my back, butt or legs. You talked and teased in a sexual language while being paid to work on me.

These are all the bad men I remember at this time. I know there could be more.

Today I wish to thank Jonathan, my sponsor, and my friends for all they have done to put this Humpty Dumpty together again. I also have to thank my HP [Higher Power] for letting me see this a little at a time so I could handle it. Thank you God.

A history of childhood trauma and abuse is one of the single greatest obstacles to abstinence and serenity an alcoholic or addict can face and poses many challenges to an already recovering person's sobriety. Because of the number of women addicts and alcoholics in my practice, I find myself listening to many abuse stories. For trauma survivors, abuse issues often surface with sobriety. Therapists committed to providing a safe space for people to do recovery work should prepare to help people cope with these experiences and feelings as well. Clinicians will also find that these issues show up in much greater numbers within this population than they are accustomed to seeing in the rest of their practice.

Both trauma and addiction originate in shame. Many of the experiences associated with an individual's addiction and home life are laced with guilt and shame. To distinguish between the two feelings, we usually experience *guilt* over something we've done to others; *shame* stems from feelings of inadequacy about who we are or, in the case of an alcoholic or abusive home, from whence we come.

This chapter, along with a brief one that follows it on eating disorders, will explore some of the connections between trauma and addiction through the eyes of Cara and two other women, Karen and Sophie. Parts of Karen's and Cara's stories have already been told in previous chapters. Sophie's experiences are described here for the first time. The current discourse on memory, incest, sexual abuse, posttraumatic stress disorder, and other disassociative experiences is a heated one. Regardless of how one weighs in on these issues, these women's narratives provide those of us in the therapy and recovering communities with three authentic voices and qualified front-line correspondents. They also conjure up the words of anthropologist Veena Das (1997) when she observed that denial of others' pain is not about the failings of the intellect but the failings of the spirit.

THE "FORGOTTEN WAR"

The truth is more important than the facts.
—FRANK LLOYD WRIGHT

Karen's second letter to alcohol (readers will find this part of her story and her letters on pp. 19–27) written in response to her relapse, was an angry one. Its strong words conjure up powerful images and emotions. In the letter's closing paragraph, Karen wrote: "To me you are a slow death—a rapist that takes my pride, self respect, and future. To castrate you is my goal—you will not have power over my life unless I allow it by accepting you back into my life with that first drink."

Many thoughts come to my mind when I reflect on the fragments of Karen's story she chose to share, as well as the language she chose to describe her experience. However, prior to sharing my thoughts, it might help the reader to have more background on Karen's life—to hear more about her story and the narrative I sit with and hold when I think about what Karen's choice of words says about her life and how it may have impacted on the direction of her therapy. When Karen first got sober she experienced panic attacks and nightmares. She said she had a particularly difficult time when her husband, whom she described as a gentle and unassuming man, needed to discipline any of the children, even when it was warranted. Her nightmares were of men trying to kill her "or worse."

Karen understood both the panic attacks and her overprotectiveness of her children as stemming from her first marriage to a violent, physically abusive, and drug-addicted man. As described earlier, Karen was able to wrest herself away from this abusive relationship with the help of women's services, restraining orders, and eventually police intervention, because her ex-husband continued to stalk her and the children at home and at the children's school.

Because of the sketchy nature of Karen's recollections of her childhood and family life, her story reads more like a collage of memories, dreams, and reflections than a chronological case history. Her gaps in memory span years. After she became sober, Karen began remembering more and experiencing what she called flashbacks of things that happened to her when she was a little girl. As she explained, "That was the purpose of the alcohol, to forget all that."

One of eight children from an Irish American working-class family, Karen described her father as a physically imposing man who "always had a beer in his hand." She said he was a "jolly drunk" who always gave the kids sips of his alcohol and used to pass out in front of the television. This image was juxtaposed with memories of her father chasing Karen and her brothers and sisters around the house with a belt:

> "When he was pissed he would just reach for his waist [gestures toward her buckle]. We knew what that meant and to run for it. We'd scramble upstairs to where the bedrooms were. He would be right behind us with that belt cracking at our feet. If you made it to your room you knew you'd be okay."

When I asked where her mother was at these times, Karen responded sarcastically, "probably at the hospital having another baby."

Karen recalled with great sadness that when she reached puberty her father stopped relating to her: "It was like what little relationship we had just ceased altogether."

Karen describes her mother as never having time for her. Karen's sense of her mother was that she was always saying the right things but was never there: "I think I was the kind of baby who cried and cried and never was heard." As an adult, Karen felt this pattern repeated over and over again. Tearfully, she confessed that after the birth of her first child her mother didn't come to see her or the baby for a month and that her father didn't come at all. "That never would have happened with anyone else in the family," she said.

Karen's sense of abandonment and rage at both her parents, as well as the absence of her mother's voice in her life, is captured in the following story from adolescence: Karen woke one night to the sound of fighting. When she opened her bedroom door she saw one of her brothers standing in the middle of the kitchen, too drunk to speak or move. Her father, laughing and yelling, was punching him in the face, while her mother, standing to the side, looked on with a pained expression on her face. When Karen shouted at her father to stop it, her mother told Karen not to interfere.

Karen's earliest conscious memory is of being 5 or 6 years old and contemplating suicide. She recalled one episode where she had gotten into a tackle box in her basement, found a hunting knife, and held it to her stomach, wanting to die. Karen remembers the look on her father's face, who walked downstairs at that moment. "He was pale as a ghost," said Karen, "and what he saw in my face must have really frightened him, because he didn't yell at me. He just took the knife out of my hands and walked silently back upstairs."

An equally disturbing memory that Karen recounted was of having slept with her father until the age of 9 or 10, whenever her mother's parents came to visit. On these occasions, her grandparents would sleep in Karen's room, her mother would sleep on the couch, and Karen would sleep in her parents' room with her father. She remembered:

> "I hated the way he smelled. Sometimes he used to wrap his arm around me like I was her. I'm not sure when this stopped, but looking back it doesn't make any sense, there were so many other possible arrangements. Why didn't I get put on the couch with a sleeping bag or something?"

In sobriety, Karen also remembered having fainting spells throughout her childhood:

> "I forgot about that. I used to pass out without explanation. It used to happen once every month or so. My mother took me to a physician. He said it was from low blood sugar. I had medication but recently learned from my mother that they were placebos. My grandmother used to tell me how much it scared her. It happened

to me for the first time when I was at her house. I was standing by the stove and she carried me into the bedroom. I must have been 6 or 7 because I was always big for my age and she was already an old lady then. One of the last times, I was in church and collapsed on top of some aluminum chairs. I know I must have been 14 or 15 because I was dating some guy I was in high school with at the time."

As a young adult, Karen recalled hanging out with delinquents, "Nam vets," and runaways on the steps of her Town Hall, "with my army jacket, old clothes, and my fuck you attitude." This experience was emblematic of her family history and the dynamics of her childhood trauma and abuse: Karen standing in her tattered battle fatigues, getting stoned with veterans of a war the community wanted to deny ever took place. When I shared these thoughts with Karen, she said it was painful to think of her life as a war: "But it was a war, certainly a war inside myself, and no one told me it was okay to feel that way, no one responded to my anger."

When Karen turned 17, she left home. "I just crawled out my bedroom window and never looked back." This image was a metaphor for this chapter of Karen's life. In her therapy she kept checking back to it, as to the North Star to orient herself. Karen felt intense guilt and shame as a consequence of this action. Her guilt stemmed from the sense of loyalty she felt to her parents. She felt it was a terrible thing to do to her mother and father: "I rejected them." Her shame came from imagining what awful things she could have done or may have happened to her that would cause her to leave home in such a way.

Reflections

In therapy, theories, like maps, should be used selectively and not confused with the actual territories they're trying to explore. In my work with Karen I found myself using, like any good cartographer, more than one kind of map to help us find our way. What follows is a brief examination of Karen's written correspondence to alcohol, created early on in our work together (presented in Chapter 1), and some alternative readings of it.

Karen's letters had both some immediate consequences and some longer unforeseen ones. Using the framework of narrative family therapy, I viewed Karen's communiqués as a declaration of independence from alcohol and drugs, a "(w)rite of passage" from addiction to sobriety. The letters provided an opportunity for Karen to reauthor her relationship with her addiction; to rewrite the terms of her contract with drugs and alcohol, using language that emphasized her needs and self-interests.

These ideas shed light on other concerns in Karen's life. Because of the constellation of problems and kinds of dissociative experience Karen struggled with, this telling or version of the events of her life caused Karen to fear that she might have been sexually molested as a child. After many conversations in sobriety and therapy with little change in her dissociative experience, Karen participated in a women's group for survivors of sexual abuse as a way of exploring her fears and concerns. She found the group helpful. The group validated her concerns that something awful happened to her, offered strategies to help her manage and contain her fears and terror, and loosened the grip these fears had on her life and relationships.

In our work together, we viewed the possibility of Karen having been sexually abused as an unfinished manuscript, so to speak, a story she could put down and return to as needed. However, we did conclude that as the result of the abuse of alcohol and violence in Karen's family, boundaries were significantly blurred. Together with the sexual assault and violence she endured in her first marriage, there seemed more than enough ways to make sense of her experience without assuming the existence of some undiscovered "truth" about her life.

In this sense, Karen's letters served as flashbacks to various unsettling aspects of her past, as well as "flashforwards" to conversations she and I would be having in the future. Karen was writing about both the seen and unseen aspects of her experience.

Psychoanalytic narratives, especially Schafer's "storylines" and hermeneutic investigations, allow us to further explore the invisible aspects of our experience. One feature of the analytic dialogue, Schafer (1992) observes, is the way it shows us that dialogic experience, both in the past and in the present, is never limited to two people present to one another physically. These analytic conversations make us aware of the multitude of voices arising from our inner world, as well as from our interaction with others. It illuminates and gives voice to what Deena Metzger (1992) calls our unconscious, unarticulated, unenacted aspects of self. Once these voices can be sorted out and heard more clearly, we can begin to trace them back to their origins, personal or cultural, to reduce their grip on our lives and actions.

When, for example, I asked Karen what it meant to her to see alcohol as "a rapist," she described an incident from her first marriage. Karen's ex-husband used to take her to pornographic movies and want her to perform acts from the movie in the theater. Karen would refuse, but one time after the film they went to a secluded place in a park and, she said, "I tried to please him and act the way the women in the movies did." Karen said she was actually enjoying her "role" and the sex, when her husband pushed her away and called her a "whore." Karen was devastated by his comment. She feels she continues to move through the world with his voice in her head telling her how "pathetic" and "disgusting" she is.

Karen and I talked about the episode as Karen having been "verbally raped." The twisted and perverted aspects of this experience were not the acts themselves or the feelings of pleasure or disgust Karen felt or did not feel about them. It was the way her ex-husband's words destroyed the connection she felt between the two of them and severed her relationship with her own desires.

From a narrative point of view, Karen's letters demonstrate two visions of reality, the romantic and the tragic.[2] Her letters helped us explore both. On the one hand, Karen's writing reflected the heroic task of becoming sober and reaching for her "higher goals." They assisted her in removing the obstacles in her life that kept her from realizing her aspirations. On the other, it gave Karen courage to face the tragic events and aspects of her life. It helped her sit with the absences and silences in her life, the broken pieces that always seem in a state of disarray without much hope of mending.

Cracks in the Mirror

This close-up look at Karen's letters also highlights some of the tension and differences between individual and family therapy perspectives. We shouldn't have to choose between the two.

The family therapy concept of "reflexivity"* urges us to look at how our experience impacts upon our clients' stories, as well as explore how our clients' knowledge shapes and colors our own narratives. Psychoanalytically oriented therapists call this "countertransference." Countertransference is a term (with its companion expression, "transference") I've never been comfortable using, as both seem to suggest that the client is solely responsible for the kinds of spells we fall under, in the intense emotional states that surface in the therapy relationship. They

---

*Readers unfamiliar with this term will find an in-depth discussion of it on pp. 223–225.

create false categories that divide therapy relationships into observers and subjects. This book may be making a case for the role of "counter-transpondence" in psychotherapy. Regardless of what one calls it, it is crucial that therapists remain open to exploring *both* their own experience *and* their clients' experience of the therapy.

I found it useful to listen for Karen's and my own "transference" in the therapy. Oftentimes, during our conversations about her drinking, Karen transformed the language of AA into the tyrannical and punishing voice of her father. She experienced her father as a man who withheld love and approval until she complied with his understanding of who she was supposed to become. Sometimes Karen would experience the ideas and slogans of AA, such as "One day at a time" and "Easy does it," as directives and orders she had to comply with, rather than suggestions to help her stay sober.

Despite its difficulties, Karen derived a great deal of satisfaction from her relationship with her father. However, those good feelings came at the expense of contorting herself into painful and unacceptable descriptions of herself. She had a deep longing for his acceptance and love, and a deep sense of hurt and rage because of his abusive and violent treatment of her and his other children.

In her therapy, and especially in AA, it was important for Karen to avoid the tendency to transform a potential community of allies who offered some helpful guidelines into voices of authority with set rules and commandments. At those times in her therapy and recovery, Karen would experience a sense of disconnection in our relationship that felt similar to the way she often felt judged and mistreated by her father or abandoned by her mother.

Other ways that Karen remembered past experiences within the context of our relationship included what Davies and Frawley (1994) call the "eroticization of her fear"—that is, Karen's concern about my becoming aroused and no longer being able to maintain the professional boundaries of our relationship, or my exploiting her sexually. Like the episode described above, this is another example of my representing—standing in for—the perpetrators of abuse in her life.

Another kind of traumatic transference involved Karen seeing me as what Miller (1994) terms the passive nonprotective bystander. In this instance, Karen might become angry with me for not anticipating when she was going to drink or get high and for not intervening and stopping her when she did. Conversations about these ideas with Karen early in her recovery led to discussions of Karen's fear of her desire and impulse to drink. We talked about her need, at that time, to foster a healthy dependency on AA and a relationship with a Higher Power that could be present for her unconditionally, without many of the dangers she associated with an intimate one-on-one relationship.

Finally, Karen's story also brings to the fore Spence's observations about the merits of narrative, rather than historical truth, as a basis for interpretation in psychotherapy. Interpretations are meant to capture the spirit or essence of a person's experience, not provide evidence of it. The fate of an interpretation is determined by a client's experience of it. Does it speak *her* truth, not *"the"* truth? How an interpretation helps a person do this is more important than its correspondence to an actual happening or the details or "facts" of an event.

Karen's Voice

This story would not be complete without making space for Karen's voice. Karen read a draft of the chapters of this book related to our work. The following are some of her reactions. For Karen, writing made her experiences feel more real:

> "I hadn't looked at those letters in years; the feelings were so intense. I remember how hard it was to write them; it took me forever just to sit down and put my pen to the paper. Writing it all down like that made it seem more real. Once I put the words on paper it felt like I couldn't take them back. Even though I could hear you saying, 'This is just a snapshot or journal entry from your life, it's about where you're at today, this moment, it's a place to begin,' I was terrified because it felt like I had started something that I was now committed to finish."

Karen voiced amazement at how much had changed in her life, "at how far I've come, and what a different place I'm at in my life with all these problems." She found particularly useful the discussion of "identifying" at an AA meeting as being, for most people, a trauma in and of itself. She was especially moved by excerpts from the story of Sophie, who she knew from a group. However, most difficult for her was reading about my experience of my own mother's alcoholism. She said it made her "incredibly" sad knowing that I had to deal with the absence of someone so important to me because of her drinking.*

When Karen shared her feelings with me, I worried that reading even a little about my own experiences with these issues had made her question my ability to be present for her in our relationship and continue to help her with her concerns. However, after reading those passages, what upset her most, she said, was her imagining me sitting and listening to her all those years, judging her, and thinking, "Why doesn't this woman just get her act together and take care of her children?" She said she knew that I didn't ever feel this way and that if I did—revealing just how well she does knows me—"I know you would read a bunch of books and talk to someone so you would no longer feel that way."[†] Karen reported that my disclosure still brought up a lot of shame for her about her parenting that she said she doesn't talk much about anymore but still feels all the time. I said I understood that she was grieving over events in her life that had already happened and could not be undone, and there was nothing anyone could say to undo what had happened: the years lost to her drinking and the time stolen away from her children. However, because of what she was choosing to notice about my life, I said that she needed to realize that our work together was beneficial for me as well. It was no coincidence that one of the things I find myself doing a lot, because of the kind of therapy I practice, is helping parents get sober. In this respect, I said that her recovery was a gift in my life, as well as her own children's lives. She said she had thought of this as well, but still her feelings of shame and grief over what she'd put her children through seemed inconsolable.

Finally, I asked Karen if she could imagine her own mother "in recovery," suggesting to Karen that they try and help one another gain a better understanding of some of the grievous events that happened in their home and resolve some of the pain it still caused them. Karen responded that she couldn't imagine this—"It would be unthinkable." This, I reminded her, was the experience she was providing her children. She said she understood.

Karen's struggle to arrive at this point reminded me of the first order of business following a massive trauma caused by violence, addiction, and abuse. It is to restore hope.

Making these connections and listening to Karen's voice helps me remember that prior to developing what Shafer calls "the sense of an answer" for my client, I first need to locate myself in the process and try

---

(footnote from p. 155) The discussion of my own experience to which Karen is referring can be found on p. 85. The discussion of "identifying" at an AA meeting as a trauma in and of itself can be found on p. 38.

[†]I used to feel some abashment of my own about Karen's observation until recently when I was reminded of Edward Hirsch's words that "Love, for Jews, is nothing if not bookish."

and determine where I fit in a person's story. Karen's reflections helped me appreciate how my attitude has gradually shifted from one of disappointment to one of concern. I am also beginning to foster that same capacity for concern in my clients, especially regarding their drinking and other forms of self-harm.

Carl Whitaker (1981), one of family therapy's great originals, said that clients do not require a completely adequate or effective therapist to heal. What people need is for the therapist to make available all the adequacies (and even some inadequacies) he or she has available; in other words, in order to work properly, therapy demands the total participation of the therapist, including the latter's "immaturities."

At one point in the conversation about our work together, Karen and I began discussing some of my harsher and less-than-therapeutic reactions to Karen's relapses, and her anger at my responses. Karen and I shared a moment of laughter when I pointed out that my reaction to my own mother's drinking is still disappointment, but because of the way I've grown and matured in my work with Karen, there was still hope for me!

In order to discover how I can be useful to my client and how the person needs to use me, I often find it helpful to start with Bollas's (1983) question, "How do I feel used?"[3] I try and let the response this question generates inform my search for an answer. As Bollas writes, "In order to find the patient we must look for him within ourselves. This process inevitably points to the fact that there are two 'patients' within the session" (p. 3). The therapist, advocates Bollas, should approach herself—as well as her associations to her own and her client's experience, feelings, and intuitions—as the "other" patient. Therapy, Bollas writes, creates a space in which therapist and client "live a 'life' together." He cautions us not to "close down this internal space and replace it with some notion of absolute mental neutrality or the idea of scientific detachment" (pp. 3–4). It is our capacity to express this aliveness to our clients, not our ability to function as an inanimate object or mirror for life, that helps them develop a passion for knowing themselves and the world around them.

Karen's efforts to get to know herself and to better understand her desires, as well as the conflation of her desires with violence and alcohol, led to her wanting to discuss her intimate feelings for me and fantasies about our relationship. When Karen first shared these feelings in therapy, she said she felt awful and ashamed for having them. She thought that I would tell her that she would have to leave therapy. Her imagining an intimate sexual relationship in place of our caring professional one upset her. As she explained, she felt she was using me in "the same way I was used." We discussed the differences, the most crucial one being that she was not exploiting me, that it was okay with me for her to use me in this way, and that it didn't seem like an awful place to be at all.

Our understanding of the meaning and timing of Karen's feelings (i.e., why we found ourselves having these conversations at that point in our relationship) underscored Karen's need for a safe space to have her desires without having to act on them; her worrying about the other person finding her desires unacceptable or inappropriate; or her overwhelming the other person because her feelings were too much to deal with. Most importantly, we talked about Karen needing to have her desires and wishes without something awful or destructive happening to her as a result of having them.

In one of our meetings, Karen said she thought that sometimes she chose to say things just to make me uncomfortable, "even though I know there is probably nothing I could do to rattle you." I told her that wasn't true, that I was sure she could and may still think of things to say that would embarrass, upset, or unnerve me. However, as in all of our previous conversations, I had faith that if that happened, we would muddle through those moments together as we had all the others.

Following our discussion of Karen's sexual feelings and desires, Karen had a dream that she shared during our next appointment: "In the dream, you and I are just sitting together at my dining table talking. That was it, that was the whole thing," she said. I asked Karen what she thought the dream meant. Karen responded:

> "In my sleep, watching the dream unfold, I remember thinking how comfortable and relaxed I felt. It was a good feeling. I think the dream is about the connection I experience us having and my wanting to see us as friends. I think that's all I've ever wanted from another person. It's what I was searching for in many of my relationships with men. It wasn't sex that I wanted, it was connectedness, respect and caring."

Erich Fromm said that our deepest need as humans is to overcome our separateness, to leave the prison of our aloneness. Safety, intimacy, and connection are often the grails we find at the end of our search for physical and sexual closeness with another person.

The significance of these discussions was not that they allowed Karen and me to arrive at some definitive meaning or absolute truth about the dream, or her experience of our relationship; rather they allowed us to explore many different readings and all the possible meanings the dream and our relationship held for her. The Kabbala says an uninterpreted dream is like an unopened letter. Karen and I tried to bring the same type of insight to our explorations. For example, a psychoanalytic reader might interpret the dream as Karen's reaction to and defense against my rejection of her desire for a sexual relationship. As rejection and abandonment were such prevalent themes in Karen's life and relationships, she and I entertained this reading of the dream as well. This led to a conversation about longings and what it's like to desire something you know you can't have but to want it anyway. These feelings often surface when something we want in our present reminds us of something in our past that we needed and never received.

These are very important conversations for persons in recovery. Fulfillment of desires and longings is at the heart of the addictive experience. Desire is not the same as craving, and addicts often confuse the two. Clients in the throws of an addiction may find their feelings and desires unacceptable in a fashion that leaves them feeling flawed, or unacceptable as a human being for having them. Cravings for drugs and alcohol are often confused with the longing and desire for unconditional love and connection with others; they ward off painful feelings and help us forget unmet needs. When the void and emptiness these absences create become unbearable, we become desperate to fill them. Cravings stem from a state of disconnection from ourselves and our feelings. In desire we experience a connection to our spirit. A successful therapy relationship demonstrates the capacity to hold both.

Prior to turning to a discussion of the development of a narrative context for understanding addiction and trauma, I want to say a little bit about what this account of Karen's story left out. This version did not discuss Karen's attempts, some successful and some not, to reach out to her parents, her mother in particular. Nor did it focus on the stories of pride that Karen feels about her family and childhood.

I did not present the upsetting news of Karen's minister's decision to leave her congregation and move to a new city, and what a profound experience and loss her leaving was for Karen. Her departure was the first time when Karen, faced with an important ending in her life, didn't drink or "crawl out my bedroom window and run away." Her minister's leaving provided an opportunity to talk about what our not meeting any longer would be like, and for Karen to imagine what kind of an ending she would want for her therapy. This discussion led to conversations of how one can hold onto people and relationships in a positive way, even when they are no longer physically present in your life.

This telling of Karen's story did not talk about the joy Karen receives from music and the profound impact Melissa Etheridge's songs have had on her life. It didn't recount how music has given voice to many unspoken aspects of Karen's experience, or explore the reverberations of what seemed like a relatively small decision to travel to a rock concert by herself because she couldn't get her husband to go with her, leading to much bigger unforeseen changes in how Karen sees herself. These are aspects of herself that no one realized were there. They have led to a more fulfilling relationship with her family and to Karen's enjoyment of her own company.

Some of these themes were explored in earlier chapters, others not. In sum, Karen's letters, like the narrative voices I used to illuminate them, generate more possibilities and questions than proofs and theories. However, one sparkling fact of her therapy is that Karen is no longer "writing for her life," she is living for herself.

SOPHIE: "A STORIED THERAPY"

> What is to give light must endure burning.
> —VIKTOR FRANKL

Sophie, a 44-year-old woman, had 10 years of sobriety when she overdosed on antidepressants, Valium, and alcohol. A gifted poet and writer, Sophie used her talents during the course of our work together to document and reauthor her experience of childhood trauma. When Sophie was 11 she was raped by her 16-year-old brother (although she is pretty sure the abuse started when she was younger). The abuse continued into her early teens.

One way Sophie coped with the traumas of her childhood—like many survivors—was through self-harm and abuse. During her adolescence Sophie recalled biting her hands and wrists and cutting her arms and body. When she discovered alcohol, she discovered the only thing that seemed to arrest the cutting:

Sophie's Story

My mother was always coming home drunk and hitting us. One night she smashed my head against a porcelain sink. I was still bleeding when she passed out. I made up a story about falling off my bicycle, and a neighbor took me to the hospital. I needed seven stitches. When I got older I started hitting her back. When I was 15 she sent me to live with my father. Even though I barely knew him I was relieved because it got me away from my brother. My father was an alcoholic and a con-artist. He gambled a lot and got by on his wits. It was either feast or famine, and we ended up on the streets a number of times living out of dumpsters when we couldn't get into a shelter. It was around this time that I discovered liquor. From that first drink I could never get enough. Alcohol made everything seem okay. I finally stumbled onto something that made me feel better about myself. I was desperate to find something to like about myself. Drinking helped me control the cutting and other self-harmful behaviors. The cutting didn't stop completely, but things improved enough so that people stopped noticing it. When I was in school the counselors were always threatening my Dad that they were going to send me to the hospital, but he always convinced them not to. He could talk a canary out of a cat's mouth. I remember wishing they would send me somewhere, but I couldn't let my father know or he would get mad, so I pretended to hate the idea and threatened to run away.

When I was just sixteen I became involved with one of my Dad's gambling buddies. When I turned eighteen we got married. He was an older man. I never had the chance to meet anyone my age because I was always with my father. He took me everywhere with him. I think he thought it made him more sympathetic. Having a kid with him made it easier for him to talk people out of their money. Dad wasn't happy about my getting married, but I think he owed my husband a lot of money so he never said anything about it to me. My father never molested me, but until the day I left him we always slept together. He treated me more like his girlfriend or wife than a daughter. I remember he didn't come to the ceremony. He said he had to meet someone important at the track who was going to help turn things around for him. He said now that he knew I was going to be taken care of he could concentrate on his life and gave me a hundred dollars. That was it. I was married by a justice of the peace in the city gardens, which is all I remember about that day because I was so trashed. My husband thought he was rescuing me from the hard life I'd had. He was very kind and made very few demands of me. In retrospect I don't think I knew what to do with a man who didn't mistreat me. So I started hanging out in bars, which is where I met my second husband. He was a heroin addict. I was hooked on smack for a while too. I smoked it while he shot up. That was the last straw for my marriage. My husband said he could handle the cheating but not the drugs.

I had all three of my children with my second husband. It didn't take long to figure out that if I stayed with him one or all of us was going to die. We were living in the South in a camper on some land that belonged to a friend of his. He was okay when he was high, but when he drank he became violent. One night he broke my collarbone. He was standing over me while I lay there on the kitchen floor trying not to scream out in pain because my two older children were huddled in the corner crying. He said he was going to score some drugs but when he got back he was going to kill me. I believed him. We left him and the state.

That was the first time I tried to get sober. I had nowhere to go. I had only seen my mother a couple of times since I was 15 and my brother was still living with her. So I went back to my Dad's. He had recently quit drinking and was living in a small efficiency. He gave me five hundred dollars to help us get into an apartment. After we moved in he brought over a small black and white television and some groceries and gave me another two hundred and fifty dollars in cash. I'll never forget that. He had never been a father like that to me before. It meant a lot. He's been in AA for going on twenty years now. I wanted to stay sober, but I had no support and was trying to do it all on my own. A year after we moved back north I was back in the bars again. My oldest child would come and get me and tell me it was time to go home. She was ten.

One night I went on a real bender. By then I was a blackout drinker with the beginnings of alcoholic neuropathy, losing sensations in my hands and feet. Slicing my feet on broken glass and not knowing it. I wasn't eating or sleeping. Everything was just drinking, drinking, drinking. I remained in drunken blackout for a month. When I came out of it I found myself 700 miles from home in a detox center in Pennsylvania. The Social Worker had been in touch with the authorities in Massachusetts and my kids were put in DSS [Department of Social Services] custody and placed in foster care. When I returned to Massachusetts I wasn't allowed to see them unless I agreed to enter treatment. I went through the motions, but I still kept going out. Until one day during one of our supervised visits when I said to my baby (I still called her that even though she was seven), "Come to Momma" and the other two children just looked at me and said, "You call yourself a mother. Please, you're pitiful!" That was it. That was my bottom. Prior to that I managed to put together a year or two of sobriety, I did that several times. But I couldn't sustain it. I'd slept in the streets when I couldn't make rent, something I swore I would never do again, and I slept with men to get drugs or so they would buy me drinks. But that's what it took for me to get serious. And, when I did, I was able to put the 10 years together.

The first five years I did it with the help of AA. I went to meetings morning, noon, and night. I did service, went to conferences, sober dances, I lived and breathed program. My life was AA and my kids. Then I reconnected with my mother and my siblings, and my life became family and children. I stopped going to meetings. For several years I read literature and stayed in touch with my AA friends, but eventually I let those relationships go as well.

The habit of cutting followed Sophie into the present, while her description of her relations with men continued to be one of taking undue risks that put her in dangerous and compromising positions, often leading to further violence and exploitation (e.g., exchanging sex for closeness and staying with physically abusive and alcoholic partners). As a consequence of the assaults on her body and physical self perpetrated by the incest and rape, Sophie's relationships with people were heavily weighted toward sex, drugs, and alcohol—the only means by which Sophie felt safe being close, touched, and nurtured by others. After she got sober, Sophie said cutting was the only thing left to control painful emotions. These incidents began occurring more frequently when she became sober and stopped going to meetings. Sophie used her self-inflicted wounds as markers to commemorate the painful episodes in her life. She said of her own wounds, "I'd look at different scars and I'd think, yeah, I know when this happened, so each one told a story. When they started to fade I became scared, it felt like a piece of me was disappearing along with them."

Sophie's comments support Muller's (1996) observation about clients who cut and mutilate themselves using their scars as indexes. Within the chaotic and fragmented existence created by her mother's violence, the sexual assaults perpetrated by her brother, and the incestuous relationship with her father (during the years he was drinking), Sophie's cutting seemed more about binding feelings than releasing them. When Sophie cut herself, it was as if she was setting a marker at the edge of herself so she could experience a limit—that is, some sense of order and understanding of where her own boundaries lay that she could rely upon.

The events that led to Sophie's suicide attempt happened prior to our work in therapy together. Sophie's brother was brought up on charges of sexually abusing his children—Sophie's niece and nephew. Sophie planned to testify on behalf of her sister's children but decided not to when it looked as if her brother would be convicted without her testimony. Following her brother's conviction and sentencing, Sophie began experimenting with controlled drinking again:

"I had to force myself to keep the alcohol down. My side ached and I could feel it burning the lining of my stomach but I made myself drink. That probably doesn't make a whole lot of sense to someone who isn't a drunk. Part of it was that I was drinking and my life wasn't coming unraveled like it had in the past. I felt like I had it under control. I'd never drunk like a normal person. I know it's not normal to forcefeed yourself alcohol when your body is rejecting it, but at least I wasn't blacking out or doing crazy things. I became intensely depressed. I went to see a psychiatrist. He gave me pills (Valium and Prozac), which I took whenever I felt down. The depression lasted from morning till night. The sleeplessness and constant crying without reason. I couldn't see a way out of it so I kept on those pills. If I ran through my prescription too quickly, I bought more on the street. The Valium made all feeling, not just the depression, go away. I started taking it with alcohol because by itself it took longer to work. One evening thinking about my brother's children, knowing they went through the trial and that whole ordeal without me or anyone else in the family standing up for them, I took the whole bottle. I woke up in the hospital."

More than any other client with whom I've worked, Sophie's was truly "a storied therapy." During the first 12 months of our work together, each week Sophie would bring a new poem, dream, or letter to read in session. Soon there was a sheaf of poems:

"The times I succeed in trusting are moments when I write. Sitting at my typewriter the wheels of my mind quiet and slow to a hum, and my hands and unconscious take over. Writing has been a harbor for me. A place to lay down my sword, to let go of action, reactions, and the need to save myself from self-inflicted pain."

Early on in the work, I asked Sophie to "contract for safety." She created a document for us both to sign. The contract was Sophie's first effort at developing the sense of a protective presence in her life. The page was divided in two. On one side, under the heading "Ideas for Taking Care of Myself," was a list of activities:

Ideas for Taking Care of Myself

Write
talk to a friend
exercise
take a bubble bath

listen to music
go to a 12-step meeting
call my sponsor
paint
go to the movies
walk at the ocean
hike in the woods
ride my bicycle
rent a funny video
cry
hug a tree
pet my cat
meditate outdoors
meditate indoors
pray.

On the other side, under the heading "Ideas for Releasing Anger," was another list of activities:

Ideas for Releasing Anger

Journal
write an angry letter
throw rocks
hit the ground with a stick
beat up a pillow
tear up newspapers
cut up a photograph of my brother
scream at the TV
yell under a railroad bridge
call my sponsor
go to a 12-step meeting
meditate
curse god
pray.

Sophie agreed to try these ideas whenever she felt overwhelmed by the urge to drink or hurt herself. If, after trying them, she still felt self-destructive or craved alcohol, she promised to call her sponsor, my answering service, or a crisis line, and to keep calling until she reached someone. If all else failed, she said she would go to the hospital emergency room.

Miller (1994) talks about the importance of trauma survivors internalizing a protective presence in order to establish a sense of safety and self-coherence. A relationship with a therapist, a 12-step group, or a Higher Power—or another important relationship—can stand in for this presence until the client has developed this capacity within herself. Objects can sometimes help people feel more connected to this protector. An amethyst rock borrowed from my office served as Sophie's transitional object. Sophie later explained to me that to the ancient Greeks amethyst had healing powers that could ward off the intoxicating effects of alcohol.

Sophie and I discussed how her sobriety had cleared the way for her traumatic memories to surface and that in her case we had to work on her abuse and drinking issues together. Because her trauma history was so deeply etched into the story of her alcoholism, taking a more conventional approach to Sophie's recovery—where therapy for her sexual abuse issues would be put on hold until she achieved some ongoing sobriety—wouldn't work. Sophie was also interested in exploring alternatives to AA. She read Charlotte D. Kasl's book, *Many Roads, One Journey: Moving Beyond the 12 Steps* (1992). After finding out more about Kasl's approach (she also authored *Women, Sex, and Addiction: A Search for Love and Power*, 1989), Sophie sought out Women for Sobriety meetings. This is a group that supports a lifestyle of abstinence for women alcoholics but feels that many of AA's ideas about recovery are based on male experience and not applicable to women's lives. Members of this group take particular exception to the way the concepts of admitting one's powerlessness and helplessness over alcohol are conceived in AA. Many women, they argue, are already undermined by misogynist and patriarchal culture, and need programs of "empowerment" not "surrender."

While Sophie continued to participate in AA, mostly attending women's meetings in her community, she found the Women for Sobriety groups a useful component of her recovery. Sophie also complained that AA had changed. She felt it was warmer and friendlier when she first got sober. I find that many clients are voicing the same concern who have been away from AA for a long time. The changes these clients are noticing are real. I see the change, in part, as another example of a general growing discomfort with face-to-face contact in the global computer age in which we live. Also, many people have complex social identities and myriad allegiances in today's multicultural society. However, perhaps Sophie and others are also mourning the loss of a time in their lives when their recovery was simpler because it had such a singleness of purpose. Looking back, people remember focusing on their sobriety to the exclusion of everything else in their lives, and remember with huge gratitude being given the space to do so.

It's harder getting sober if you relapse after you've been in recovery for years. Others' expectations of you are greater and your life is often fuller. The assumption is that because you did it once before it will be easier the second time around. However, for Sophie, as with many survivors who are getting in touch with past abuse, this was not the case. Returning to meetings after a relapse can be a humbling experience. This feeling can be exacerbated when long-term sobriety is lost. Sophie also experienced shame at having kept her self-mutilation a secret from others in AA, people who looked up to her for guidance and support. As she contemplated returning to AA meetings, these feelings weighed heavily on her.

The pressure Sophie felt was not imagined. Once you have that kind of sobriety even people in AA come to rely on you more. Regardless of your chronological age you are considered an "old timer"—what Overeaters Anonymous (OA) affectionately calls a "long-timer." Sometimes people relate to the veteran members of their 12-step groups more as symbolic figures than as individuals. I fell into my own version of this dilemma in my work with Sophie. Many years prior to her relapse Sophie participated in a psychotherapy group with me for persons in recovery. The focus of the group was on adult–child and other family-of-origin issues. Sophie was one of the group's self-appointed leaders. The other members appreciated her knowledge about what it took to stay sober and looked to her for guidance. I too held an inflated image of Sophie's recovery. Sophie was an AA "success story," and it was very difficult for me to let go of that image and allow her to be who she needed to be, a newly sober person in pain. Sometimes I found myself deferring to her experience in recovery when what she needed was a therapist willing to confront her rationalizations and challenge her denial. However, whenever I found myself relating more to Sophie's recovery in the past, her cutting brought me abruptly back to the present.

Sophie's self-abuse remained the most trying and frustrating aspect of her therapy for both of us. She continued to disassociate and cut herself in ritualistic fashion on her arms, hands, and legs. Sophie and I both recognized we were at an extremely fragile juncture in our work together. In therapy Sophie was uncovering many alarming and disturbing things about herself and her life. We discussed how this process might be easier and safer to facilitate in an inpatient hospital setting. However, we both remained invested in keeping her out of the hospital.[4] Sophie worried about the impact such an event would have on her daughter, who because of a debilitating illness counted on Sophie to help her with her children. Because of Sophie's drinking history she felt that going into the hospital at this time would be like abandoning her daughter all over again. She also felt that her grandchildren really needed her. I voiced my concern that a hospital setting would make it easier for her to organize her identity completely around her cutting and her view of herself as a helpless victim and patient. During one particularly rough period in her therapy I suggested that Sophie write herself a "letter of encouragement." Here it is:

Letter of Encouragement

Dear Sophie,

As you make your way through this mess, try to remember the love and forgiveness, the fulfillment that's at the other end. Right now, you feel hopeless and sad; that's okay. You need to feel that pain. As a child, you blocked out the pain along with the memories. You never cried for yourself, but now it's time. It's okay and necessary to cry, to comfort your child, to forgive her and transfer the anger to him. As awful as the reliving is, you must live it, finish it, and then you can move on. It will never be completely gone, but it will become manageable as you become strong.

I understand how you feel. Loneliness is like an anchor on your heart. The alcohol and drugs are gone. You want someone to love. Someone to make the pain go away. Hopefully when you get through this it will be the last big addiction. You need to remember that you will not always be alone and that someday the universe will bring the right relationship to you; when you're mature enough to have a mature relationship.

You are one of the lucky ones: lucky to have discovered the source of your pain, lucky to have survived this far, lucky to be brave enough to face it. You will make it! As time goes on, you will learn to laugh and cry, to express all feelings, and to let go of the guilt, doubt, hatred, and fear that seem so real now. You will be able to heal. You deserve it. Remember, it is never too late to resolve past pain. Congratulations! You're on your way!

After writing the letter, Sophie seemed to have a more hopeful vision for her therapy and a less despairing outlook on life in general. The letter crystallized for her some important changes already underway in our work together. It signified a shift in her attitude toward herself and her therapy, from one of uncovering painful memories and traumas to one of recovering from this experience. Sophie, like Karen, also found the concept of the triadic self, described in my therapy with Karen, a helpful adjunct to her healing.

Although these interventions coupled with her contract for safety resulted in a lessening of her self-abuse, Sophie's skin continued to be the terrain or battleground upon which her struggle for self-preservation and self-determination was waged. In one session, Sophie shared that after cleaning up some broken glass, she had taken one of the shards into the shower and carved the outline of a women's symbol on her leg. Sophie's observation that this image was, for her, a sign of strength and unity represented a shift in meaning from cutting as only a symbol of abuse and terror to cutting as a way for Sophie to leave her own "mark" on her body. For Sophie this incident was not just a regression to or repetition of past trauma. It represented a progression of sorts and was part of her ongoing search for a protective presence in her life.

Miller (1994) discusses some of the dilemmas presented when a survivor's story of trauma is told by an act of violence against herself:

> Clients and therapists alike strain to find language to express the secrets of the abuse victim, but we are almost mute when it comes to expressing the secrets of those who commit acts of violence, including those who commit acts of violence against themselves. In exploring our attitudes toward women who hurt themselves, it may be useful to consider them as women who are inflicting abuse, akin to those who perpetrate violence against others. We may not easily accept this double description if we are angry, frightened, or judgmental about anyone who inflicts violence against children and women. (p. 72)

Most of us don't want to listen to the story of the perpetrator because it challenges our image of these men and women as "criminal," "inhuman," "sick," or "deranged." Also, many survivors have actual memories of reenacting their own childhood abuse on other children or playmates. Any harsh attitudes the therapist harbors toward sexual offenders and other perpetrators of violence and abuse may be misconstrued by the survivor as a condemnation of her actions and behavior. In fact, similar to the anorexic who looks in the mirror and sees obesity regardless of the image in front of her, in her own mind the survivor may see no difference between her abuse-reactive behavior as a child and the adult offender who abused her. Dusty Miller challenges us to attend to the voice of the woman who acts against herself in the role of the abuser; otherwise we risk silencing her experience as it was silenced in her childhood. I still find these dilemmas that people face in therapy challenging and at times scary to witness. However, Sophie taught me a lot. I will always be extremely grateful to her. As a result of our work together, I now have much more courage as a clinician to engage in "cutting" conversations.

Sophie then sought my help creating a ritual. Sophie and her sponsor had gathered from her home all her prescription medications—past and present—and threw the contents away. Sophie then brought all the containers with her to her next therapy session. She carried them with her in a plastic garbage bag and dumped them on the floor. It was a formidable collection. She then packed them up in two separate boxes. As she placed each container in the box, she looked at the date on the label and tried to recall her emotions and circumstances at the time she had the prescription filled. Had she cut herself? Did she wash the pills down with alcohol? Was she trying to forget how lonely she was without a man, or was she with a man she was trying to forget? Sophie shared these thoughts:

> "I was meditating last night and thinking about all the harmful things I've done to myself, habitually over the years, alcohol, drugs, unwanted sex, cutting, all that stuff. Then I thought about my ex-husband and all the abusive partners I've chosen over the years. And I realized they were just middlemen for my self-abuse. It's almost like me hitting myself except that they were doing it for me. It was just a convenient place for me to put my self-hate. I was able to place it on all these violent abusers, but it all stems from my own deep desire to hurt myself. It was just an indirect root to self-harm."

After she finished this exercise she took both boxes with her. She mailed one to her brother, along with a note saying that she was no longer willing to keep his secrets or take these or any other poisons to make it more palatable for her to do so. She planted some flowers in the other and took it to the cemetery where her ex-husband was buried. He had died of a drug overdose in prison. Sophie had chosen not to attend the funeral and had never been to his gravesite. She placed the flower box besides his gravestone along with the medallion she'd received in AA when she celebrated her 10th year of sobriety: "I told him that I no longer live my life in fear of him or anyone else, said a brief prayer, and told him that I was leaving the medallion with him because I felt he needed it more than me now."

After Sophie performed her ritual, the only subsequent incident of self-harm happened approximately 3 months later. Sophie cut herself superficially on the arm and called my answering service, extremely distraught. When I spoke with her she was in tears, repulsed by the sight of her own blood, and even more upset that, for the first time, she was in touch with her feelings and experiencing discomfort, not pleasure or relief, from the physical pain caused by her wounds.

For all trauma survivors, finding some way to confront their abuser is an essential aspect of healing.[5] These do *not* have to be face-to-face confrontations with actual family members and do *not* have to include forgiving the perpetrator. These are very personal decisions every client must make for her- or himself, along with the help of a therapist and/or supportive community.

Sophie's effort at resolving her past pain took the form of poetry and a letter to her brother. Sophie wrote many drafts before she felt the letter was complete:

Sophie's Letter to Her Brother

Dear Blaine,

I'm sure there are things you don't want me to remember. Like you, I repressed a lot of our childhood. For years I have lived in fear. I forgot some things and attributed others to nightmares. All my life I've had terrible dreams of awful things happening to me, but now I know that some weren't dreams. My childhood depression was caused by real events.

I am finally getting help for myself after a lifetime of alcoholism, depression, self-hatred, night terrors, suicidal thoughts, self-mutilation, and marred relationships. Those things didn't come out of nowhere; they are the direct result of what happened between us.

I remember trying to avoid you when we were older. I was afraid of you, hated you, without understanding it. Since we fought so much when we were growing up I think I somehow justified the abuse as your getting back at me for something I'd done to you. That somehow I deserved it. It was my punishment for wishing you dead. I felt guilty for hating you, and at the same time I felt sorry for you because of the way Mom and Dad treated you. Treated us. I tried to believe what you said about it being for my own good, and that you were just trying to protect me from your friends. That you loved me. None of this had anything to do with love at all. It was about power and your need to control people.

My deepest fear was that I could never be loved by any man. That I was dirty and ruined and that no decent, honest man would want me. And, guess what? I found and married four different men from the time I was 16 and all but one treated me as if I was damaged goods and undeserving of true love and affection. The one nice husband I had, as well as several nice men I didn't marry, I got rid of fast. I just remember feeling if they really knew me, and what had happened to me, they would not want me. No matter how hard I tried to change, I was overcome by self-loathing and disgust and the only men I allowed in my life supported this. These thoughts I had about myself, however buried they were at times, almost killed me.

For years I rationalized that what you did to me was the result of the physical abuse you endured. But how many men who have been beat up by their fathers and mistreated by their mothers respond to the abuse by raping and torturing their sisters? And what about your children? You were no longer a victim of child abuse, you were a grown man. How do you explain that!?! They showed such courage standing up to you. It's what I should have done years ago. If I had they may have been spared all the suffering they had to withstand. The hardest thing I've ever had to do is find a way to forgive myself for that. Then, I realized that if I didn't it would be just one more way of allowing you to continue owning my life.

It is very hard for me to say these things to you and to admit that despite everything I still care what happens to you. But it is important for my own recovery. I wish that you would get some help for yourself, too. Whatever happened between you and your children is still festering inside you and needs to be addressed. You will have no peace in your life until you face it. I wish you would seek and accept counseling from someone who knows how to help sexual offenders, and perpetrators of other types of violence and abuse, heal.

It would help me to know that you are in therapy. It would help to have an acknowledgment from you that this happened. It would help to have you accept responsibility. But I do not expect any of those things to happen. I know that most abusers remain in denial and continue to act out and hurt others; I hope you will be different.

After much thought, Sophie decided to send her letter. She also contributed one of her poems to a multimedia exhibit of survivors' writing, photographs, sculpture, and artwork that took place at a local gallery, so her story would have a larger audience and serve as an inspiration to other women.

REWRITING STORIES OF TRAUMA AND ADDICTION*

> Recovery doesn't end with the telling and hearing of the story. . . . What finally renews people is the belief that their own capacity to love has not been destroyed.
> —JUDITH HERMAN

Trauma comes from the Greek word meaning a wound or hurt. As Sanville (1991) writes, "It refers not to what inflicted the injury but to the effect on that person. What is wounding to one person may not be to another, or what is hurtful at one age might not be at a later age"

(p. 151). When retelling traumatic stories about our lives in therapy it is inevitable that we also revisit some of the painful and frightening feelings associated with those experiences. This is particularly true when the constellation of gender, age, and sex of the client and therapist parallel those of the abuse.

Pearlman and Saakvitne (1995) use the phrase "vicarious traumatization" to describe the range of emotions and feelings that therapists experience when collaborating in therapy with clients trying to rewrite stories of sexual abuse and trauma. Sexual abuse and incest often leave women and men survivors desperately trying to change something about their past that is not changeable. They're trying to resolve what was an impossible situation, such as trying to love someone or something that seems to be causing their spiritual death. Often this results in a person seeking out impossible situations—what family therapy theory refers to as "double binds"[6]—in adult life that re-create these feelings and the dynamics of the abuse. It explains in part what kept Karen and Sophie both trying to master and control their drinking and Sophie her cutting.

Against the overwhelming onslaught of dehumanization, devaluation, and degradation of her body, each woman's act of self-harm can be seen as her own existential strategy to cope with the insanity of her life and the human condition. As Karen wrote in her second correspondence to alcohol, "To me you are a slow death—a rapist that takes my pride, self-respect, and future." When I asked Sophie why she continued to cut herself and to force her body to keep alcohol down, she replied that she preferred the uncomfortable sensation caused by physical pain to the anguish of contemplating her spiritual death. Toni Morrison in *Beloved*, her monumental story of slavery, characterizes black women's search for ways to resist similar abuse and terror and the process of "dirtying you": "That anybody white could take your whole self for anything that came to mind. Not just work, kill or maim you but dirty you. Dirty you so

---

(footnote from p. 172) While this chapter and Chapter 8 (on food addiction) make some important connections between trauma work and addiction therapy, the reader should be cautioned that a book on narrative approaches to trauma would tell a very different story. There are issues particularly regarding the nature of the therapeutic relationship, boundaries, and managing disclosure and memories of abuse that, while alluded to here, would be addressed differently and in more detail there than they are presented here. Some of these themes were addressed in the preceding passages and are discussed further in Chapter 8, but as they are not the primary focus of this book they have not been given the attention they deserve or require. My not doing so should not be interpreted as my belief that this is all I feel a clinician needs to know in order to assist clients in overcoming traumatic experience, nor do they comprise all the ideas that inform my work when addressing these concerns in therapy.

bad you couldn't like yourself anymore. Dirty you so bad you forgot who you were and couldn't think it up" (1987, p. 87). In the inhuman and twisted climate of slavery Morrison's novel takes this dilemma to its logical conclusion—that people's flight from the horrors of genocide may lead to the murder of those loved ones who are candidates for the "dirtying" process. The black mother, Sethe, kills her daughter, Beloved, "to outhurt the hurter," as an act of resistance because she loved her daughter too much to allow her to live and die this way. Literature has long recognized that for many of earth's inhabitants death is the only liberator from suffering and evil. For Sophie, Karen and many survivors of sexual abuse, cutting, bingeing, purging, drinking, and other forms of self-harm, even suicide, can be seen as their own attempts to "outhurt the hurter."

Miller (1994) talks about a "transitional period" in a person's recovery, where the therapeutic relationship "substitutes" for the client's symptoms. The client then develops a myriad of feelings toward the therapist, feelings which previously had been attached to the client's symptoms. These might include making impossible demands on the therapist's time, demeaning his or her work, or subjecting him or her to intense bouts of anger and rage. These phases of therapy do not have to be destructive to the client, the therapist, or the relationship, and they can strengthen people's resiliency and resolve to put the trauma behind them, so long as the therapist is aware of the impossibility of the requests and doesn't get into an impossible situation by trying to resolve the client's dilemmas.

On occasion we may find it necessary to respond or set limits on people's aggressive and sadistic impulses. Sometimes we have no choice and may find ourselves reacting out of a sense of self-preservation. These retaliatory and very human moments can offer us a glimpse into the sort of frustrating feelings or painful rages and dilemmas that a client may be struggling with. Challenging as it is, it's important that we do our best to stay present and not react in anger. I often find myself making excuses when my own anger or sadism enters the room or the therapy: "Her behavior was out of control and needed to be kept in check" and "He's never had the experience of having someone stand up to his bullying" are some of the thoughts I use to rationalize my behavior when I respond defensively to clients in a session after having been shamed by them. It's difficult for me at those times to remember that, more often than not, clients' humiliation of us is their way of asking us to be strong for them.

These dramas are always already present in the therapy relationship. It is what Winnicott was referring to when he talked about therapy being a "search for a cure"; or, as T. S. Eliot's "Little Gidding" put it, "to make an end is to make a beginning. The end is where we start from" (1943/1962b, p. 144). Sophie expressed fears early in our work that she had never experienced an intimate relationship with a man that had not been sexualized or exploitative. When Sophie first disclosed her sexual abuse history, I asked her if she would be more comfortable meeting with a woman therapist. She said she would not be comfortable working with a woman, "because women are weak and vulnerable. A man is more powerful, and even though he might hurt you, at least he can protect you."

I told her that her reasoning made me feel like a Doberman pinscher or junkyard dog tied to a chain to protect his owner's property. The animal's job is to scare off anyone who comes near his territory. The owner and the unpredictable beast get along so long as the owner remembers to feed him. The relationship is tenuous at best.

Sophie and I both had a good laugh at this imagery. This was perhaps my first effort at what Bollas (1995) calls "cracking up" Sophie's self-deprecating image of herself and women. Humor often created a safe space where Sophie and I could use our creative imaginations to crack up seemingly immovable objects and fixed stories in her life and replace them with more affirming ones.

While "comic relief"—an indispensable part of any serious or tragic drama—helped us through many trying moments in the therapy, it could not crack them all up. Sometimes the silence, what Bollas (1995) calls the "blank nothing" created by trauma, can be deafening. Sophie's poetry, as well as the dreams she wrote down and brought to sessions, sometimes had this kind of traumatizing effect on both of us. Often brutal in their imagery and starkly graphic in their descriptions of violence and torture, Sophie would stay up late into the night in a dissociated state, editing and refining them. She would come to therapy the next day, tired and exhausted, and become angry if she did not have time to read and discuss them all. Although usually a cathartic experience for her, in these instances the readings were traumatizing for both of us. I would often find myself not knowing what to think and having to look away for a moment as Sophie's narratives presented the facts of the deeds done to her.

For survivors, therapy is what takes place after the fact. It is a process of unpacking the trauma and wrapping a story around it. "Profound facts," writes Bollas, "are wrapped in their own traumatic space" (1995, p. 114). They are shocking and arresting. Neither the client nor the therapist can stop thinking about them when they're presented in sessions, so a client's recurrent telling of them and a therapist's recurrent noting of them become important stages in both the client's and the therapist's recovery from the shocking facts of the person's life.

For Karen and Sophie the act of writing helped facilitate this process by putting words to previously indescribably terrible events and feelings—what Melanie Klein (1984) called our "unthinkable agonies." No activity is more essential to a person's recovery from pain and trauma than the act of naming and putting words to that traumatic experience.

Rewriting My Own Story

In my work with Karen and Sophie, I often found it difficult to move away from the addiction and trauma framework in which we usually discussed their experiences, to a more open-ended conversation about the nature of their sexuality, desires, and needs. When bearing witness to and discussing specific aspects of a person's abuse, I try to create a safe structure in the session where the client and I spend considerable time "talking about talking" about the events. The emphasis, especially when any details are recounted of the story a client wants to share, is on safety and staying present and in touch as much as possible with herself and others in the room—therapist, companion, group, or family members.

Due to their work in therapy, both Sophie and Karen expressed the need to begin exploring what they wanted and needed from adult relationships, including sexual intimacy. They needed to reclaim this aspect of their lives. What was required of me at these times was to stay present and connected to my client. I found myself reluctant to participate in these dialogues without the safety and security provided by the narrative frame of trauma. In the family therapy speak of the 1970s and 1980s, it was as if "the system" formed by the therapist and client required that all "communication" and stories told in therapy involve victims of trauma and abuses of power. But Sophie and Karen had begun to heal, and with that healing came the awareness that not all of their experience fit neatly into categories or boxes labeled trauma or addiction. With my clients no longer "functioning," in this mode, I found myself returning to these "old tapes" in order to maintain "homeostasis."*

My discussions both in supervision with a consultant† and with Sophie and Karen provided a rich repertoire of alternative narratives for addressing these issues. In supervision, I talked about the awkward and uncomfortable feelings that discussions of sex and intimacy brought up for me personally, and my fears that this discomfort would color my interactions with clients. Because of Sophie and Karen's trauma histories, I worried that these conversations might retraumatize them or cause a rupture in our relationship.

Dialogues in therapy about sex and intimacy, and the "erotic transferences" that often accompany them, can be powerful opportunities for learning for therapists and clients alike. Transference relationships and other unconscious experience, as demonstrated in the previous chapters, can be invaluable sources of knowledge about past relationships and provide future opportunities for healing. Although dismissal of the classical analytic concept of transference in contemporary postmodern and narrative literature is in vogue today, this in my opinion is a mistake. Diagnosing and policing people's sexual desires and preferences is what therapists should take issue with. Exploring our sexuality in therapy as a way to help us better understand and express ourselves can be an incredibly helpful exercise. In the work Karen and I did together, exploring these feelings served as a kind of relational time capsule that offered insight into her past traumas and experience.

Consultations with a knowledgeable supervisor also helped me recognize that this was for both women the first time in their lives that either had experienced a man with any kind of authority and power in their lives scrutinize the effects on them of his feelings and behavior. Bringing these issues to my supervision with a female supervisor was important also in that it reinforced the message that I always tried to give to Karen, Sophie, and other women clients: We needed another female presence and voice in our work.

This message about a woman client needing another female presence and voice in her therapy can be reinforced by helping clients develop a close working relationship with a woman sponsor. If father–daughter incest and other forms of sexual abuse have been present, the client's relationship with a woman sponsor can be a first step in mending her feelings toward her "nonprotective parent." The broken relationships between women in a family can be some of the most hurtful and enduring casualties of the abuse. Identifying with a strong and powerful woman whose job is to provide mentoring in the context of a safe, reliable, trusting, and loving relationship can provide the client an important opportunity for healing.

---

*(*footnote from page 176*) A term family therapists borrowed from general systems theory to describe the gravitational pull of a family to return things to the emotional status quo, as it were, following a crisis.

†(*footnote from page 176*) My consultant during this period of my work with Sophie and Karen was Dusty Miller.

The Personal Is Political

Another important aspect of Karen and Sophie's healing, and that of many of the other women in this book, was their development and involvement in an active and politically conscious social network. Political activity was another way for each woman to develop a stronger sense of self and connection to the community. The Mosaic Group, for mothers of girls who have been sexually abused, at People's Bridge Action in Athol, Massachusetts, emphasizes the oppression and political struggles clients face. These women, in addition to serving as a support group for other mothers, started a newsletter, created a video, and used their resources to raise the community's consciousness about child abuse. For Karen and Sophie, the growing awareness of their own political consciousness culminated in their participation in a Take Back the Night March to protest violence against women they attended with other members of their support group.

Parenting, Trauma, and Addiction

These ideas about trauma and addiction carry over to generational issues of abuse and neglect in families as well. Some of the most eloquent writing on this topic is found in Louise Kaplan's *No Voice Is Ever Wholly Lost* (1995). Kaplan has drawn from psychoanalyst Judith Kestenberg's (1972) work on the unconscious cross-generational transmission of massive trauma. Based on her research of Holocaust survivors and their children, Kestenberg calls this phenomenon "transposition." Summarizing Kestenberg, Kaplan (1995) writes:

> Transposition describes the uncanny experience where the past reality of the parent intrudes into the present psychological reality of the child. Transposition is an anomalous version of the ordinary psychological process whereby the wishes, desires, fantasies, ideals, and experiences of a parent are unconsciously transmitted to a child. . . . What makes transposition so much more awesome than ordinary generational transmission is the amount of psychological space the parent's past occupies in the child's ongoing existence. (pp. 223–224)

Transposition also effects the temporal dimension of people's lives, causing a reversal of ordinary time whereby the temporal positions of parent and child are exchanged: "Since the parent's past occupies the psychological space that would ordinarily belong to the child, the child must give up her right to exist in her own present" (Kaplan, 1995, p. 224).

The kind of massive trauma Kestenberg is talking about is, in a word, "unwitnessible." A client's mother who was dying of cirrhosis used to spit up blood and bodily fluids all over her bedroom walls. The woman continued drinking herself to death even while her teenage son made a daily ritual out of washing his mother's blood off the walls. In such cases alcoholism becomes a child's or family's own personal Holocaust.

Addiction that is manifested in later generations, even in more mild and less dramatic forms, often represents the transposition of family trauma. And what about circumstances where addiction skips a generation, showing up in the grandchild of an alcoholic? Family and other genetic research indicates that this is very common. In this case people's silence serves as a monument to the traumatic experience. Mothers and fathers who, in response to their own parents' addiction, say "I don't want to talk about it" or, to borrow Claudia Black's expression, "It will never happen to me," help pass on the trauma to their children. In the face of this kind of silence, the substance abuse of teenagers or younger children may be the only way that generation has of maintaining the dialogue and remembering what happened to their parents and grandparents. In this instance, addiction keeps the alcoholic's legacy of pain and suffering alive. Karen, like many other adult children of alcoholics, reenacted both her own and her parents' past trauma through her relationship with alcohol and drugs. Remembrance that takes the form of addiction allows children of alcoholics to simultaneously memorialize or mourn for their dead, and maintain the hope that their parent may one day get sober. The refusal to let go of the past is often why people keep using substances that are killing them, returning to people who are abusing them, or remain in other relationships that no longer sustain, nurture, or support them.

Destructive and unhealthy parenting styles are also passed from one generation to the next. Finding good role models for parenting is essential to arrest the cycle of abuse and addiction in families. Karen, Sophie, and Gere (Jesse's father; see Chapter 2) all needed help with these issues. At times, all three experienced envy and anger at their own children because they received from them a kind of caring their own mothers and fathers could not provide.

As bad as Gere's behavior was toward his son, it was still a vast improvement over the way Gere was treated by his father. His worst rages were often triggered by his sense that Jesse (who had no reason to feel otherwise) did not appreciate what he had and therefore took his parents' love for granted. Gere's inability to accept and grieve for the violence experienced at his own father's hand was keeping him from stopping the physical abuse he was perpetrating on his son. This is what Michael Balint refers to when he writes of the need for therapy to help people change "violent resentment into regret" (1968, p. 183).

For Karen and many other survivors, coparenting was difficult because of her mistrust of any man's ability to parent appropriately. She had intensely vigilant and fiercely protective feelings for her children. These feelings were fueled by her own history of violence, betrayal, and abuse. Also, as a result of these same histories, many women have difficulty coping with their children's emerging sexuality. In therapy, Karen needed to hear that it was important for parents to talk to their children about their bodies and their sexuality. She needed to hear that these are challenging issues for all parents—not just survivors of sexual abuse—and that she need not be ashamed of her feelings. In sessions with her husband we talked about how important it was to find other parents and couples with whom they felt safe talking about their experiences.

Karen worked hard to transform her anger and shame about her parenting. Gradually she held more compassion for herself as a mother and a daughter:

"It's difficult with my mother. I don't know what to do with that relationship. The distance used to be emotional, now it's physical too. I need the distance sometimes, but when it happens it hurts. We go for months at a time without talking. She lives 30 minutes away. I called to invite her to dinner and she came over. If I hadn't called I think it could have been three months. That hurts. It hurts when she's around and it hurts when she stays away. She's getting old. She'll be turning sixty soon and I don't know if she'll be around by the time I get around to reaching out, if she'll be there [starts to cry]. I don't know if I should just forget everything that's happened and forgive her, forgive each other. Or if I should be truthful and say, 'I've been in therapy for almost two years trying to sort out all the awful things that happened to me when I was little and I need your help.' I don't know how she'd handle that. I don't want to make her feel bad.

"I tried when I was a kid, when I was a teenager. I did reach out in a very difficult way. I used to try and hurt myself. I would cry and scream and run to my room and slam the door and sob for hours. No one came. I can't imagine doing that to my daughter or any one of my kids.

"Sometimes my daughter will come home and be upset about something and when I try to help she'll shout at me and say, 'You don't understand. You've never been a kid!' Occasionally I won't have the energy. I'll just be too exhausted, but most of the time I can look her in the eyes and look beyond all the anger and that stuff and say, 'I know it hurts sometimes, and I don't seem to get it—I'm only human—but if you can just be patient, I'll try, and you know I care. You know this is me, Mom.' And she'll come back and we'll work things out together. I can't imagine my mother saying that. It was really hard. I remember when I left home I felt so alone. I didn't think you could ever depend on someone. Now I know I need people. I need that connectedness. It hurts and infuriates me to say that, but it also feels good. I'm still learning that it's okay to have needs. It's a process. I'm getting better at taking care of myself, at letting others in."

The process Karen is describing is a painful one. It requires a lot of nurturing to nurture and parent others. It is hard for a woman to provide mothering to her children in the absence of a strong maternal presence in her life, or for a man who has lost his father to parent his children. Regardless of the reason for a parent's absence (alcoholism, abandonment, divorce, death, or depression) these experiences leave a terrible void in a person's world, one that stays for a lifetime. Sometimes the hurt and pain people feel is so real that it feels like the missing person is with them. People have a hard time letting go of these feelings and may find themselves consciously holding onto their pain. This is understandable. Even when Karen's anger and sadness about what she lost, or lost out on, was making things intolerable for her, she continued grieving for her relationship to her mother in this fashion. Agonizing as this experience was for her, in a moment of bare attention Karen observed, "It's the only way for me to feel close to her or have her present in my life at all." The gift Karen's awareness offered her is what psychoanalyst Adam Phillips writes of in his book *On Kissing, Tickling, and Being Bored* (1993): That it is exceedingly difficult for any of us to maintain so powerful a sense of *absence* without turning that absence into some kind of *presence*.

The long-term effects of trauma and addiction are not the physical or even the emotional scars they leave but the way in which these patterns prevent people from participating fully in their parenting, work, family, spiritual, and sexual relationships. Not all trauma leads to addiction, but all addiction causes trauma. It blocks people's capacity for intimacy and ability to grieve. The therapeutic process, then, is one that encourages just this kind of grieving. As Hans Loewald (1980) said, "Your goal is to help people transform the ghosts that haunt them into ancestors."

An unhealthy relationship to substances doesn't just cover up pain, it embodies and memorializes it. This is why it can be traumatic for addicted persons to imagine a future absent of alcohol, drugs, gambling, cutting, anorexia, bulimia, sexual obsessions, or compulsive overeating. What is required is the divestiture not of just a trusted ally or companion, which is difficult enough, but a part of herself.

CHAPTER 8

Reality Bytes
Narrating Food Addictions

Compulsive behavior, at its most fundamental, is a lack of
self-love; it is an expression of a belief that we are not
good enough.
                                            —GENEEN ROTH

At an open meeting of Overeaters Anonymous (OA) for men and
women in a local town in Western Massachusetts, the format is to select
a topic and to write about it for 20–30 minutes. Participants then share
what they've written with one another. There is no direct response to
people's sharing—or critique of their writing—and individuals have the
option to pass or not read. The group helps participants confront the
way their fears and desires are intimately bound up in their relationship
with food. One individual read the following entry from his OA journal:

> In my family-of-origin so much emphasis was placed on looks
> and appearances—image was everything. This was captured in
> my mother's penchant for gourmet cooking and meals. Feasts for
> the eyes and pallet that inevitably ended up the first battlefield of
> the evening for the ongoing war my parents called a marriage.
> This is one reason I have such a difficult time making a home
> with regular meals. Too much trauma. We were a family of
> carnivores. Steak, chicken, tongue, pastrami, corned beef—Jewish
> soul food—we had bloodied meals to go along with our bloodied
> relationships.
>   My body image was also shaped by this emphasis on
> appearance. By the time I was ten or eleven my father and
> brother had me convinced that I was fat regardless of what I

looked like or weighed. It was just another outlet for everyone's sadistic rage at having so many of our needs for love and intimacy go unmet.

My mother did not participate. She was oblivious to it all, drinking her dinners and trying to avoid my father's abusive outbursts. I, for the most part, did not let their words affect my relationship with food. I enjoyed it too much, and being Jewish the connection between my body and eating was not a strong one. "Essen, essen, essen" was the mantra of the New York Jewish intelligentsia from which my parents came. Food soothed everything. Bodies just happened. Their cruel barbs did come back to haunt me eventually. The shame and hurt, stored in my fat cells, surfaced when I left home and still colors my eating habits.

The tension between my mother and father at the dinner table was so thick you could cut it with a knife—you wanted to eat and get the hell out of there. I can still finish a twelve-course meal faster than most people can open a can of soda. Slowly these patterns are changing as I gain more understanding and acceptance of the idea that I was not responsible for the violence and abuse that plagued my family nor, hard as I tried, could I have prevented it.

Mostly I find myself at the mercy of an aging metabolism and a compulsive exercise regime. Everyday is my own Jimmy Fund run for food where I earn my calories. Sometimes it feels like a vision quest, moments when I can find true happiness on a trail in the woods early in the morning just me and the dogs—my Irish soul mates. Other times it feels like home. A race against time in which I have to hurry or something bad will happen. Most of the time it did.

Acceptance of all these things and a new 12-step program is helping me revisit some of these memories in a different way. The most painful thing for me to accept is not how awful things were but how much better they are now. And hard as all of it is sometimes—the pain and the recovery—it allows a new kind of acceptance of my life, my family, and, most importantly, myself.

*   *   *

It's said a disciple once remarked to Socrates that he knew a man so brave he knew no fear. Socrates responded that if he knows no fear, then he's not brave. Chemicals provide people a false sense of courage by removing their fears. It gives them the sense of being in control when they're not. Earlier, I suggested that at the core of all addictions is *control*. Addicts depend on substances to manage feelings, manipulate the environment, and avoid pain, and most people rely on more than one substance to get the job done. As Knapp (1996) points out:

> For women, the path often winds around alcohol and heads straight to food. You hear about women who became bulimic or anorexic in high school or college, then established some kind of equilibrium around food when or after they start drinking. For men it's usually other drugs, most often pot or cocaine, or it's gambling [or work]. Sometimes it's a more obscure behavior, like self-mutilation—you'll hear about people with compulsions to cut themselves with knives, which sounds horrifying and bizarre until you think of self-mutilation as a way to physicalize the pain the same way lots of addictions do, the way anorexia creates the physical pain of hunger, the way drinking creates the physical pounding of a hangover. (pp. 134–135)

Although bulimia, anorexia, and other compulsive relationships to food have much in common with other addictions, there is one crucial difference. What separates food addictions from other compulsive behavior is what, for lack of a better term, we'll call *the abstinent event*. When making peace with an addiction to alcohol or drugs, it's possible to abstain from these substances altogether. Similarly, when it comes to gambling or overspending, you can make the commitment to stay away from the track "one day at a time" or throw away your credit cards. But you can't live without food.

People who are struggling with a food addiction and integrating some form of 12-step work in their healing will need to establish their own definition of abstinence or sobriety. Recovery from any addiction is best thought of as a daily reprieve rather than a once-and-for-all accomplishment, but in the case of recovery from an eating disorder this is paramount. It does not mean clients should be left or abandoned to come up with these ideas on their own—that is what sponsorship, meetings, and therapy are there for—but it does place more responsibility on people to establish and stay connected to a strong and safe circle of caregivers and supportive people in their lives. They can not quit "cold turkey," "coast," or afford to go through periods of time where they merely stay away from dangerous substances—"people, places, and things"—and do what AA calls "white knuckling it." Although not ideal strategies for any person in recovery, at least for the alcoholic these stopgap measures are plausible. For the food addict they are not.

There are an exhaustive number of sources in the literature and the professional community to help people struggling with an eating disorder. These map out the importance of having a sound and disciplined nutritional plan, a good rapport with a dependable pediatrician or primary-care physician, an ongoing relationship with a safe and trusted therapist, and—especially in the case of children and adolescents—a supportive home environment and family therapy to help family members openly discuss their concerns and channel their support in constructive ways. My comments will be limited to the challenges clients face when taking on these problems within the context of sobriety or another addiction.

A TALE OF TWO RECOVERIES

A clean vowel
is my morning,
Latin pronunciation
in the murmur of confused time.
With rational syllables
I'm trying to clear the occult of my mind
and promiscuous violence.
My linguistic protest
has no power.
The enemy is illiterate.
—NINA CASSIAN

Cara began her session with the following insight: "When I am mad at myself or anyone else, I take it out on my body. . . . And when I am angriest at my body, when I hate it the most, is when I feel most suicidal." After 6 years of sobriety and active participation in AA, Cara finally decided she had to do something about her compulsive relationship to food: "If I don't, it's going to kill me," she said. She wasn't exaggerating. More than 40 pounds overweight, her body was rebelling against the abuse she put it through. Cara had all the early warning signs of adult diabetes. She did not eat nutritional meals, exercise regularly, or get adequate rest. Cara's physician was growing increasingly concerned about her inability to keep her high blood pressure and cholesterol levels in check. (It is worrisome that nowadays Cara's physical and emotional profile is becoming increasingly common, not only within the recovering community, but among the general population as well.)

What's more, Cara's overfunctioning was a liability, not an asset. At work, if it could be done, she did it. A good provider and mother to her teenaged children, she didn't fit the stereotype of the overweight American "couch potato" who watches too much television and refuses to walk any further than the mailbox. She got up at 4:30 every morning to begin her first of three jobs. She stayed active in both children's lives (attending all their school activities and sporting events). She made it to three, sometimes four, AA meetings a week. She stayed in close personal contact with her AA sponsor, and sponsored many others herself. However, at night, exhausted from the day's events and alone with a depression that refused to quit despite years of antidepressants, she ate. Sometimes she soothed herself by eating a pound and a half of M&M's in one sitting. That sugar "high" was her reward for having survived another day without giving up or giving in to alcohol and drugs. At other times, having skipped dinner in an effort to impose *her* will, rather than *food's,* over her life, she would find herself standing in front of the refrigerator—her deprived and worn body about to provide safe refuge to any items that had not found a home or been claimed by anyone during mealtimes.

In an attempt to help Cara better understand the nature of her food addiction, I suggested she write a "good-bye letter" to compulsive overeating and her tortured relationship with her body.

Cara's Letter to Her Obsession with Food

Dear M&Ms, Compulsive Overeating & Bulimia,

I'm giving you up to survive. But how can I nourish myself without the nourishment I gave myself with you? The first bag is always a treat, something sweet to help stave off the anxieties caused by not drinking. I deserve seconds of my favorite food for working so hard and not complaining to anyone. The third is to comfort myself during an evening spent home alone. The fourth is self-pity; the fifth, sabotage.

The 10th has the sickly taste of too much sweet. My mouth is numb to flavor; my senses are numb to feelings. My stomach aches from the strain. The rolls of fat remind me that all these candies keep me hungry for affection and physically unappealing. I know I can't keep them down now.

I make myself vomit. In college we called it "scarf 'n barf." Why do I still do this to myself? Why do I stuff myself with hatred and shame? Why can't I control myself? I'm like a human garbage disposal brimming over with my own anger and waste. Sometimes I pretend each bite is a different person who hurt me in the past: "Good-bye, husband repulsed by the sight of me. How does that feel, neighbor who told me I was fat and ugly and then molested me. Bite me, cute little fitness instructor in the ass-tight lycra shorts who can't make eye contact with me in aerobics class." I clean the toilet for the third time in a day. "Yup, Mom has the flu again." Why can't I get over my obsession with food? I find it difficult calling it that. It's partly right because this is about being obsessed with food and weight, but it is also much much more. These are the things that I think about as I eat something to soothe my raw throat and get rid of the awful taste in my mouth. "Why do I hate myself!" I cry as I swallow a handful of laxatives and return to the refrigerator and begin eating compulsively again.

I only know one prayer. I say it every night hoping for some relief "Help me, help me, help me."

Love,

Cara

In a phrase borrowed from her AA recovery, when it came to her relationship with food, Cara was "sick and tired of being sick and tired." Cara was mad at herself, feeling she should have had the insight and perseverance to take care of her problem before this. She assumed that knowledge and recovery in one area of her life ought to have made her denial-free in all others: "Me, of all people, should know better," she lamented. There are many reasons Cara's assumptions were misguided. We shared a good laugh together at the idea that because she was, in her own words, a "recovery Diva," problems would lay down in the presence of her "stardom." Cara was operating under a delusion many recovering alcoholics subscribe to: that going to AA meetings and living by the 12 steps should be enough to control their obsessive relationship with food or any other compulsions. Many doggedly hang onto this belief in the face of horrendous weight losses or gains. To paraphrase Hollis (1986), they insist that since they practice AA principles in all their affairs, they shouldn't have to attend OA meetings, for example, to relearn what they already know. Though this belief seems reasonable, people often continue to eat compulsively. Cara and I both agreed that if any of the approaches she had already tried could be effective in arresting her overeating, they would have worked some time ago.

Regardless of the spiritual or knowledgeable program she adopted in AA, Cara and I discussed her need for contact with people living out similarly troubling relationships with food. As Hollis (1986), speaking to fellow alcoholics and overeaters, asks: "Isn't that what initially worked and attracted us to AA? Didn't it seem like a miracle that so many of those people were actually living a life totally free of the comfort of alcohol or other drugs? That's what we need to grab hold of in OA! We need to be with people who can say, 'We know how hard it is' " (p. 4). When it came to food, *powerlessness* was Cara's dilemma—not lack of knowledge. She needed to realize that all the work she had done had in fact gotten her this far. There was no wasted effort, no failure. Success for persons in recovery is not the contrary of failure. They are two dimensions of the same world. Success is the achievement of a goal known, open, given. Failure is the achievement of a goal not known, hidden. Everything she had learned in AA had prepared her to walk through the doors of OA and extricate herself from her maddening power struggle with food.

When AA's Go to OA[1]

Like AA, OA isn't for everyone. While many find its message inspiring, others don't. In Cara's case, however, her successful track record in AA and the positive attachments formed there were promising signs that she might be able to establish an equally effective alliance with OA. Cara had been to some OA meetings before and expressed some fears about returning. She recognized that some of her concerns were particular to her story. Other concerns voiced by Cara were of a more universal nature and frequently surface when AA members go to OA. In this chapter's closing passages I will name some of these more universal concepts as well as the strategies Cara employed to overcome them.

Cara's first protest was, *"I don't wanna diet!"* Dieting felt too much like trying to be in control: "God removed my obsession with alcohol just through prayer and meditation; why shouldn't this apply to my relationship with food?" This sounds reasonable and there is, as Hollis (1986) says, no possible rejoinder. The problem with this argument is that it doesn't work. As with most paradoxes which people face in recovery, balance is key. There is a middle ground between fanatic dieting and uncontrolled bingeing. Learning to eat in a satisfying way is not the same as eating whatever you want. OA actually stays away from the term "dieting," as too often it implies a quick fix. But abstinence, as defined in OA, does require a radical change in attitude and behavior toward food. More often than not, this includes making more rational decisions about nutrition and eating habits. There are many in OA who have discovered healthy and peaceful relationships with food. Making a commitment to a safe and disciplined food plan is, for some, the first step on a person's path to recovery.

The use of food plans and other tools for monitoring people's caloric intake are controversial in OA and among therapists who treat eating disorders. The strongest argument for what OA calls "weigh and measuring 90-day meetings" (where, in addition to carefully planning every meal, members are not permitted to speak until they've achieved a mini-

mum of 90 days of abstinence) was made by my client Larry,* who, after reading a draft of this chapter, offered the following remarks in a
correspondence sent me:

> I read the section about OA and although it is accurate, I found
> it incomplete. I am talking about the weigh and measuring 90-
> day meetings. These fanatics (I was one of them so I can make
> this judgment), helped me with their structured meal plans. Now
> although I surrendered my food to a scale and not to God, I did
> lose weight and I felt like I needed this success to stay in the
> program. . . . I think a scale (and structured meal according to
> the Gray Sheet[†]) can be beneficial to some neurotics like myself
> who need the structure to get started. To be able to lose weight
> and begin to actually feel their body. I liken the scale to
> medication for clients who are unable to respond to therapy and
> need to stabilize their symptoms. After the condition stabilizes,
> one can be weaned off the scale and replace it with grace or
> prayer or whatever works.

For others, it is important not to become fixated on setting weight-
loss goals and to throw away the scales and other tools that have become part of the obsession with weight and body image (this principle
does not apply to negotiating minimum body weight requirements for
anorexics under close medical supervision). These expectations can be
dangerous because of the despair that sets in when the scale does not respond as quickly as people would like. As Hollis points out, "Sometimes
the weight has to wait until the psyche is ready" (1986, p. 9). Clients
need to surround themselves with people who can applaud their recovery one day at a time. Who can appreciate that just eating normally in
public without shame or embarrassment is a major achievement regardless of whether a person has gained or lost any weight in any given
month. In addition, for people confronting serious obesity even a large
amount of weight loss over a safe period of time may not be noticeable
to others. So, having goals that are grounded in a change in their *rela-*

---

*Correspondence and feedback for Larry Takki, MA, LRC (Licensed Rehabilitation
Counselor), can be e-mailed to ltblues@javanet.com. I'm very grateful for his input and
feedback on this and other parts of the book. Additional aspects of Larry's story can be
found in Chapter 3.

[†]The first sanctioned food plan used by OA in the 1950s. Following several lawsuits, it
was dropped and replaced with the words, "OA does not sanction a food plan or diet.
Consult your food plan or nutritionist."

tionship to food and their body, rather than changes in their dress or pant size, is crucial.

Most important is that clinicians and clients not confuse emotional or physical health with weight. For many compulsive overeaters, changing eating behaviors does not necessarily result in weight loss, and it is important that we not set up this expectation and instead concentrate on people's emotional and spiritual well-being. For some, long-term damage to their bodies is just one of the many casualties they have to mourn as a result of a lasting war with food. One way that therapists working on food issues with people can adapt some of the ideas in this book to their practices is to ask clients to write good-bye letters to their bodies. This might help them to grieve for the loss of the body they think they should have—or may once have had. This can also be a useful way to help people begin the arduous task of looking at their relationship with food in the first place or to say good-bye to the excess weight that has been preventing them from experiencing certain kinds of intimacy with others.

When caught in the throes of her compulsions, for Cara, as for many women struggling with an eating disorder, food is love. In recovery, Cara, like many others, discovered that food is more like a best friend that betrays you. When alcohol was no longer in her life, Cara's relationship with food became paramount. Rather than being vulnerable and allowing people to be close, Cara felt safer alone with her food. She said that despite her complaints about her body she felt that she held on tightly to her extra weight because it kept her from being seen. She remembered how anxious her mother became when Cara started to develop breasts, grow body hair, and menstruate. Like many women, she remembered that her father stopped talking to her altogether at this time. The message she received about her body and her sexuality was that they were dirty. Instead of celebrating her emerging womanhood and the changes that were taking place, her parents feared them. Their fears were quickly twisted into concerns about her weight. Cara learned fast that breasts, hips, and bodies in general got you in trouble. They got you yelled at, pushed away, and abused. Better to eat and gain weight than have the people you love push you away—or worse. The teasing she took for being overweight was a small price to pay for the sanctuary she got from the grabbing, groping, and betrayal of neighbors/friends/ uncles/fathers/brothers and other men who were supposed to take care of her and whom she was supposed to trust.

When Cara first got sober she tried going to OA meetings. Sitting in a room with many other women present, who shared all or parts of her story, Cara's feelings about these events caught up with her. The experience left her feeling too vulnerable, so she left. It was too early in her recovery from alcoholism. Cara wasn't ready to deal with the emotions OA meetings brought up for her. Neither was she prepared for the kind of intimacy and other types of experiences she encountered there. Part of what appealed to Cara about the kind of camaraderie she found in AA meetings is that it allowed her to bond to a *group* of people without having to get too close to any one individual. In OA there was more direct sharing and talking among members. Also, many OA meetings had a less celebratory and more somber tone. Some of these differences have to do with OA being a much younger fellowship than AA, and so without as much long-term sobriety there is less structure and role modeling to guide newer members. But some differences are explained by the earlier-mentioned fact that OA operates less like a "fellowship" and more like a "sisterhood." As OA offers a more woman-identified space, there is often a greater level of comfort in the meeting rooms when people are talking about feelings and more open expression of intense emotion and tears.

However, bringing more gratitude, jubilation, and sense of joy to the kinds of things people share about themselves at OA meetings is more difficult than it seems. In AA people receive public acknowledgment and acclaim when they admit to being an alcoholic. This doesn't happen when people admit to being anorexic or bulimic; the shame is too thick and stigma too entrenched. Part of what accounts for these different attitudes is that, in spite of all the clinical evidence which refutes popular opinion, alcoholism is still viewed as a predominantly male disease, whereas eating disorders are associated with women. In our culture, men who overcome personal adversity are viewed as heroes, while women—especially mothers—are seen as "fallen angels" despite overcoming adversity. Furthermore, men who overeat and lose large amounts of weight may be congratulated, but they are not seen as courageous. The rewards for a radical change in one's weight and appearance have more to do with absence than celebration: gone are the ridicule, torment, and discrimination. Though you are the same person on the inside, you now look more socially acceptable and "normal" on the outside and hence people take you more seriously. Rarely are the difficult steps it took to get there or the painful reasons for your overeating acknowledged. Finally, not only is the path of the recovering alcoholic often seen as a more heroic one, but the illness itself (i.e., alcoholism) is often valorized in literature and films. The notorious binges and drunkenness of authors like Ernest Hemingway is the stuff of story and legend, stories told and retold with bravado. People don't brag about eating two bags of Oreo cookies. They confess to it.

Addressing her food addiction, Cara and I talked about what was different for her this time, as well as what we could do to help her cope better with whatever feelings surfaced during OA meetings. The most obvious change was that Cara was no longer in early recovery in regard to her alcoholism (i.e., neither she nor her sobriety was as fragile). Also the food issues that she wanted to tackle with the assistance of OA were not a surprise to her this time around. Cara had been discussing them in therapy and making connections between her body image, childhood trauma, and abuse of alcohol for years prior to her decision to "finally stop talking about my feelings about my body and actually do something about it!"

Surrender

The hardest thing Cara had to face at this juncture in her therapy and recovery was the realization that even though she was free of mood-altering chemicals, she was still longing to be filled and was looking to external substances to do the job. For Cara, as with many others in recovery, creating a more gentle and peaceful relationship with food means giving up the idea that something out there can fix her. If a person has already surrendered that idea, it can be disheartening to face the possibility that she may have actually switched substances and may not have surrendered at all. When Cara felt most despairing about this, it was helpful to remind her that giving up the last addiction is hardest because it is the *last,* and self-destructive eating is perhaps the core addiction for many women. There was no substance left to fill the emptiness or ease the pain. She had no recourse but to face herself and her life.

Trying to be present for people in these places poses a difficult challenge to therapists who endeavor not to abandon people in the pain and despair but, at the same time, do not want to rescue them from "hitting bottom" because to do so would deprive them of the opportunity to discover their own inner strength and courage. This is the central dilemma confronting therapists in their work with clients suffering an addiction. In this later stage of treatment, I often find myself thinking about clients' early attachments and childhood experience. A client who has had her basic needs for love and safety met at an early age will need a different kind of emotional support during these *healing crises* than a client who for whatever reason—sexual trauma, physical abuse, poverty, illness, loss, neglect, or abandonment—has not.

Creating a developmental context and understanding of the effects of early childhood trauma on our clients enhances our understanding of their plight and deepens our relationships with them.[2] In situations where clients have been subjected to severe trauma, accessing the feelings of helplessness and surrender needed to take the first step in OA, AA, or any other 12-step program may restimulate aspects of past abuse. In the case of trauma and addiction, accepting their powerlessness over food or alcohol may leave some women clients feeling humiliated and depleted rather than humbled and rejuvenated. As Dusty Miller (1994), echoing B. A. van der Kolk's (1987) sentiments, writes:

> Many childhood survivors of trauma share the experience of crying out to "Mama" in the agony of the traumatic moment and discovering that she does not appear to rescue, protect, comfort, or hold and rock the wounded child. This terrible disappointment and disillusionment becomes the central confounding dynamic in efforts to help victims of childhood trauma. (p. 67)

Growing up without the experience of being shielded or safeguarded from harm by a safe and caring adult guardian or parent, these clients have a fierce longing to be rescued and protected. At the same time, because of the abuse and neglect, they have difficulty allowing others—friends, family, sponsors, 12-step groups, or therapists—to function in that protective role. Just as drinking, bingeing, or cutting can be understood as a client's attempt to remember and restory the original trauma, a person's failed attempts at using the help of a group or a therapist to stay sober or abstinent can be heard as a person's cry for the shelter and protection she never received as a child.

This dynamic often sets in motion a cycle of abstinence and abuse. The most common and frustrating situation that therapists who see clients with drug and alcohol issues encounter is the client who appears unable to sustain any real change or recovery over time. However, if a person never internalized the sense of a safe protective presence in her life, or has been betrayed whenever she tried, she's not going to know how to use supportive relationships. As a consequence, being asked to "admit defeat" in the face of an addiction may be interpreted by the trauma survivor as yet another admission that there is something fundamentally wrong with her. In the case of chronic relapse, clients with trauma histories are particularly prone to blame themselves for not "working the program" right rather than looking at the limitations of the program. Although AA and other 12-step programs can be useful allies to people with severe abuse histories, they are not designed to meet the myriad needs of trauma survivors.[3]

Drugs, food, and other such substances offer people safety, security, and pleasure, usually with more consistency and dependability than any other person or presence in their lives. As Miller (1994) describes it:

> In the trauma-centered environment of childhood, violation and pain come from the same person as food, shelter, and care-taking. It makes sense that the small child will grow up assuming that pain equals connectedness. Self-harm becomes the most familiar and most dependable form of feeling relationally connected that the adult woman knows. Her symptom and her pain protect her and she feels less. Her symptom becomes the relationship in which she feels seen and understood. She can only begin to move away from this relationship with her pain when there is the possibility of being understood by someone outside herself who can fathom the complexity of her self-harmful patterns. (p. 67)

Cara and I talked about her need to use therapy, OA, and other supports to form a more positive connection to her body. Cara expressed some fear that looking more rigorously at her relationship to food and her body would stir up feelings about her capacity to parent, as well as her feelings about the mothering she received as a child. She and I had talked about how her drinking was, in part, a way of identifying with her father's alcoholism and a way of maintaining a relationship with him after his death. However, her associations to her body and food were, in her mind, more closely linked with her role as a mother and daughter.

Cara resented her mother for not teaching her how to take better care of herself and protect herself in the world. Yet, at the same time, she felt strongly that losing weight and feeling better about herself would be a terrible betrayal of her mother, who faced many of the same health problems and food issues as Cara. She also questioned whether she could still mother effectively if she lost weight, even if it made her healthier and gave her own children less cause for worry and concern. Finally, Cara felt that she related to me as another healthier mothering figure of sorts, including sending me cards and presents on mother's day and other holidays, and she worried that our connection would be threatened by her efforts to accept and let go of her food addiction. At this point in her treatment, Cara felt our relationship was in a strong place and "I don't want to mess that up," she said.

Recovery

Cara and I understood that by staying stuck in her relationship with food and abandoning her body in this way, she was in a sense re-creating the aspects of her trauma in which her mother was not there for her or able to adequately protect her. However, I invited Cara to consider the possibility of her "bottoming up" in response to her food obsession rather than feeling she had to arrive at her bottommost place before she could act or change. For Cara this meant returning to OA but listening at meetings for stories about different sorts of mother–daughter relationships in an effort to establish a more compassionate and loving connection to her mother and her own body. As with most of us, Cara's relationship with food was closely tied to her earliest experiences of love and nurturance. Our relationship with food is fundamental in that it is one of the first arenas in which we test out how and if the world is going to respond to our needs. It is important that we not reinforce in therapy the message that "food is bad" or contribute to any other negative messages about eating that a person may have received as a child, especially someone who grew up overweight or was teased and tormented because she was fat. On the other hand, as one recovering member of OA put it, self-love is not the same as self-indulgence, and once these connections to childhood experience are made, "You don't want to let the baby run the show."

Because of her experience with her alcoholism, Cara already knew how to "work a program." This was part of her problem. No longer the naive newcomer, Cara had no delusions about the hard work and pain that lay in store for her if she decided to make significant changes in her relationship to food and her body. Consequently, she was comforted by my recommendation that she only take that step when she was ready. In the meantime, I suggested that she view this crisis as an opportunity to create, in both OA and therapy, a new and different kind of healing presence in her life. This proposition was both scary and exciting because she saw that her two recoveries—one from food addiction, which she strongly identified with her mother, and the other from alcoholism, which she felt she'd inherited from her father—didn't have to be at odds but could work together.

Much of recovery is about making peace with the tension and conflict between the needs of competing addictions. The relationship between our compulsions often reflect past family conflict and trauma. This is just as true for people's issues with food and their bodies as it is for alcoholism and drug addiction. In most cases, the obsessions and angst about food represents pain in a significant relationship. The goal of therapy is to help people be more aware and present in these struggles.

Cara worked hard at her recovery. Often showing up was more

than she could manage. Cara kept a recovery journal that helped her when she found herself too worn out to get to a meeting or even make a phone call. The journal also became a way for her to affirm her progress in therapy and sobriety. Writing helped her discover her own voice and create her own story. Many of the passages in her recovery journal dealt with her understanding of abstinence as practiced in AA and OA and her sojourn from addiction to sobriety. Here are some of Cara's own words:

Cara's Story

During the course of my lifetime, I have experienced trauma after trauma, as have many of us. I am without a doubt an alcoholic and suffer from a grave eating disorder as well. All my life I felt like a smashed mirror broken into small pieces and fragments. Last week I celebrated 8 years of sobriety in AA, 2 years in OA and saw my daughter graduate from high school. It was quite an emotional time. The sense of gratitude I experienced was overwhelming and I wept openly throughout the week. My co-workers kept asking me what was wrong with me. They thought they were tears of sadness, but they weren't. I told them they were tears of joy, but only my sponsor, therapist and fellow AA and OA members knew how hard I'd worked to get to this moment. It was the culmination of years of painful and joyous work and I was celebrating all of them—the sober years—in which I grew with my daughter. During my drinking years my children were a reflection of my addiction. For example, my daughter's third grade picture in which she looks so unkempt and disheveled took place when I was hitting my bottom. She would get herself up in the morning and off to school without my help because I was too hung over to get out of bed. Now I could celebrate her march down the aisle because this time I had been with her every step of the way and all the days leading up to it. The report cards, soccer games, and stage shows. I laughed with her at the all the absurd rules and eccentric people high school throws at you and helped her through the difficult times with her boyfriends and her father who is also a drunk but not in recovery.

When I first came into AA I thought I was cured. I had found a new life and nothing and no one would hurt me again. I was truly humbled and ready to get out of my own way. I did everything I was asked. If someone said get to "90 in 90" I went to 120 meetings in the same period of time. I didn't always agree with what they said but this is what I needed to do to get sober. If I had to do it over I would do it the same way, although one time this approach did get me in trouble.

I was feeling so depressed I didn't want to leave the house, not even to go to meetings. I was scared because it reminded me of how I used to feel before I got sober, but I didn't want to drink this time. I said I would kill myself before I would let that happen. My therapist suggested I try antidepressants. My sponsor said I shouldn't rely on "drugs" or "pills" to help me feel better. I didn't know what to do. I came close to throwing it all away. I knew I needed something and if what I was going to do was considered using I figured I might as well go for broke and drink. The next night I found myself in my car on the way to a package store when I ran out of gas. Because of what I planned to do I'd taken a back road that led to a small country store in another part of the county. It was getting late and not one car had come by. I was starting to get desperate, when a woman stopped to pick me up. I couldn't believe it, the woman was my sponsor's sponsor. She was on her way to a meeting and asked if I'd mind going with her and getting my car afterwards. What could I say, she was going out of her way to help me. Besides the whole thing was too weird. So I went with her. On the way I told her everything and asked her for help. She told me she'd used medication to help her overcome severe panic attacks, and that AA is very clear that taking medication for another "illness" under a doctor's supervision does not interfere with recovery. Looking back, I don't think what happened was chance, it was providence. Either way, it was an important lesson for me. I realized that by refusing to question my sponsor's advice and doing what I knew was best for me, I was behaving like the dutiful daughter I'd been growing up.

My father was alcoholic and my mother was always angry and exhausted from picking up after him and six children. What I remember most about childhood is being made to feel bad whenever I needed to ask them for anything, so I learned to fend for myself and eventually stopped asking all together. It hurt too much and if one of them was willing to help the other got mad. Their fighting was horrible and often became violent. Everyone would leave the house and hope it was safe to come back by nightfall. As a result, I often found myself in dangerous situations with no one to turn to. Physically hurt, and sexually abused by men (some strangers, some neighbors, and once by my best friend's father), I usually dealt with these problems all on my own. But if my parents found out, there was hell to pay. Somehow it was always my fault. Throughout it all I drank, which is one reason why I don't remember much. So in AA when I found this wonderful family of people who loved and accepted me, I listened. Initially things got better, but they didn't stay that way. When I stopped drinking lots of painful memories came up. This time instead of drinking booze, I ate. Most of my life I'd always been in a battle with food and my weight, but this time, without alcohol there was nothing to keep me in check.

Three years ago I hit rock bottom. There was nowhere left to turn—I couldn't believe what I'd done to myself and my body. My second year in AA I lost 75 pounds. People talk about how when they are newly sober they feel like they're going to crawl out of their own skin, well I nearly did! I am 5'7" and I went down to 112 pounds. I thought I should weigh 105 pounds because I weighed that once when I was 12 years old. I became quite ill—I came down with what is now called Chronic Fatigue Syndrome but was referred to as Epstein–Barr virus. I was anemic and run down. The bottom line was that I was not eating enough to stay healthy. I never thought I would find myself on the anorexic side of an eating disorder but there I was.

I used to derive pleasure at how little I could get away with eating and still call it a meal. I considered nausea and fainting spells the price I had to pay to look the way I did and I thought women who weren't willing to do this were lazy or wimps. It was a very macho thing. I was obsessed with losing weight. My first sponsor in AA was the first person to say something to me. She also had an eating disorder and recognized all the signs. She got me eating healthier and less destructively and said that I needed to get counseling. I did. I put all my faith in her and then she drank. After she relapsed she never returned to program and I never saw her again. It took me a long time before I was willing to trust another woman that much, or ask someone to be my sponsor again. When I started therapy my therapist didn't know about the eating disorder. He knew I was in early recovery but I had already gained all the weight back I had lost plus another 40 pounds. I looked better, at least I didn't look as though I had walked out of a Nazi concentration camp. Of course when the weight came back so did all the feelings and the low self-esteem. All the wild swinging up and down wreaked havoc on my body and I became very sick again.

It was my therapist that recommended I go to OA. He and I had been talking for several years about my issues with food and my body. At first I said no because I had been before and didn't like it. But then, after I became frustrated that nothing seemed to control my eating and I found myself considering diuretics and laxatives—total suicide for a diabetic—I decided I had no choice. I had to try something or I was going to die.

Abstinence from compulsive overeating is different from abstinence from substances—from alcohol or other drugs—since there is not a healthy way to cease eating altogether. I knew when I came to OA how to do something fully or not do it at all—which, for me, is the way it has to be with booze. But, to do a thing in "appropriate moderation" was a totally foreign concept. To me abstinence in OA is the act of refraining from compulsive eating—including overeating, undereating, starving, purging, and bingeing, and any other obsessive or compulsive relationship with food I've left out. To do this requires a disciplined food plan but OA is not some kind of diet fad, I know because I've tried them all. Sobriety and abstinence in OA has to be defined by each individual the same way the third step of Alcoholics Anonymous asks each person to define the Higher Power for him- or herself. After much soul searching in therapy and program, I looked to my Higher Power to help me apply this important concept to my life. I decided to take my definition of abstinence from the 11th step. Step 11 tells me to seek through prayer and meditation to increase my conscious contact with God as I understand God. Praying only for knowledge of God's will for me and the power to carry that out.

This is how I apply this principle to abstinence. I borrowed this idea from a woman whose story I heard in OA. Each morning I meditate and ask my Higher Power to tell me what I should eat that day. Then I do my best to do so. During the day I try to stay conscious of this. I find that taking a break to meditate or read some literature in the middle of the day helps me keep focused and stay on track. Sometimes I plan what I am going to eat in great detail, other times I have a more general idea of what my eating will look like and use the plan as a guideline. Prayer works as both my spiritual and nutritional compass. Some days circumstances require me to substitute other food choices than the ones I had in mind. I try to remain flexible, and take it a day at a time. Every evening I look back at the day to see how I've done and how closely I followed my Higher Power's will, admit any character defects that got in my way and make a note to work on those or talk about them with my OA sponsor. This practice has kept me abstinent, going on three years.

One obstacle that got in my way was my obsession with my looks. Would this make me look like the culture's standard of a cover girl? I didn't like that I still cared about such things and feel these images have caused terrible harm to women and their bodies. In recovery I've had to learn what it means to be abstinent from approval seeking not just food, drugs, and alcohol. Eventually I gave up that question and concentrated on a question I found in a piece of OA literature, "I wonder what my Higher Power wants my body to look like?" I started exercising regularly. Everyday I get to the gym or outdoors on a walk is a victory. Even when I miss a day at the gym or should my eating habits get a little sloppy it's okay so long as I do not use these momentary setbacks or failures as excuses to beat up on myself, and use them to help me refocus my program. I learned a new prayer; it's very simple, "Thank you, thank you, thank you." I try to say it at least once a day.

Sometimes I still hear the voices of all the people who have doubted me and men who have mistreated me telling me I am not good enough or that I am ugly and fat. But today I am surrounded by too many people who believe in me and shower me with love to let these voices in. Their words still bother me, but they no longer penetrate my bones. Through my recovery I've learned that while smashed mirrors can't be mended, people can. And, unlike objects, when people heal we become stronger in the broken places.

"KEEP IT COMPLICATED"

> If there are two courses of action, you should take the
> third.
> —JEWISH PROVERB

Public radio's Terry Gross once asked jazz singer Joe Williams about a Star of David pendant she noticed he was wearing around his neck. He said it was a gift from his wife along with a Saint Francis of Assisi medallion with the words "watch over my career" inscribed on it. When she asked him if either he or his spouse were Jewish, he laughed and replied, "No, we just don't like to take any chances."

Watching over someone's recovery I feel the same way—I don't want my client or me overlooking any resource that offers help or relief from their suffering. OA is not perfect. It is, like NA (Narcotics Anonymous), GA (Gamblers Anonymous), and other programs based on the 12 steps of AA, a relatively new fellowship. As a consequence, there are going to be individuals and groups whose activities contradict the program philosophy or what's considered, by professionals in the field, sound therapeutic practice. AA went through similar growing pains in its early years. Many recovering alcoholics are still told that if they apply AA's principles in all their affairs they shouldn't need any additional help including therapy or other 12-step programs such as Al-Anon or OA. While this may be true for some people in AA, for most it is unrealistic and counterproductive for most. Therapy can also become isolative and reductionistic in its thinking and approach. People need to heal in the context of community and with their bodies not just their minds.

Nearly a century after the creation of the "talking cure," helping people understand the mind–body connection is psychotherapy's future.

When it comes to revealing the mysteries of addiction we cannot afford to take any chances that our way is the only one. Like Cara, we need to embrace and value different approaches to recovery and not shy away from asking tough questions that muddle things up and expose life's complexities. In order to do this, clients need therapists who can tolerate contradictions, have compassion for their own and their clients' frailties, and who appreciate the diversity of human experience. This means accepting and celebrating people's spiritual beliefs, including their faith in the existence of a Higher Power or divine presence in the universe and their lives.

CHAPTER 9

Writing Home

Applications to Family Therapy

> I believe that if one goes deep enough into the experience
> of powerlessness one naturally discovers a spiritual reality
> that is beyond conventional notions of cause and blame.
> Conversely, if one stretches the boundaries of system
> thinking far enough, one encounters the experience of
> higher power.
>
> —DAVID BERENSON

As Augustus Napier observed in his and Carl Whitaker's book *The Family Crucible* (1978), the first family therapists were distinct individualists: strong, creative, and thoroughly rebellious. However, despite its reputation as a maverick profession, initially family therapy was heavily influenced by psychoanalytic concepts and ideas. Early proponents looked at how unconscious family scripts and other emotional processes left out of Freud's theory added a multigenerational perspective to our understanding of human behavior. Spurred on by developments in cybernetics, communication theory, and evolutionary biology, a second wave of family therapists and researchers provided a new grammar to depict the process of change in families. Circular notions of causality replaced causal explanations of problems and social relations. Where treatment was once looked at as finding an "etiology" of a so-called illness arising from either biological or psychological causes, problems were now understood as being embedded in patterns of communication rather than sealed in the envelope of the skin.

Looking at families through this lens required therapists to abandon any clear linear markers that indicated where people's problems began or ended: one event was seen as modifying another, which in turn modified the first. The recursive nature of family process meant it was no longer possible to assign one part of the system, or one family member, a causal influence vis-à-vis another. Another important implication for therapy was that the therapist could no longer be viewed as the agent and the client could no longer be viewed as the subject of change. They are both part of the same larger system.[1] This was welcome news for therapists in the addictions field, who found that the only thing more difficult to change than the alcoholic's drunken behavior was the way people responded to it.

An illustration of circular causality and alcoholism in action can be found in Antoine de Saint-Exupéry's *The Little Prince* (1943), a wonderful saga of a boy's journey around the cosmos and his encounters with life's lessons. The second planet the adventurous hero visits is occupied by "the tippler" (a "drunk"), and the following conversation ensues:

> "What are you doing there," he said to the tippler, whom he found settled down in silence before a collection of empty bottles and also a collection of full bottles.
>
> "I am drinking," replied the tippler, with a lugubrious air.
>
> "Why are you drinking?" demanded the little prince.
>
> "So that I may forget," replied the tippler.
>
> "Forget what?" inquired the little prince, who already was sorry for him.
>
> "Forget that I am ashamed," the tippler confessed hanging his head.
>
> "Ashamed of what?" insisted the little prince, who wanted to help him.
>
> "Ashamed of drinking." The tippler brought his speech to an end, and shut himself up in an incomprehensible silence. (pp. 40–41)

Systems thinking offered a way of interrupting these enigmatic patterns of communication and taking the toxicity of cause and blame out of conversations about addiction and other problems. Unfortunately, in practice the emphasis merely shifted from one type of what Hoffman (1993) calls "clinical hate speech" to another. Psychosis and other forms of psychopathology (e.g., "borderline" and "narcissistic" personality disorders) give way to "enmeshed" and "dysfunctional" family systems. Embedded in these diagnostic categories is the suggestion that there is some buried truth or secret that lies at the core of a person's character. The therapist's role becomes one of uncovering its hidden dynamics or—when applying systemic methods—of decoding their dysfunctional patterns of communication. Either way, clients are dependent on the expertise of professionals to help them understand and make meaning of their behavior and actions. Nevertheless, in cases of addiction as well as many other presenting problems, the need to help families develop clear, consistent, and nonaccusatory communication skills is obvious and all therapists owe these early systems thinkers and therapists a considerable debt.

A SPIRITUAL ALLIANCE: BUILDING BRIDGES BETWEEN FAMILY THERAPY AND AL-ANON

From the standpoint of narrative therapy, helping families suffering from addiction heal is about giving people the opportunity to restore a sense of safety, integrity, possibility, compassion, and faith in their lives. Family members who are unable to transform or extricate themselves from their relationship with an alcoholic and his or her self-destructive behaviors are not "codependents" or "enablers"—they're blocked. Their creative dreams and yearnings are siphoned off by the drama and chaos surrounding the addict's lifestyle. When a person's child, parent, spouse, or significant other is impaired by alcohol or drugs, just performing the minimum daily routines necessary to maintain a household can be draining, if not impossible. It is difficult to sustain a nurturing and healthy home life when so many of the family's emotional resources go into keeping up the pretense of denial and propping up the addict's depleted sense of self. During a writing activity for a children's therapy group, one 11-year-old boy, Josh, wrote the following lines:

> My dad drinks too much sometimes. My dad wouldn't hurt anybody but he likes to just drink. He stopped smoking a year ago. He's on a cholestrol diet. So he's healthy. He drinks once a week. He gets drunk about every 3 months. But not too bad. A little while ago he got drunk. He just wants us to not pick on him. In the morning he doesn't really have a hang over. It's not a real big problem. It just he likes to have a drink once in a while.

Another group member the same age, Jamilla, wrote:

> One time my mom and dad were fighting because my dad drinks a lot. They got into a fight and he left. He was gone for one week. I went to my sister and I told her what happened and we

tried to find him. When we found him, we tried to get him back and to stop drinking and smoking.

By showcasing two clients' stories, the Kelly family and a young man named Peter, this chapter offers strategies that individual as well as family therapists can use to strengthen their own and their clients' connection to Al-Anon and also to improve the effectiveness of their interventions with alcoholics, addicts, and their family members. An "intervention" is when family and friends concerned about someone's drinking or drug abuse gather together and make that person feel more loved, embraced, and cared for. If they do their job well, the person often feels worthy of self-respect and self-love and shows it by pursuing help. It is, by anyone's standards, a success if either an increase in love or sobriety occur; it's a miracle when both happen.

During my work with the Kellys, my ideas about therapy were informed by family systems thinking. By the time I met with Peter, the field of family therapy was witnessing the emergence of new metaphors and frameworks for practice and I had begun to employ narrative techniques in my practice. Both stories connect my thinking about therapy, Al-Anon and recovery. They are by no means complete but provide therapists and other readers an adequate place to start when shepherding their own or a client's recovery, or attempting to establish a partnership between family therapy and Al-Anon or another 12-step program.

While use of the term "system" to describe families is currently out of fashion, it's important to remember that some therapists' conception of family systems were more organic than mechanistic. Murray Bowen, one of the profession's pioneers, received inspiration for his ideas from nature and astronomy rather than general systems theory, which borrowed metaphors from rocketry, computers, and other man-made systems. Bowen tried to connect his odyssey into the world of human emotional systems to the evolution of the cosmos and described the human emotional system as stemming from the same life force connecting all life on the planet. Bowen said that "a theory that proposes to move towards science must somehow be in harmony with the sun and the earth, and the tides and the seasons" (Kerr & Bowen, 1988, p. 35). My image of Bowen, one he undoubtedly wouldn't especially appreciate, associates him with the early founders of modern science such as Copernicus and Galileo, who were unabashed about combining religion, mysticism, and astrology with their new discoveries. Psychotherapy, according to Bowen, is a combination of science and art: the scientific aspects deal with our increased knowledge of how people evolve and change; the art with the application of that knowledge.

THE KELLYS: A FAMILY SYSTEMS
APPROACH TO ALCOHOLISM

Alcohol travels through families like water over a
landscape, sometimes in torrents, sometimes in trickles,
always shaping the ground it covers in inexorable ways.
—CAROLINE KNAPP

Ten years ago I met with a 15-year-old and his parents.* The young
man, Mark, had been arrested for disturbing the peace and possession of
alcohol by a minor. This was particularly disconcerting to his parents
because Mark's father was a district attorney. In our first meeting
Mark's mother, Cynthia, expressed dismay at her son's predicament and
seemed desperate to find help for him. She indicated that she felt she had
done everything she could to keep him out of trouble, including paying
his court fines, driving him to and from baseball practice, and helping
him with his homework. Mark's father, Jim, felt guilty because so much
of the parenting of Mark and their 6-year old daughter, Jill, was shoul-
dered by Cynthia. Jim explained that he worked long busy hours and
was often called out of bed in the middle of the night to help obtain a
warrant or prepare someone to testify before a grand jury. Although
physically a large and imposing man, Jim always looked to his wife before speaking and let her do most of the talking in our sessions. He did,
however, say that he was also concerned about Mark's trouble, particularly the embarrassment it was causing the family. He said that to a certain extent he understood Mark's behavior, because when he was that
age he used to go out in the woods with some friends and a case of beer.
But his behavior never led to so much trouble. When asked about his
drinking now, Jim said he spent his leisure time at Eagle Lodge, "a private drinking club for guys who don't like to hang out at the bars." His
time at the Lodge was a source of tension between him and Cynthia. He
reported drinking beer on a fairly steady and regular basis. In fact, he
candidly labeled himself an "alcoholic" but made it clear he did not view
his drinking as a "problem" because it caused him no difficulty at work
or at home. He felt he drank as a way of helping him cope with the stress
of his job and that he would drink less if he were in a less intense and

---

*During the therapy with the Kelly family, I was joined, periodically, in sessions by my su-
pervisor and cotherapist at the time, Samuel Muri. I wish to thank Samuel for his insight
and guidance during our work together, and for his help documenting and reconstructing
the events of this therapy.

high-profile line of work. This last point was contested by Cynthia, who felt her husband was so tired and depressed all the time because he drank so much rather than from his work.

Alcoholism ran like a river through both Jim and Cynthia's families. A brief family history revealed that Jim's father died of his drinking and Jim's mother and all his brothers were described as "alcoholics" or "heavy drinkers." Cynthia's father was an alcoholic, and her brother Brad was in rehab at the time for cross-addiction to heroin, cocaine, and alcohol.

Cynthia and Jim urged me to meet with their son. I agreed but told them I believed the problem was not only Mark's. I said I felt it would take a great deal of effort on the entire family's part to turn things around. During a series of conversations with Mark, several things became apparent to me. The first was how much Mark loved and admired both his father and his mother. Mark expressed concern about the toll his father's drinking was taking on his father's health and his parent's marriage. He also expressed his fear over how much difficulty he was having controlling his own alcohol and drug use. Following my discussions with Mark, I presented my assessment to him and both his parents. I offered the family several options, including referring Mark to a drug rehabilitation center. Cynthia was surprised and began to cry at the suggestion of inpatient work. She had thought that Mark was not doing as badly as her brothers. I said why wait for matters to become worse with Mark? Why wait until the courts intervene and send him away without giving the family an opportunity to consider this treatment option?

While Jim expressed a clear preference to participate in outpatient counseling, Cynthia said she trusted my judgment. She asked my opinion about what they should do. I responded that she, Jim, and I would not be seeing Mark through these difficult times together. Therefore, it seemed to me very important that whatever was decided be something that she and Jim felt confident they could live with. I suggested they go home and talk about it and return the following week with a decision.

The Kellys presented a constellation of problems which I often find in families seeking help for a teenager whose substance abuse masks parental alcoholism. Because the Kellys' story took place more than a decade ago, it offers an opportunity to examine some developments in family therapy and how these have influenced my work with alcoholics and addicts. When I saw the Kellys, many of my ideas were informed by family therapists David Berenson (trained by Murray Bowen) and David Treadway (trained in Salvador Minuchin's methods). Berenson (1976, 1979) understood the cognitive aspects of addiction with his insight into its "wet" and "dry" affective states. Berenson, in his more recent explorations (1987, 1991) into spirituality and 12-step epistemology, asks clinicians to confront their ignorance of the inner workings of AA and their long-standing apathy towards clients' spiritual needs in therapy. Playing Freud to Berenson's Jung, Treadway (1989) has a firm grasp of the structural underpinnings and dynamics of addiction. He examines how different hierarchies and patterns of relationship within families reinforce drinking behaviors. Treadway brings to family therapy an intimate knowledge of addiction and alcoholism treatment grounded in his clinical consultations with clients as well as his own experience of his mother's alcoholism and depression.[2]

"Cognitive affective experience," "family structures," "hierarchical imbalances of power," this chapter borrows from these concepts but ultimately weaves them into a narrative that offers the reader insight into the heart of addictive experience.

The Bowen Family Therapist: "Standing Like a Stoughton Bottle"

Patented by an English apothecary in the 17th century, the Stoughton bottle contained a tonic made mainly with alcohol. The name Stoughton wasn't based on the contents or the condition it induced in consumers if taken as recommended, but rather on the shape of the bottle. The appeal of the ingredients notwithstanding, the bottles were even more popular because they were large, made of stoneware, and had a flat side to keep them from rocking or spilling. The image of a strong unbreakable container holding a powerful and unpredictable contents is a good metaphor for the Bowen family therapist. Bowen's (1978) view of the therapist as an impartial coach whose aim is to help people differentiate from their families is well suited to the emotional intensity and volatility often found in alcoholic families. However, therapists who use Bowen's approach must also be careful not to repeat the common alcoholic pattern of ignoring and denying feelings.

"Triangles"—their form and function—are one of the cornerstones of Bowen family therapy. When two people are under stress, they "triangulate" a third person or object into their relationship. While the most common example is the child whose symptoms or problems cover up some unresolved conflict between his or her parents, alcohol can serve this function too, deflecting deep disagreements between people to arguments over drinking. Over time, such problems can be mapped as a series of interlocking triangles in a kind of chain reaction across generations. The son of two alcoholic and depressed parents devotes his childhood to protecting his younger sister from their parent's drinking and abuse. When he's older he repeats this self-sacrificing behavior in his marriage—protecting his spouse from any upsetting interactions with their substance-abusing daughter. But this time he resents the role and becomes angry with his wife and distances himself from their relationship. Therapy, according to Bowen, is about helping people identify the way their past causes them to be emotionally cut off from the present and fused in reactive positions that keep these family dramas energized.

Another of Bowen's examples, which became a brand emblem of sorts for family therapy, is the couple that becomes entrenched in their roles as "pursuer" and "distancer." The way these roles are manifested in alcoholic couples is that one partner assumes a position of under-responsibility and the other, of overresponsibility. Coaching the non-drinking spouse to underfunction can upset the system enough for change to occur. Bowen used genograms, or family trees, to diagram these relationships for people. The genogram was, perhaps, family therapy's first real move toward a story-centered practice, helping families externalize their problems so they could get more distance from them and transform their problem-saturated narratives into stories that had, what Jerome Bruner (1986) has called "literary merit."[3]

Bowen's model is a good one for families whose members have high levels of reactivity to one another. His method parallels Al-Anon's message to its members to "detach with love"—that is, to compassionately refuse requests by the alcoholic for money, or to make excuses for him to his employer to cover for his mistakes on the job, or to apologize for his drinking to others. In this context, during early recovery, family-of-origin work makes sense. Bringing to the fore people's experiences growing up in families where adults routinely ignored or made excuses for drunken and bizarre behavior by fathers, mothers, grandparents, aunts, and uncles can help clients recognize their ability to do the same. I also find that once a genogram is complete, if I ask clients to place a symbol next to every known alcoholic or addict in their extended family and another symbol next to family members they suspect had a drug or alcohol problem, the results can be sobering. When a family or an individual completes this exercise and I stand back to review the finished product, my first comment is often the same: "It seems to me it would take a small miracle for a person to come out of this family without having to question their relationship to alcohol or drugs at some point in their life." When other addictions and compulsive behaviors are added to the drawing or diagram, this observation becomes even more apparent. The same approach can be applied to any type of substance abuse or self-destructive pattern of behavior. This exercise can reduce the amount of shame and guilt people feel about their own or their family's alcoholism. It can be extremely useful at lifting the sense of blame and responsibility parents feel for their children's substance abuse problems.

Having successfully lessened the level of shame people feel about themselves, therapists may be tempted to continue using the genograms to cull as much information about people's lives and experiences as possible. However, in the case of addiction, therapists need to be mindful about introducing too much intimacy and emotionality prior to helping alcoholics and their families establish good support and sobriety. When working with a family's genogram, we are often too quick to explore people's past traumas and personal histories when we could, just as easily, be using these tools to examine clients' reluctance to use AA and Al-Anon and their experiences—good and bad—in these groups.

Breaking the Silence

The Kellys returned ready to begin therapy the following week. My initial goal was to introduce each family member to AA or Al-Anon and get each one to discuss his or her concerns about alcohol and drinking as openly and honestly as possible.

Mark was referred to a support group for adolescents experiencing substance abuse problems that was offered at our clinic, and also to a 10-session therapy group for juvenile offenders run by the courts. In both groups he was strongly encouraged to attend AA and NA meetings. Although he did not go to meetings on a regular basis, at least he was exposed to them and reported enjoying the three meetings he attended with friends from the group.

Jim was defiant in his resistance to AA: "If I don't want to drink, I won't. I don't need meetings to tell me how to do it."

Cynthia, although more open to discussing AA and Al-Anon, was also reluctant to attend meetings. She did agree to go to a two-part family workshop being offered at the clinic. Cynthia liked the workshops. She said she was discovering a great deal about her roles at home which only made her problems worse—running interference for her son when he got into trouble at school, and not making any demands on her husband at home. These were just some of the ways she made sure her needs never competed with her husband's drinking and that her son didn't have to face the consequences of his actions. She felt supported talking about this with other women in her situation. Several months after the workshop ended, she decided to try Al-Anon and then began attending meetings regularly.

At first, I convinced Cynthia to attend Al-Anon meetings out of her concern for her son, her husband, and her marriage. In other words, I told her I felt it was the best way for her to help her family. This may seem odd, given Cynthia's overfunctioning at home, which prevented her husband from taking more responsibility for his drinking and for his relationship with Mark. However, this intervention was strictly to get Cynthia to Al-Anon. Once there, I hoped that what she learned about addiction and its effect on families would encourage her to put more energy into herself and less into her caretaking of Mark and Jim.

In family sessions with the Kellys I continued my work with their genogram, identifying patterns of abuse while also processing what members were learning in AA and Al-Anon. It's pivotal when treating alcoholism to get the family to confront each other about a member's drinking. This is not the therapist's job. The emerging struggle should be among family members rather than between the family and the therapist. I continued to honor Cynthia and Jim's need to focus on improving communication with Mark and troubleshooting his problems at school, court, and home. However, the overriding emphasis of the work was to raise the family's consciousness about the danger addiction posed for everyone. I wanted them all to learn as much about alcoholism and recovery as they could.

One way I encouraged this learning process was to get Jim and Mark to agree to a "no drinking contract" for the duration of therapy. Sometimes I tell people this is a condition of therapy, and other times I simply argue its necessity if therapy is going to be effective. However, I never approach these contracts with the expectation that people are going to be able to stick to the agreements. Mostly, they allow me to focus on people's alcohol and drug abuse without policing their personal conduct and behavior or working harder at exploring their addictions than they are.

This is accomplished by allowing clients to decide for themselves how long they're going to abstain from alcohol or in some cases what is a reasonable amount of alcohol (or, say, pot) to consume before the person is willing to acknowledge their use is a problem. Allowing the drinker to establish the parameters and limits of the contract places responsibility for any abuse squarely on the alcoholic. When the agreement is broken the drinker can't use the excuse that the volume of alcohol determined to be a sign of a problem—or the amount of time needed to abstain in order to demonstrate self-control—was unreasonable.

Under these circumstances, if the alcoholic tries to rationalize or minimize his or her use, the absurdity of that position becomes evident to others.[4]

In my conversations with the Kellys, for example, we would discuss each family member's effort to maintain abstinence and what it meant if he or she could not do so. On one occasion Jim had a few beers at his sister's house but insisted, "That's not drinking. I haven't been to the Lodge for weeks!" Mark, in turn, admitted to smoking marijuana but said his parents should see it as a blessing because "pot mellows me out and keeps me out of trouble." At times, Jim did in fact make a genuine effort to abide by the agreement. This experience also held valuable information for the family. Complaints about Jim's edginess and irritability highlighted the significant role alcohol played in his life as well as Mark's.

"The Drinking Pact"

These conversations exposed what I called at the time the covert "drinking pact" between father and son. It is a common theme in many relationships between substance-abusing teenage boys and their alcoholic fathers. Such a tacit agreement between an addicted father and an addicted son has many functions, the most apparent being to support each other in their respective addictions. It allows the father to take the stance of the disapproving parent, while the son plays the role of the "sacrificial lamb" keeping the heat and attention focused on himself and off his dad.

The pact also serves to cover up any real expression of feeling between the father and son. Alcohol creates a kind of pseudointimacy between family members. In my therapy groups with substance-abusing teenage boys, there is inevitably a session where each member talks about a special evening or event at which he got drunk with his father. These episodes often result in meaningful conversations about the "purpose of life," stories about first sexual encounters, or physical fights that according to these young men brought their fathers and them "closer together." I find, however, that beneath this pseudointimacy is a myriad of angry and hurt feelings which their drinking or substance abuse keeps buried.

These same issues reached an emotional peak between Mark and Jim in therapy when, after an argument about the quality of their time together, Mark shouted, "I can't talk to you anymore, Dad!" In this meeting Mark was able to express his despair at having to spend most of his time relating to his mother because his father was physically and emotionally unavailable to him.

Cynthia's tears bore witness to Mark's anger and disappointment. She tried very hard, with encouragement from me, not to buffer her husband from Mark's anger and pain. Inspired by Mark's courage, Cynthia said how powerless she felt over both Jim's drinking and Mark's problems. It seemed to her that the more she tried to improve the situation the worse it got.

Cynthia told Jim how embarrassed and alone she felt when he passed out at family gatherings. She said that for years she felt there was something terribly wrong with her because Jim preferred getting drunk rather than spend time with her: "Now I understand you're the one with the problem, not me!" Al-Anon, Cynthia said, was helping her recognize how similar and counterproductive the roles she was playing with her husband and son were. She knew she had to learn to "let go" at home and in her marriage but was frightened of what would happen, especially to Mark, if she did. In response to this, Mark said he felt his parents were still together only because of him. While reassuring Mark she had no plans to divorce his father, Cynthia admitted that she had sometimes considered leaving.

When asked about the mixed messages his drinking must give his wife and children, Jim responded that he realized it must "adversely affect" them but made it clear that he nevertheless felt he was "okay." He said if the family could just "stay the course," paying a little more attention to Mark, they would all be fine without Jim himself having to change. I told him I thought he was playing Russian roulette with his family.

Mark's comment that his parents were only together because of him seemed to identify a crises in the parents' relationship while averting one at the same time. His insight united his parents in response. I told Mark that saving his parents' marriage seemed like an awful responsibility for a 15-year-old boy to assume and maybe he should let others share it with him. I then asked Jim and Cynthia to imagine what it might feel like if Mark left home for a year. What kind of home would he return to?

In retrospect, it was much too early in the therapy for me to introduce these kind of questions and ideas. For Jim to have any success working on his marriage, he would have to let go of his drinking. Clearly, he was not ready to do so, and my question only served to distract us from that crucial task. Furthermore, I was duplicating Mark's parents' efforts to involve and triangulate him further in their relationship. Mark made this point even clearer at the end of the session when he requested to "not be a part of my parents marriage counseling."

When I first wrote this case up I remembered trying to imagine what David Treadway or David Berenson, my alcohol mavens at the time, might have said in such a session. A more appropriate response, borrowed from Treadway's files, would have been: "Jim, it sounds like Cynthia feels your drinking affects your ability to help the kids and meet her needs and may lead to the marriage breaking up. Can you talk it over with her and find out what's going on?" Conversely, I might have said to Cynthia, "It seems you are feeling really desperate about your situation. You are saying you can't depend on your husband anymore, and because of his drinking he is unable to help you with Mark's problems. Could you go ahead and speak frankly to him and see if he is able to listen to your worries without getting mad at you for having them?"

Despite my error, Cynthia's frank disclosure did have a significant impact on the therapy. As Cynthia's crisis worsened, an interesting shift occurred. Although Jim remained adamant in his refusal to attend AA, he became more willing to discuss the impact of his drinking on the family. Previously, Jim identified more with his son than his wife and would often join Mark in ridiculing and making fun of Cynthia for all her worrying. Now he began to take a more assertive and constructive role in sessions.

When one of Mark's best friends landed in the emergency room with severe alcohol poisoning, Jim came into our next session and said he was considering three options to deal with "Mark's problem":

1. Send him to inpatient treatment.
2. Ground him indefinitely.
3. Move.

Jim agreed with his family that options 2 and 3 were not viable solutions to Mark's troubles. When asked about following through with option 1, Jim said he would rather take Mark away with him to Alaska or Canada, where they could live together in the outdoors "without booze." Jim's struggle was painful to watch. He seemed desperate to find a way to help his son without he or Mark having to give up alcohol. His idea of taking Mark 3,000 miles away showed what drastic measures he felt it would take to separate them both from chemicals. I interpreted the hopelessness and despair Jim expressed about Mark's predicament as a cry for help with his own addiction.

This hypothesis seemed to be borne out in our next session, during which Jim invited us to talk about our concerns about his drinking and seemed genuinely interested in hearing them. We discussed our fears about his health, pointing out his high blood pressure, smoking, blood-shot eyes, and the toll alcohol was starting to take on his relationship with his wife and son. I asked all three to think about whether they thought they could handle the changes that might result from Jim seeking help for his drinking, while acknowledging that he wasn't ready to take such a big step. This was not a "planned intervention" meant to facilitate his admission to a detox center or treatment program, but the dialogue about Jim's condition that took place, and the nonjudgmental and nonblaming atmosphere in which it transpired were important developments. Cynthia, in particular, was able to express her opinions more directly and with less anger than she had at prior meetings. She credited Al-Anon for this change in her behavior. At the end of the meeting, Jim accepted my invitation to attend a session on his own in order to help him determine the severity of his problem. I made this offer to avoid any unnecessary humiliation and embarrassment for Jim, which might arise were we to discuss his drinking in front of his family.

"The Courage to Change the Things I Can"

In stories of addiction, change can be very moving and inspirational to witness. However, as in most therapy, the process of transformation is usually less dramatic. Progress, if noticeable, is evolutionary rather than revolutionary. This was the case with the Kelly family. Mirroring many past promises and well-intended resolutions that Jim had made about quitting drinking in the past, his momentum once again waned. I don't know whether he bent under the weight of this mammoth task or succumbed to the reality of the pain involved in unpacking the years of unresolved feelings and resentments.

The Kellys stopped going to family sessions as soon as Mark appeared, according to Jim, "out of the woods." After our meeting, Jim decided to lose some weight and quit smoking. Then he reported that although he was still drinking, he was drinking a lot less and trying to spend more time at home. Jim said he wanted to go it alone for a while and see how he and his family would do. He added that if he wasn't able to control his drinking or things at home did not stay on the mend, he would be willing to come back.

Mark's drug use decreased considerably over the course of the therapy. Mostly, I believe, because of the close scrutiny of it by all the adults in his life, because his parents became more effective at limit setting, and also somewhat as a result of his work in the teenage support group. At the completion of therapy, Cynthia, who said she was going to continue in Al-Anon, reported feeling less isolated and more hopeful about the future. Mark said the only thing he liked about family therapy was that his parents "stopped bugging him at home and waited till these stupid sessions to bring up problems where we can sometimes work them out without fighting." I took this as a rave review. In addition to the trust and rapport built with Mark, Jim made a small but important shift in his attitude and willingness to discuss his alcoholism and its impact on the family. The most significant step was his agreeing to make an appointment to talk about it on his own. Finally, and most significantly, the family was introduced to a 12-step program and at least one person was using it regularly. While this certainly did not represent transformation or sobriety, the potential for both was recognized, and insight and skills were gained which could move the family closer to change.

When all was said and done, perhaps the most important condition therapy provided for the Kelly family was a safe space to express their feelings about Jim's drinking. This gave Mark and his father an opportunity to engage in a more honest discussion about their relationship and led to Cynthia's involvement with Al-Anon. These are much humbler achievements than my original goals of arresting Mark's drug use completely or helping Jim get sober, yet they were important.

Helping the Nondrinking Spouse or Partner "Hit Bottom"

The impulse to treat Jim's alcoholism first was the most crucial temptation I faced in my therapy with the Kellys, and it was one misstep, or misdirection, I've tended to fall into on too many occasions. There are several pitfalls to this almost instinctual response. The most obvious is that by addressing the alcoholic's problems first the therapist is choosing to challenge the family member most reluctant to change and who has the most to lose by doing so. Another problem with pursuing the alcoholic is that the therapist's interventions and behaviors in sessions are, more often than not, going to replicate the behavior the nondrinking family members have been employing at home to get the alcoholic to stop drinking. Focusing on the active drinker exclusively reinforces the message that family members are not free to think, feel, or act independently of the alcoholic. Finally, bringing the alcoholic to a point where he or she is ready to entertain the notion of getting help prior to laying the necessary groundwork with the family members who have been caretaking him or her is often counterproductive. In other words, if the alcoholic is ready to change but the people with whom he lives are not ready for that to happen yet, the therapist may find herself swimming against the current, so to speak.

Among the Kellys, Cynthia was the person who was most upset by the drinking of Jim and Mark. Consequently, she was the person most willing to do something about it, but her rescuing behaviors had to be addressed first. I took Berenson's (1976) tack of getting the codependent to "hit bottom" before the alcoholic. I liken the goals and objectives of this approach to an oft-heard popular expression with a Zen twist: "Don't just do something, sit there!"

In Cynthia's case the situation was complicated by the fact that two relationships (with her husband and her son) were blocking her. This allowed her to move from one to the other depending on which relationship showed the most hope for change or, conversely, was the most active or "wet"—thereby offering the greatest possibility for excitement and relatedness.

To address this dilemma, I sent Cynthia to Al-Anon, where I knew she would be encouraged to stop driving herself crazy, so that life for Jim and Mark could run more smoothly. In addition, at the outset I requested that both parents attend therapy. Jim's participation was a source of contention. Cynthia explained that because of his work schedule, he might not always be able to join us. I said I understood his dilemma, but I did not feel we could be productive without his presence. I suggested that at times it might make sense for the parents to meet without Mark present, but I refused to meet without both parents. At the same time I offered to meet them evenings and/or Saturdays if necessary in order to accommodate Jim's schedule.

This practice was only tested once. After our second meeting mother and son showed up alone. I sat down with them and again explained that we could not meet without Jim. Mark was disappointed. He felt he and his mother were having the most trouble getting along, and they did seem genuinely ready to discuss their problems. I nevertheless repeated that Mark's father would have to join us if we were going to have any success tackling their problems. The family returned with mother, father, and son at the next meeting.

There were several levels of communication taking place simultaneously in this interaction. On one level, it was a "structural" intervention because Jim had abdicated his role as a primary parent and left all the parenting duties to Cynthia. It was important to press him to take responsibility for things at home, particularly Mark's situation, if his family's circumstances were going to improve. On another level, it seemed likely to me that Cynthia had become a "single parent" in a two-parent family because of her husband's drinking. Therefore, having Jim in the room was necessary to underscore the effects of drinking as we discussed why things were not working. On yet another level, the family didn't want to talk about Jim's drinking and neither did I. I had felt the tension and anxiety rise in the room when I asked about it in our first meeting, but that is what needed to happen.

If I had this interaction to do over, I wouldn't handle it the same way. I feel it would have been more respectful for me to say what was on my mind: "Jim, your presence is necessary because your drinking is interfering with everyone's ability to sort out what's really going on at home. I understand you don't agree with this assessment, but even this disagreement is causing a lot of tension between you and Cynthia. I need you here so we can get to the bottom of all this. We must figure out, if we decide it's a problem, what we're going to do about it; if not, how we can get people off your back and get Mark some help." Instead, I cloaked my "strategic" motives to expose the severity of Jim's alcoholism in a set of arbitrary guidelines or rules about Jim needing to attend sessions in order for therapy to be effective. In retrospect, this attitude seems disrespectful and dismissive of Cynthia's experience (as well as that of nondrinking parents and guardians in general). She was struggling to keep the family's head above water and had been, as Jim aptly put it, shouldering the burden of parenting on her own. Although the Kellys continued to attend our sessions, many families often drop out at this point in treatment. In the Kelly's case, they may have responded positively to the limit I set regarding Jim's attendance because of Cynthia's dogged determination to help her son. Also, Mark's legal bind gave them few options but to comply with my request. In other circumstances, they might not have agreed to these terms.

As Mark and Cynthia often found themselves alone in the house, cleaning up the mess—both literally and figuratively—left by Jim's drinking, it would have made sense for me to help them sort out their feelings about these episodes. They could also have used strategies to cope better with Jim's drunkenness at extended family gatherings. I felt strongly that both mother and son's resentment and frustration about Jim's drinking had to be contributing to the conflict they experienced in their relationship with one another.

Today, if I think trying to help "the nondrinking spouse" hit bottom is needed in order to bring about any significant change, I will more often that not share this information with the couple or family. I will explain the ideas behind this kind of thinking, sometimes giving them a copy of Treadway's book, *Before It's Too Late*, or one of Berenson's articles, for example, and inviting people to discuss the merits of these ideas. I find this especially useful if I feel therapy is keeping a marriage afloat when it's already on the rocks.

In these instances the nondrinking partner often feels therapy provides a safe haven to discuss her concerns about her spouse's drinking. On the other hand, the drinker often attends therapy dutifully but makes it clear that he feels the process is just an excuse for the therapist and his spouse to "team up" on him. Here therapy, rather than introducing new ideas or offering a different way of talking about their problems, is simply mirroring the life of the problem and reinforcing both parties' position and opinion.

It is a dilemma. If therapy provides just enough help to ease the tensions caused by a family member's drinking, or offers just enough hope to keep a woman or man from giving up on their marriage, what motivation is there for the alcoholic to change? Conversely, therapy safeguards a future for people so that when and if they enter into recovery there is a marriage to which to return.

This last point I find especially poignant is when children are involved. Again, my job is not to resolve these dilemmas but simply to put them to people in such a way that they can grapple with them in a mindful way. Obviously, if people ask my opinion, I will offer it. Is therapy "enabling" problems in the present or "safeguarding" the future? Usually both. Couples need to think things down to the bone, so to speak, and decide which description of therapy resonates more for them at that particular time in their relationship.

The Metaphysics of Play-Doh: Including Young Children in Family Therapy

Little mention has been made thus far about the Kellys' 6-year-old daughter, Jill, or her participation in therapy. Leaving out the voices of a family's youngest members is a common mistake made in both the professional literature and our clinical practices, one that I, unfortunately, did little to correct here. However, as a rule, I always seek young children's participation in the therapy, especially in the early stages of the work. I find it informative to see how a family shares information and manages problems when small children are present. Also, children don't beat around the bush when it comes to saying what's on their mind or expressing their feelings about what's going on at home.

My desire to have children present has to be balanced with a family's need to protect young members from some of the upsetting topics discussed at therapy sessions. How a family fares in such attempts to protect the young can be diagnostic as well. My belief is that if children are present for the trauma surrounding a family's addiction or other troubles, then why not invite them to be present for at least some aspect of the healing as well? If a couple is able to compartmentalize their problems and keep them out of the ebbs and flows of family life or their children's daily routines, that is usually a positive sign. And, while a couple's inability to contain their anger during a session when young children are present is usually a sign of trouble, I make sure to give people credit for being able to bring their problems into the room in such a real and honest way. I tell them it shows me that they're really invested in getting help.

In the case of addiction, therapists need to be aware that sometimes drunk and crazy adult behavior becomes so ritualized in children's lives that they come to expect parents to have one set of behaviors when drinking, or at home, and another for when they are sober and in public. These codes of conduct are communicated to all family members. Again, the participation of young children can sometimes cut through this kind of denial because they don't always honor these behavioral codes or communication protocols.

In the first family session Jill attended with Mark and her parents, I asked, "Why do you think you are here?" She answered, "Because Mommy doesn't like it when Daddy drinks too much, and Mommy and Mark fight too much." When asked how she felt about Daddy's drinking, she said it didn't bother her because "He just falls asleep and I can watch what I want to on TV." She added that sometimes she wished Daddy wouldn't sleep so much so they could play more together. When asked what she thought of Mommy and Mark's fighting, she said, "It's loud." I asked her if their arguing bothered her, and she replied, "Only when it makes Mommy cry." Finally, when I asked Jill "If you could change one thing about your family, what would you change?," she answered, "Mommy and Daddy would have more fun together." Jill was sitting on her father's lap when this exchange took place. Jill was not fielding any job offers at the time, but she'd already helped me enormously with mine.

When seeing families with small children I try to have toys, art supplies, Play-Doh, etc. in the room or available to let parents know it's a safe place to bring children. I also learn a lot from how families play together. Are parents comfortable getting down on the floor with their children when a child asks them to draw with them? Do the children relate to both parents and vice versa? Do families, when using a messy material like Play-Doh, regress together or does one family member separate him- or herself from the group or get left out of the play? Does the play become angry and aggressive, and when it does how do parents respond?

I always encourage parents to bring small children to at least one or two therapy sessions as well as a couple of Al-Anon or AA meetings. I do this to enlist children's support for therapy and recovery, and to keep parents from undoing their progress in treatment in an effort to protect their children from "family secrets." I find children respond to parents' need to go to AA/Al-Anon/NA/OA/etc. similar to their need to go to work. When the reasons for these changes in their lives are explained and they know where their mom and dad are going, they feel more connected to family life and taken care of. Such meetings can also become a fun ritual if child care is offered, as children can develop friendships, experience safe and healthy play, and express their feelings with one another. In other words, the children have their own meetings. If it's not possible for children to attend meetings, I encourage parents and children to sit down with books such as Jill Hasting's and Marion Typpo's *An Elephant in the Living Room* and Claudia Black's *My Dad Loves Me, My Dad Has a Disease,* and tell children what the meetings are about.

The introduction of stuffed team members can be invaluable in these sessions. They're great interpreters of young children's thoughts and feelings, and often make it easier for adults to find the courage to say painful things for which they're having difficulty finding words. I have a gifted group of these interpreters in my office that I have been working with for years. The senior members of my team consist of Mr. Lion, Mr. Elephant, Mr. Wizard, and Anemone Witch. I always make a point of letting clients and other curiosity seekers know the stories behind each team member's career and how long each of the puppets has been part of the practice. I say that because they are puppets they are especially sensitive to the issues of control that often accompany problems associated with trauma and addictions.

Clients in crisis seem to appreciate these particular team members most. I think it's because these puppets have witnessed people experiencing so many different kinds of worries and problems without judging them, and they're also so good at keeping confidences.

Closure Is Hard to Come By

Unfortunately, the Kellys' lives did not proceed without further calamity. Seven years after our meetings together Jim died of a massive coronary. Cynthia sent me a card informing me. In it she wrote, "The death certificate did not say alcoholism, but it should have. I hope it's a wakeup call for Mark, who's started a family of his own now and is already showing signs of Jim's old habits. He is also following his father's foot-steps in more positive ways as well, pursuing a career in criminal justice." Cynthia said she would be in touch about finding someone Jill could talk with about Jim's death, and my heart went out to a 13-year-old girl who would no longer have her father.

While I realize now that I wasn't responsible for Jim's death, I certainly entertained those feelings at the time. Now, looking back, I see my response as an indication of just how much I joined with the family during our work. I shared their collective wish that something could have been done to change the course of events so that Jim could still be alive. One of the most frustrating aspects of this work is that even if you do everything right you may still not be able to avert this sort of tragedy.

Even so, Jim's dying felt unnecessary and probably could have been avoided. Ten years later I still get sad thinking about it. It reminds me that my zealousness about Jim seeking help for his drinking, while not always effective, was not unwarranted. Eventually, addiction always becomes a matter of life and death.

"TAKE WHAT YOU NEED AND LEAVE THE REST": REFLEXIVITY AND REFLECTING TEAM WORK WITH SUBSTANCE ABUSE

> What is invisible to us does matter. Sometimes it drives us, sometimes we are deprived by it.
> —DEENA METZGER

In AA, Al-Anon, and other 12-step recovery meetings, after participants share their drinking or substance abuse history (or, in the case of family members, their own story of recovery), how they got to the program, and what life is like sober, members are encouraged to "take what they need and leave the rest." The use of the reflecting team in family therapy as a way of offering families an array of ideas, thoughts, and reflections about their problems from which to choose is a therapeutic version of this same principle and complements AA's approach.

An innovation in the use of the two-way mirror in family therapy, this technique, pioneered by Norwegian family therapist Tom Andersen (1987, 1991, 1992, 1993), was adapted and expanded in this country by Lynn Hoffman (1990, 1993), Bill Lax (1992), and their colleagues at the Brattleboro Family Institute, as well as by Harlene Anderson and Harry A. Goolishian (1988, 1992) and the Galveston Group in Texas. Andersen offers the following definition of reflexivity as it is applied in this context: "Reflecting refers here to the same meaning as [that of] the French word *réflexion* (something heard is taken in, thought over, and the thought is given back) and not the English meaning (replication or mirroring)" (1992, p. 62).

In this practice, after observing a consultation between a family and a therapist, the team and the family trade places, and family members have the experience of observing and listening to the therapists share or reflect upon their thoughts and feelings about the family's predicament. The two groups trade places a second time, and the consulting therapist facilitates a conversation in which participants sift through the team's offerings and pick and choose (reflect back) those they found most useful or that resonate with their own experience (i.e., those ideas that fit with their own experience and story about themselves). The process may be repeated several times during the course of an interview. As a result, family members often describe feeling a strong sense of connection—what White and Epston (1991) call "communitas"—with therapist and team members.

In my own experience, therapy which employs reflections regularly takes on the call and response of a jazz concert. Ideas are shared in a give-and-take process that avoids methods which cause us to "practice down" to the people we see or that organizes our thoughts in a hierarchical fashion which weighs the therapist's ideas more heavily than the client's. Hoffman (1993) feels the process dramatically alters the family's position in relation to the professionals they come to see by introducing more equality between consultant and client, as well as generating more freedom for clients to accept or reject an idea. Hoffman describes a process that creates more "horizontal" and positive ways of working with families:

> People talking in front of a family had to abandon the clinical language that was usually used to describe family or individual dynamics. Phrases like "enmeshed family," "over-involved mother," "projecting," "controlling," and the like were not appropriate to this situation. Thus, the use of a reflecting team was as much of an influence on the professionals as on the family. For the first time in the history of psychotherapy, as far as I knew, a constraint against this blameful in-house discourse was put into place. (1993, p. 59)

In cases of alcoholism and addiction, when team members do their hypothesizing and thinking about the troubles of a family out in the open, it is good role modeling. Sharing their concerns with each other and the therapist and bearing witness to one another's grief and hurt is very healing. For many, this is their first experience talking about a loved one's addiction without using a currency of shame and blame.

Salman Rushdie said every act of writing is an act of censorship, as it prevents the telling of other tales. The use of the reflecting team in consultations with people provide clients and therapists with opportunities to tend to both the said and unsaid aspects of therapy. For example, a team observes a conversation between a newly sober alcoholic, his spouse, and their therapist. The couple is excited about the growing sense of intimacy in their relationship, which they attribute to their recovery in AA and Al-Anon. When it's the team's turn to reflect, one member might comment that because of her experience growing up with an alcoholic parent, whenever she received good news about someone's progress in AA she found herself waiting for the other shoe to drop— and wondered if either spouse ever found these sort of gloomy feelings interfering with his or her enjoyment of the relationship. Another member might ask whether the couple had any plans to celebrate this wonderful development or whether there were other people in their lives they could share it with who could appreciate what a significant achievement it was for them. Finally, another might ask whether in the midst of this type of intimacy the drinker and/or his spouse felt pressure to keep any doubts or fears they might have had about the alcoholic's ability to remain sober to themselves. Did they worry that raising these concerns might "spoil the moment"?[5]

The use of letters and other types of writing in therapy also allows for the exploration of these kinds of dialogues, offering therapists another way to attend to the unspoken aspects of a person's experience. Both innovations challenge the binary logic and "all-or-nothing thinking" which both clients and therapists alike can succumb to when trying to resolve painful problems in their personal and professional lives.

Seeing therapy as a collection of cultural narratives and personal stories encourages therapists to view their role as a process of moving from the center to the edge, rather than moving up and down a hierarchy (i.e., being "one up" or "one down"). Sometimes we are more central characters in the drama of people's lives; other times we rest at the perimeter of their stories. There is no canon, no story, that applies universally to all clients' experience.

These ideas have strongly influenced my work with families and individuals. In the Kellys' case, use of my cotherapist as a "team member" made it easier to introduce difficult material in a nonthreatening manner in the therapy, as well as allowing me to share it earlier in the work. They were also at play in my letter to Andrea (in Chapter 2), as well as the one to Sylvia and Jeff (in Chapter 5); although I was working alone, without the benefits of a reflecting team, I decided to share my thoughts with my clients as though we had one, thus allowing them to pick and choose the ideas that they found useful.

I also find letter writing a refreshing change from the conventional "discharge summaries" written in the cryptic discourse of our field. When I have had to write these documents to meet the requirements of a client's insurance plan or agency regulations, I try to write with my client as the audience.

Working with problems of substance abuse in therapy almost necessitates thinking systemically and viewing the whole family as the client. It also means defining success in less dramatic and more subtle ways. Seeing the alcoholic or addict become sober is not the only yardstick for measuring one's success when working with alcoholism or addiction. Therapists who work with alcoholism and addiction must be ready and willing to accept that they may only be present for part of a person's story, and not necessarily the most rewarding part. In fact, as said, too much attention focused on the alcoholic or addict and his or her drinking or drug abuse is often counterproductive, as it mirrors many of the family's failed efforts to get the person to stop or quit using.

We need to broaden our concepts of sobriety and success. Helping a 5-year-old child understand and cope better with a parent's alcoholism and/or seeing a family member find her or his way to Al-Anon are outcomes no less meaningful than helping someone get sober, and can lead to profound changes in people's lives and the life of the problem.

DETACHMENT WITH LOVE:
THE LEGACY OF VIRGINIA SATIR

Another popular metaphor for alcoholism is the story of the elephant in the living room whose presence no one wants to acknowledge. This metaphor highlights the shame and secrecy associated with the experience of addiction. It shows how certain family rules and practices—"Don't talk, don't trust, don't feel"—constitute alcoholism's life-support system. Sharon Wegscheider-Cruse (1981) and Claudia Black (1985) have applied and extended Virginia Satir's (1964, 1972) typology of family roles to the alcoholic family. These have included, in different incarnations, the family hero, the codependent or enabler, the lost child, the mascot, and the scapegoat. Satir's unabashedly loving and caring style was ideally matched to counter the rigid rules and role-play found in many alcoholic families. She also had a knack for transforming experiences of shame and derision into areas of radiance and pride.

While other therapists talked about the importance of people learning how to detach and differentiate themselves from their families, Satir showed us how. Also, when she demonstrated her techniques she never appeared to be fostering acts of independence that separated people; instead, her view of detachment seemed to foster more loving connections between family members. Hers was a healing voice to conjure up when working with addiction and other shame-based problems.

I honor Satir's legacy by sometimes discussing with families the creation of what I call a "no shame zone" in which we can talk about their experiences, problems, and concerns. While striving for an atmosphere of shame-free acceptance is an important goal in all family work, it is imperative in the case of addiction. If someone in the room feels unsafe talking about his or her feelings about alcohol or drugs, the discussion then proceeds to focus on what needs to happen in order for everyone to feel safe doing so.

In certain stages of recovery and therapy, therapists need to work extra hard to avoid interpreting, blaming, and judging family members' behavior. In my conversations with the Kelly family, for example, I ran into a lot of denial from Jim during the early phases of the work. During this period, I kept reframing the therapy away from him and back onto the family. I did this because Jim was not ready or able to look at his own drinking problem. At these times I would say to him, "Jim, it seems like you are feeling shamed and hurt, like you, and in turn, your father have done something terrible that has harmed the whole family. I don't want you to try and come to terms with this stuff or your feelings about your drinking or your father's drinking right now. It seems when you do that you feel attacked and then need to retreat and protect yourself. Then I end up trying to chase you down, and so we go around and around. I want you to try to stop kicking yourself and take some credit for allowing a forum in which we can discuss these issues."

IT TAKES A FAMILY OF WOMEN TO RAISE A MAN

Director and playwright Stanley Brechner (1997), when describing his work with the American Jewish Theater, once said:

When you hang your shingle out, and say you're the American Jewish
Theater there are certain people, including a portion of the American
Jewish Community, who don't want to come. They feel uncomfortable, like there's chicken fat on the seats. They think: "Why do I need
to go back and deal with this stuff? It's issues of the past." So when
somebody walks through the doors, there's a drama that's already begun. (p. 5)

Whenever I sit with a new family and hang out my family therapist
shingle, I'm reminded of Brechner's words. Family therapy is theater. It's
a form of human drama. Like theater, it's a way of remembering and retelling the past, and, like the themes taken up by the aforementioned
repertory company, therapy often brings up unpopular topics. This is
only one of the many things that Al-Anon and psychotherapy have in
common. People enter both looking for a common sea of experience,
and their objectives, once they find them, are often the same. Therapy
and Al-Anon allow family members to air their feelings and experience
one another's pain and perspective without judgment and blame.

For this reason I sometimes find it helpful to suggest that adult children attend an open AA meeting to listen for their parents' story, or send
the parents of clients to AA for similar purposes. Often I'll suggest to clients that they bring a photograph of their child or family member with
them to the meeting and place it on a chair beside them. This practice
doesn't necessarily lead to forgiveness, nor is it intended to, although it
may facilitate people's healing in this area. Rather, its purpose is to increase the amount of insight and compassion clients feel toward themselves by deepening their appreciation of the alcoholic's predicament—in
other words, to make them more aware of just how difficult are the challenges they face in recovery.

Peter, an 18-year-old with a serious drinking problem, said he'd
brought a picture of his alcoholic mother to an AA meeting so he could
feel like they'd gone to the meeting together. He said it made him cry because he was pretty sure this was as close as he would ever come to doing so with her.

Peter's Story

Peter was an inpatient in a dual-diagnosis program whose temper always
seemed to get the best of him, especially when he'd been drinking. Peter
was admitted to the hospital for depression. One night after coming
home drunk, Peter flew into a rage and threatened to kill his mother and

himself. Peter lived with his mother, but because of their fighting and his mother's alcoholism he spent much of his childhood moving between her house, his grandmother's house, an aunt's home, and more recently his sister's house. His father, a recovering alcoholic, hadn't had regular visits with Peter since his 10th birthday, even though his parents' divorce agreement allowed for it.

In the hospital groups, Peter described his estrangement from his father as a source of anguish and pain for him. He said he understood that his parents didn't get along and his mother continued to drink, so his father didn't want to see his mother. However, Peter couldn't understand why this affected his relationship with his father. He felt his father was "a real bastard for abandoning his children that way." I couldn't argue. I did, however, challenge Peter's insistence that his father no longer mattered and that he never wanted to see him again. Peter used his individual therapy sessions to express his anger and disappointment at both his parents for their drinking throughout his life. They were emotionally unavailable, and his father was literally gone after their divorce. This dynamic was painfully repeated during his hospitalization. His father refused to visit him and didn't respond to any of my requests to attend family sessions or participate in any kind of meeting related to Peter's care.

Toward the end of Peter's hospital stay I organized a family session attended by his mother, Dorothy; his sister, Sally; his aunt, Florence; and his maternal grandmother. At the beginning of the meeting, Sally said how angry she was with their father for once again leaving his son alone to sort out all his problems. Peter's grandmother also expressed her concern that he didn't have a man in his life to help him make decisions about his future. I said that I thought Peter took out his disappointment in his father on the women around him who, despite whatever shortcomings or limitations they might have had, were there for him when he needed them. The idea of Peter having had, in essence, four mothers standing by him through some very difficult times who had managed to raise an independent and strong-willed young man was a description that appealed to Peter and the rest of his family. It also helped Peter appreciate what a special kind of person he was to have such a powerful constellation of women rally around him. Peter was still despondent about his father's absence, but the image of his being raised by four strong women helped him understand that he wasn't any less of a man because of it. In fact, the opposite was true: these female role models appeared to be the source of Peter's sensitivity to others and his gentle way with his niece and other children.

Midway through the meeting Peter read a farewell letter to alcohol that he had written in the chemical dependency group:

Peter's Good-Bye Letter to Alcohol

Dear alcohol,

    I am finally confronting you as a sober person. I am writing you a letter to tell you how I feel. I am very pissed off at you, because you have affected my father in a negative way. But he has realized that he doesn't and never needed you as a friend. I hope that my mother finds out soon that she doesn't need you either. I would not like to see her get hurt or hurt anyone. I have also realized that I do not need you as a friend. That's why I have not talked to you in six weeks. I want you to know my niece is five years old and when she gets to be my age I hope she has more sense to stay away from you than I did.

Peter

When Peter was finished reading there wasn't a dry eye in the room. His mother said it took a lot of courage for Peter to share what he'd written and that she was proud of him. She also said she knew that she had a drinking problem and was aware that everyone else knew this about her as well. This led to Peter's grandmother and aunt (Dorothy's mother and sister) echoing Peter's concern about his mother's drinking. With her son grown up and needing to move on, they worried that the few "speed bumps" that existed in Dorothy's life to slow down her drinking were now gone. Peter's aunt said she had not talked to Dorothy in years because of her anger over her drinking and her abandonment of Peter and Sally when they were little. Dorothy responded that she only felt torn down and shamed in the presence of her family—never supported. It always felt, she said, that in order to accept their help she had to admit she was a total failure as a parent and a person. She didn't feel this was fair and pointed to her successful business as evidence of what she was saying.

Families are more willing to take risks and ask for help in hospital settings. It is important to take advantage of these openings without exploiting people's vulnerability, as family members have to live with the consequences of their actions and conversations long after their inpatient therapist and other caregivers have closed the file on their case. In these situations it is important to assess whether a family is capable of maintaining change as well as initiating it. This is particularly true when it comes to exposing family secrets such as parental alcoholism. While it is essential to validate a child's experience of a parent's addiction, it is not always necessary or wise to confront the parent. With younger children, it can result in their being blamed and punished for telling family secrets. With older children, if the confrontation has not been planned carefully and doesn't provide enough support for the alcoholic and other family members, the results can be even more disastrous. In both cases the child ends up feeling responsible for making the situation worse and may have difficulty feeling safe speaking to others about his or her concerns in the future. Sometimes simply coaching adolescents and younger children in ways to look out for their own safety is the most prudent tack. Needless to say, in cases where a child's personal safety is in question—when, for example, physical or sexual abuse is suspected—the therapist has no choice but to intervene promptly to protect the child.

In Peter's case I would have preferred his family to witness rather than join him in confronting his mother's drinking, but there was nothing I could do to stop it. Instead I shared with the entire group the concept of the "no shame zone" (used earlier in my work with the Kellys) and praised Dorothy, the way I did Jim, for having the courage to show up for this conversation and for allowing it to take place.

At the end of the meeting, Peter and his family agreed to meet again but this time to focus on where Peter was going after he left the hospital. Following that gathering it was decided that he would live at his grandmother's home in order to finish school and then get a job and live with Sally, his sister, until he decided to get a place of his own or go into the service.

"When You Come to a Fork in the Road, Take It"

Therapy with Peter revolved around a letter, not a genogram. Both are props. Neither tool replaces the trust earned within the context of a safe, caring, professional relationship. Nor do I see them as mutually exclusive. Often I use both, at different times, in my work with the same client or family. However, I prefer the tone set in consultations with clients when a letter is the centerpiece of the therapy rather than a genogram. A letter seems to capture more of people's lived experience without sacrificing their connection to their past. Letters also help me view the ideas I share with families as alternative stories about their predicaments rather than competing theories about what they should do about their addiction.[6]

Thinking about therapy as a collection of narratives or stories about people's experience makes it easier for me to accept the choices my clients make for themselves as the best ones possible at the time. This is preferable to seeing all disagreements as acts of resistance or noncompliance. Although words like "resistance" and "noncompliance" may, however infrequently, accurately describe specific clients' behavior in therapy, these terms, along with genograms (and the language used to interpret them), tell me more about the story of family therapy than stories about families. To put it another way, I find it easier to change my own or clients' stories about their experiences than to bend their experiences to fit my own or someone else's theories about them.

My therapy with Peter's family felt more fragmented than my work with the Kellys, perhaps as a consequence of an unconventional model of change. Of course their circumstances were somewhat different. But in addition, my own approach to therapy has changed. In my work with the Kelly family I saw therapy as something that we prescribed for people. If the medicine wasn't working, my job was to tinker with the dosage until I got it right. Or, again using the thespian metaphor, at the time of my work with the Kelly family I saw therapy as a sort of performance in which I was the director. In my work with Peter's family I was just another actor in the dramaturgy, and a supporting one at that.

Following the session in which Peter read his letter, I met with his mother to help her with her drinking. She attended some recovery groups at the hospital's day treatment program so she wouldn't miss work, but dropped out shortly after. She did call to tell me about her decision and said she intended to go to Al-Anon because she felt more comfortable there. I told her if she stuck with it I thought she would end up where she needed to be. Dorothy's mother (Peter's grandmother) came to see me on her own and with Peter. Both meetings were Peter's ideas. His grandmother talked mostly about her guilt at having not tried to do something to help Peter's mother sooner and for not realizing how awful things had been for Peter and his sister when they were younger.

After his discharge from the hospital, I continued to see Peter in my private practice. He managed to stay abstinent with the exception of a few slips while living at his grandmother's and attending school. Most importantly, he stayed out of trouble, passed all his classes, and received his high school diploma. After he moved to his sister Sally's home, at her insistence he started going to AA. He put together a year of abstinence and sobriety, held a steady job, paid his share of the rent, and started a savings account for college or to get his own place. During this period Peter brought Sally with him to a number of our meetings and they attended some ACOA (Adult Children of Alcoholics) meetings together.

Eventually Sally asked for a referral to see someone on her own to discuss some of the cutoffs and other experiences in her life that were causing her pain.

Peter also spent some time living with his dad–which he longed to try but had never spoken of because he didn't want to hurt his sister's feelings. Ironically, Sally told Peter she wanted him to spend some time with their father. She said that while she didn't feel she was ready to reestablish a relationship with him, she thought it was very important for Peter to try. She felt strongly that Peter was at an age when he needed to know more about his dad and that even if things didn't turn out the way he wanted, he would learn important things about himself. Sally's last point was a very wise one. It raised an important truth: *Just because a relationship might be damaged or broken doesn't make it any less important.*

Some of my favorite personal artifacts are faded, broken, chipped, or flawed in some fashion, such as the clay "tigerocerous" I made in second-grade art class that made its home in my father's office until his death. With the glaze now showing the effects of time—its blue and yellow stripes having lost some of their sparkle and luster—it has been missing a horn for as long as I can remember. This mammal (at the top of the endangered species list) now takes sanctuary in my living room. Like these treasured objects, both Peter's story and the Kelly family therapy serve to remind us that we don't need families that are undamaged, "perfect," or haven't lost any pieces in order to feel more whole, connected, and cared for.

HONORING OUR FOREBEARS

Every man is a quotation from all his ancestors.
—RALPH WALDO EMERSON

Many therapists express concerns that the contents of narrative and postmodern therapies represent, as the saying goes, "old wine in new bottles." In an effort to avoid having a similar complaint raised about this book, I want to close this chapter by paying homage to some of the profession's most treasured "objects" and honor some of the thinkers whose ideas I consider the precursors of many of narrative therapy's most salient concepts.

Harry Aponte (1976) championed the needs of the poor and people of color long before that concern was recognized as a "paradigm shift" in our thinking about therapy. He made the choices that he did in therapy not because the family therapy theories of his time advocated for clients' rights to self determination (they did not) but because he believed it was the right thing to do. Bateson, Jackson, Haley, and Weakland (1956)* and Carl Whitaker were challenging our thinking about language and traditional mental health constructs long before what sociologists call the "interpretive turn" took place in philosophy, psychology, anthropology, and other disciplines. Murray Bowen (1978), whose ideas were well represented in my work with the Kelly family and with Peter, said, "When the environment refers to the patient with 'sick' words, the patient tends to act as if he's 'sick.' If the environment can treat the patient as an adult, there is a chance for recovery" (p. 359). Most strikingly evident are the challenges feminist family therapists, who came of age in the women's and gay liberation movements, have posed to established and entrenched relations of power. Their efforts continue to bring issues of racism, sexism, gender identity, sexual orientation, and homophobia to the forefront of family therapy concerns.

My role in therapy with families suffering from alcoholism and addiction is to help their members examine and explore the significance of alcohol and drug abuse in their lives. While this is initially an educational process, helping people own the intense feelings of anger, despair, and hopelessness alcoholism and chemical dependency generate is paramount. People's affective experience must be dealt with in therapy because a purely cognitive approach perpetuates the process of having feelings deadened or ignored in a fashion characteristic of chemically dependent families in general.

More important than the specific theory or clinical approach we employ is the attitudes we model in session. What clients see us doing and how they experience the feeling and affect in the room is as important as what's said. This is reminiscent of Carl Whitaker's (1981) words that for therapy to be successful, clients must always have an emotionally meaningful experience in therapy, one that touches the deepest level of their personhood. The process is scary, exciting, immensely rewarding, and requires the therapist's intuitive and deeply personal involvement. It is the stuff of which intimacy is made.

---

*Although Whitaker was not listed as the coauthor on this work, he was an intricate part of the Symposium on which this collection of papers was based.

CHAPTER 10

Sobering Up Ophelia

Therapy with Children and Adolescents

Every Blade of grass has its Angel, that bends over it and
whispers, "Grow, grow."

—THE TALMUD

I met with a 17-year-old young woman, Katie, after she'd been released
from the hospital following a suicide attempt. Katie told me about a
night of doing crack at a stranger's house a month before she was hospitalized:

Katie's Story

It started with a glass of vodka and then he offered me the crack.
I'd been free-basing since I was 13 so I didn't think anything of
it. After we smoked the crack I started sweating and having a
major anxiety attack. I needed to go home but realized that I
reeked of alcohol and was soaking wet from perspiring so much.
He offered me a shower. I said yes but just to clean up and drive
home. The boundaries get so blurry in these places. I felt dizzy
and needed help finding the bathroom. I remember him kissing
me, and my not wanting him to. He stops and offers to help me
get into the shower, but is clearly resentful and being very
aggressive in his talk and body language. I told him I was okay
and would only be a minute. I threw up in the shower. There's
vomit everywhere it just keeps coming. I'm naked shivering up to
my own ankles in my own puke. Totally helpless. I'm just
standing there frozen, staring into space. I don't know how long
it was, but I'm guessing a while, because then he comes in and
starts to clean up, still angry. He says I can stay. He would still

235

like to be with me. Standing there naked and vulnerable I realize what a big man he is. I'm thinking how I know that his violence was part of why he broke up with his former girlfriend. I get cleaned up back in my clothes and make it home.

Nothing happens this time. I swear off hard drugs—again. And promise myself I'll stay out of the bars where I'm only going to meet people like this. But that's the only time I feel like interacting with other people, where I'm comfortable with myself, is when I'm drinking. Nice people they don't want to do that– drink all the time. So I made a compromise with myself. I told myself I'm not going to stop getting high (although I tried not to do it everyday) or drink but I'm going to stay away from bars and parties, and hard drugs—although I occasionally did heroin with my boyfriend, I never used needles or anything like that. Then I ended up in there [the hospital] following a blackout. I don't remember much but I guess I discovered that it doesn't take hard drugs to do crazy things. They told me I took a whole bunch of pills. I remember wanting to die and foraging through my parents medicine chest, but I wouldn't have had the nerve to do what I did if I hadn't been drunk.

The subject of drugs and booze never came up with the doctors in the hospital and when it did I simply denied it. A nurse in the ER asked me about my substance abuse history but I told her that it was my first time. That I'd heard if you took pills with alcohol it would kill you faster and hurt less, when it was really just the opposite. After drinking I became so depressed I couldn't imagine anything getting better, so I started looking around for a way to end it all. I don't know if I really wanted to die or not, but I was desperate to find a way to stop all the feelings and end the pain. In the hospital I would become so angry I couldn't control myself. I would get this terrible feeling in my stomach I could never explain. Now I recognize that I was in withdrawal. A psychiatrist said I was suffering from major depression and gave me massive doses of antidepressants and other drugs to help manage my anger. These helped me not miss alcohol and pot so much which, after the second or third week, was really starting to get to me. After I left the hospital I was able to trade and sell them for booze and other drugs.

I guess I didn't fit people's picture of what a dope fiend looks like so I kept flying under all their radar. After a while I started believing my own lies. I told myself that I couldn't be a junkie or a rummy even though, deep inside, I knew how much I needed my stash and that my Dad had a problem too. I was like a split personality. At school people only knew one side of me. No one ever saw the whole picture. It scared the hell out of my straight friends that I would even think of trying any of this shit. And to the druggies I was like "little miss perfect." They would never think to worry about me, even though I was doing way more than they were. I was always the one taking care of them when they were sick or in trouble. When I got into one of my rages they just thought I was being a spoiled little rich kid.

There were some secrets I couldn't keep covered up while in the hospital. The doctors felt I showed signs of sexual abuse. I was furious with them. How could they even say that to me. Abuse to me was something that happened to other kids, kids from bad families. Not me, from a good family. My parents, they were professionals with high standards, they would not let that happen to me. I couldn't remember so I figured they were wrong. I always blamed my anger on my father, who was, is, and always will be an alcoholic. He is not a "happy" drunk but a "tyrant" who would and still does abuse me emotionally. I grew up feeling I was worthless, ugly, fat, and stupid. I know now it's the alcohol talking. But a young child doesn't understand that. I had to find some way to numb my feelings.

I finally admitted to one of the nurses that I had been molested by an uncle and that I was having nightmares about it. I still can't remember everything, only segments of the abuse. I don't know the actual age it started. I was told that sometimes it takes years for survivors of sexual abuse to remember the details of what happened to them.

Looking back on my childhood, I see things more clearly now. Sometimes it's as if I'm trying to awake from a bad dream. While I was in the "cracker factory" I did some reading and discovered that women who were sexually abused as children are more likely to become addicted to alcohol and drugs. It's a way to numb feelings, suppress memories and escape pain. You know what's really pathetic—all this information didn't make a damn bit of difference. If anything it made me want to use even more. Hell, it gave me an excuse. I figured since all these terrible things happened to me I had a right to drink. I couldn't help myself!

Katie was clearly depressed, and her suicide attempt needed to be taken seriously. Whether killing herself slowly over time or in an impulsive act under the influence of alcohol, she needed help with a number of problems in her life, some related to her drinking and drug abuse, some not. However, by the time she was 12 her substance abuse was such a major part of her life that it made it impossible to sort all her problems out. Sometimes, children's identities have barely begun to coalesce when chemicals begin decaying and eroding their self-esteem and sense of self. As a consequence, there is virtually no earlier non-substance-abusing self, so to speak, or other emotional reserves to fall back on.

What do I do when an adolescent or young adult like Katie comes into my office? And what about the Katies I see who are just 13 or 14? Most teens can't reflect on their experience with Katie's insight. In either case, I contract. I contract with clients that they not get high or drink on the same day they have therapy. When they crash or try to hurt themselves, I contract with them for safety and use hospitals, wrap-around programs, and other children's services to help stabilize them. I direct them to support groups offered through my practice, their school, the Y, an outpatient clinic, or a partial hospitalization program. I refer them to Outward Bound and encourage their parents to do anything they can to enroll them in programs that will get them outdoors paddling in lakes, rafting in rivers, or climbing mountains. When they run away, I ask them to bring me something back from the place they ran to, any object that carries some significance to them, so I might better understand what they're searching for.* While they're missing, I spend lots of time on the phone trying to keep crazed and frantic parents from doing or saying something rash when they see or speak to their child next—things they may regret later. And I think about what I would do if I were in their situation. Mostly, I imagine how useless and shallow my advice might seem if it was my child that was missing.

I use writing. I ask adolescents to keep a journal and write letters to drugs, alcohol, parents, and themselves. I employ recovery literature and workbooks and recommend they read memoirs like Susan Kaysen's *Girl Interrupted*, *Go Ask Alice* (Anonymous), Elizabeth Wurtzel's *Prozac Nation*, and any other book I think a client may identify with. I look for any adult in their lives whom they admire who is trying to overcome an addiction or has had some experience in recovery that he or she can pass on. I suggest they bring trusted friends and family members to sessions who have expressed concern about their drinking and drug abuse, or others whom my client is worried about—"people who need the therapy more than me." The choices adolescents make, if they take me up on this offer, often tells me a great deal about how they see themselves and the problems they face. I listen to endless narratives about boyfriends which read like scripts of their love affair with chemicals—guys who, as one teenager put it, "made me feel wonderful when we first met and then left me feeling like 'a piece of shit.' " Sometimes these relationships are at-

---

*A gifted colleague and therapist, Ken Epstein has pointed out the following: "If you engage the runner the denial and hopelessness are befriended. If you engage the traveler artifacts and mementos can be shared and pondered" (personal communication, March 1999).

tempts to master the rejection and abandonment they experienced at the hands of their fathers, sometimes not. Sometimes alcohol and drugs mask other kinds of abuse, as in Katie's story, sometimes not.

In a word, I do anything I can to get children to reflect on their relationships and experiences with drugs and alcohol. I ask them to try favorite pastimes and activities—things they normally enjoy doing drunk or stoned—when sober. If they don't have any interests, I ask them to make a list of the three different kinds of nonchemically induced experiences that give them an adrenaline rush and terrify them most (e.g., skydiving, rock climbing, whitewater rafting, dancing, or acting in a school play) and encourage them to try them—to break the mold. The goal is to get their attention and create stories and experiences that can compete with alcohol and drugs.

Teenage girls may have an especially difficult time embracing this message about the need to take physical and emotional risks without worrying about what others will think. Preadolescence is a time when many spirited 10- to 12-year-old girls are ushered into a world of images and messages about their bodies and their personalities, most of which emphasize that the way they look and feel now is not good enough. It is, in short, a media and social hazing in which they're told what they are supposed to think, feel, look, and talk like in order to make themselves more attractive and appealing to boys and men. For many girls, substance abuse can be a way of putting distance between themselves and the demeaning messages they receive about themselves from the larger culture. In this instance, such chemicals act like a fire wall between them and the negative cultural stereotypes and impossible standards society sets for women.

Teenage boys also suffer from neglect and a lack of role models they can look up to. They may try to fill in the gaps with alcohol and other substances. Most male adolescents are longing for more physical affection in their lives and harbor a deep-seated need to feel loved and closer to others. Chemicals may provide a kind of triage for the splintered feelings caused by the lack of safe touch boys experience in their lives. Attempts at such intimacy are often met with cutting comments or labels like "mama's boy." These words are experienced as disparaging and hurtful because in our misogynist culture any strong associations with women or feelings thought of as feminine (that are not sexual) are, for males, seen as undesirable or a sign of weakness.

Homophobia is another leading factor in addiction, child abuse, suicide, prostitution, and homelessness among teens. Homophobia is also a contributing factor in the adult drinking problems of lesbian and gay couples and their families. Some adolescents may use alcohol to suppress their sexual attraction to a same sex peer or to cover up a homosexual crush on an adult mentor. Drugs can also medicate the kind of depression and suicidal feelings that stem from the impending exile or violence such teenagers anticipate should they decide to share their secret with family and friends. Or, conversely, some adolescents may use alcohol or drugs as a way to act on their homosexual desires without having to take ownership or responsibility for them. Finally, even for the most tough-minded kids, drugs and alcohol can be a way to shield themselves against the constant barrage of abuse that peers can cast because of sexual interests or orientation.

Adolescence is customarily a time when youngsters need to experiment. Discovering the possibilities and limits of their experience by pushing up against their families' established values and traditions is an important part of all teenagers' development. Teens are, in a sense, their families' cultural ambassadors to the world, venturing out into life and bringing back news of novelty and change. In the case of gay and lesbian families, children may face a paradoxical dilemma. How do young people rebel against society's established rules and norms when their parents' choices are, in the eyes of mainstream culture, more radical than their own? These teens often have to look for other means of protest—becoming, for example, more conservative than their parents or, in the case of gay and lesbian families, by using heterosexist language and adopting homophobic attitudes and ideas hurtful to their parents. Such role reversals and Faustian twists on the generation gap don't preclude other, more typical avenues of rebellion embraced by youth culture. Accordingly, alcohol and drug abuse remain steadfast ways for these and other teenagers to disrupt family life and give voice to their pain and confusion.

Some young people seem, in the course of their adolescence, to experience this entire laundry list of challenges and obstacles. Their stories have me reaching for every strategy and trick I can think of (and then some) in my efforts to help them. In these instances I often feel like I'm practicing what I call "lasagna therapy," because it has so many different layers.

SHELLY'S STORY

Shelly was a 16-year-old girl whose plummeting grades, school absences, and legal troubles alarmed her mother, Julie. Shelly had been arrested for stealing a bottle of liquor from a package store, but she maintained that she was just holding the bottle for her boyfriend. In addition, one of her best friends told Shelly's mother that Shelly had recently confided in her about having tried "acid" with her boyfriend. Shelly swore to her mother that it was the first time she'd ever done anything like that. She said she knew right away what an awful mistake she'd made and that she would never do it again. Shelly's parents had been divorced since she was a small child. Part of an agreement Shelly made with her mother was that in exchange for not telling her father about either incident Shelly would see a therapist.

In our first session Shelly asked me a lot of questions about LSD and any side effects it can cause. When I asked her why she was so concerned about the physiology of the drug if she had just used it the one time, she responded that she'd heard that in some cases just one trip could cause permanent brain damage in people or birth defects in their children. Shelly then said she'd tripped half a dozen times in the past couple of months and that she'd just found out she was pregnant. She said her main concern was for her unborn child and any possible effects the LSD might have on the baby.

Shelly hadn't told her mother about the pregnancy and was concerned that her mother would be angry with her for wanting to keep the child. Shelly said she hadn't wanted to get pregnant, but what made it especially lousy timing was that she had just broken up with her boyfriend. Her family did not approve of their relationship because of how he mistreated her. She added that she had been mad at him because he'd been cheating on her. Finding out she was pregnant changed all that. She just wanted to be with him.

Adding to Shelly's problems was her estrangement from her father because, as Shelly put it, "He got tired of my lying and stealing." Shelly had been having difficulty getting along with her mother as well. The formerly close relationship between mother and daughter had been strained of late, and not just because of Shelly's troubles. Following a long period of being on her own, Julie had begun a new relationship, and Shelly had many of the usual jealousies. For example, even though she liked her mother's new partner, she also resented the relationship because she felt it consumed altogether too much of her mother's time. However, Shelly was also angry with her mother because her mother's new lover was a woman.

This wasn't her mother's first lesbian relationship, but as Shelly had become older she'd become more aware of her classmates' snide and hurtful remarks. This made life harder and more unpleasant at school.

Because she lived in a small rural community where few supports existed for gay and lesbian families, there was little shelter for Shelly from this kind of prejudice.

Shelly complained that her mother always seemed to make the most difficult choices possible, drawing unwanted attention to herself and her kids. I commented that if it was Julie's standing out in a crowd Shelly was concerned about, it seemed to me she'd certainly found a way to "one up" her mother.

My next meeting was with both Shelly and her mother. Shelly was right. Her mother was very concerned about her decision to keep her baby, but not for the reasons Shelly imagined. Julie didn't blame Shelly for getting pregnant; rather, she worried about Shelly being able to finish school and whether she was prepared for the responsibilities and burdens of motherhood. Julie was concerned about her own future as well. Having already parented three children, mostly on her own, Julie was afraid that the lion's share of the responsibility for raising Shelly's baby would fall on her shoulders. With her own children mostly grown, Julie was just starting to feel "like there was life after parenting" and was looking forward to putting more of her energy into her relationship and career. Julie looked forward to eventually being a grandparent; it just wasn't a role she'd imagined assuming this early.

Shelly's crisis felt as though it had the potential to either unite or break apart mother and daughter. My hope was to build on the feeling that Shelly and Julie were in this together. D. W. Winnicott's (1965, p. 39) well-known aphorism that "there is no such thing as a baby" underscores the intense dependence of infants on their mothers and rings just as true for the relationship between teenagers and their parents. We might paraphrase Winnicott by saying that there is no such thing as an adolescent because so many teenagers who come into our offices have anxious and concerned mothers, fathers, or guardians in tow. The bonds that hold them together may be more tenuous than the infant–mother bond, and the feelings of affection and closeness between them are often more frustrating than tender; nevertheless, as suggested in Winnicott's words, "if you set out to describe an adolescent, you will find you are describing an adolescent *and someone*," and the two parties often seem like one.[1]

I find Shelly's case useful for teaching purposes because it doesn't follow any of the usual trail maps. For Shelly and her mother what initially felt like one of the worst scenarios they could imagine facing ended up being the best thing that ever happened to them, but the road to that "happy ending" was a bumpy one. While Shelly's pregnancy rallied mother and daughter and temporarily took the focus off Shelly's other problems, the "miracle of birth" did not make Shelly's troubles disappear.

Using People's Natural Helping Networks

Shelly tried to get her boyfriend, Brandon, to attend therapy with her after she discovered she was pregnant. Brandon refused, but he did agree to come in for one meeting. Brandon made it clear that he didn't agree with Shelly's decision to keep the baby but said he respected her feelings and wanted to take responsibility for both Shelly and the baby when he was able to get back on his feet. Shelly said she didn't want to wait that long to be a family. With my support Brandon was able to convince Shelly that she could not come live with him since he was, as he described it, homeless, sleeping in the woods, and barely managing to take care of himself. He said that by Shelly making the care of herself and their unborn baby a priority, she would alleviate some of the stress he was experiencing in their relationship. This, he explained, would allow him to focus on taking better care of himself. I offered to help him find a bed in a shelter and other assistance, but he refused—saying he preferred to work out his problems on his own.

Six months later, Shelly had a healthy baby girl, Ariel. However, like many young parents, she struggled with the tension of having to be a mother and still feeling like, and needing to be at times, a child herself. While pregnancy and a commitment to bringing a healthy baby into the world had provided a creative solution to Shelly's drug problem, it wasn't permanent. Shelly went back to getting high and to an abusive relationship with Brandon, whose efforts to turn his life around were floundering even though he now had found a place in town to live.

One of the most difficult tasks I faced was the conflict between my desire to support Shelly's emerging identity as a young mother and my agreement with her mother that some of Shelly's choices were not in the best interest of Ariel. Shelly had an agreement with her mother that she would spend a certain number of nights at home with Ariel, which meant limiting her contact with Brandon. Worried that Brandon would give up on their relationship if she didn't make herself more available, Shelly began bringing Ariel with her when she went to see him. This unfortunately resulted in Ariel being exposed to Brandon's drinking and drug abuse and to the volatility of their relationship.

Prior to contacting social services, Shelly's mother asked for me to help intervene in Shelly's life without involving the courts or an outside agency. Even though she felt the need to set limits on Shelly's behavior and protect her grandchild, Julie was terrified at the prospect of getting social services involved in Shelly's situation. Because of her homosexuality, involving a state agency in their lives made Julie incredibly vulnerable. Ironically, from the standpoint of the courts and society, an angry and confused substance-abusing teenager neglecting her baby's needs has more rights and power than a responsible and concerned gay parent.

Regardless of the circumstances, it's always preferable for people to use their own resources to solve their problems. Consequently, I suggested that Julie arrange a meeting with some of Shelly's family and friends. I also encouraged her to express her concerns directly to Shelly and to solicit her input about who she thought should attend this gathering. In our individual therapy sessions I invited Shelly to help create an agenda for the meeting and, when the time came, to take an active role in the discussion.

Whether I've contracted to do family therapy with a person or not, I often ask adolescents to consider bringing friends, family, and significant others to sessions. In cases of addiction, I find this helps break down clients' sense of isolation and any feelings of shame they may be experiencing about their situation. It offers me (and the clients) a perspective on their life that I wouldn't otherwise be privy to, and it helps them to consider the way their actions affect others. In other words, these networking sessions provide a context for competency, emphasizing stories of connection and support that can be built on.

Also, as mentioned earlier, who adolescent clients choose to bring with them provides insight into how they perceive their problem. If, for example, they bring individuals who are as concerned about them as their parent or guardian is, in addition to making my job easier, it tells me that my clients may be eager to get help—as it would have been just as easy to bring people who would minimize their problems and help them cover up their behavior. However, if the friends they choose to invite are, from the standpoint of alcohol and drugs, in worse shape than they are, that may represent their fears about the direction in which they're headed or help me understand what pieces of their support system are missing or need shoring up. Also, if teen clients bring drug-addicted friends in to support them in continuing to drug or drink, they may be in for a surprise. Sometimes, the invited guests talk about how their life might have been different had they had a similar opportunity, and they don't want to be responsible for someone else not getting a shot at a better life.

This was the predicament Shelly faced in her relationship with many of her friends, and, in a way, even with her boyfriend, Brandon. Despite Brandon's destructiveness to himself and Shelly, in the one session he did attend he was able to express his desire that Shelly reach for a better life than what he believed—and perhaps rightly so—was possible for him. Shelly decided not to bring Brandon to the meeting.

Although the networking session with Shelly did not forestall the necessity of involving social services, it did help create a less adversarial relationship between Shelly, Julie, and her other family members. It kept a dialogue going among them all. It also helped Julie and Shelly to feel less isolated, a challenge for any family with a new infant.

The basic issue of substance abuse and addiction is that it lacks integrity. We doubt our own integrity, so we cut ourselves off from the gifts reality is ready to heap on us.[2] Shelly was struggling with a similar quandary. She had been blessed with a beautiful daughter, and despite the concerns her family expressed earlier, they welcomed Ariel into their lives. Ariel's birth brought Shelly face to face with reality, and, like many of us, what Shelly didn't like about reality was that it respected her. Shelly could no longer hide behind a rebellious persona and blame her decision to engage in dangerous and unhealthy behavior on her family's unkindness or neglect. Being a mother exposed Shelly's compulsions, especially her desire to please men. She had to choose between a very real and exhausting life with her "perfect" child and imperfect but loving family, on the one hand, and an idealized or fantasized relationship with an abusive boyfriend and the escape from other more painful feelings that relationship provided, on the other.

When asked by Shelly's social worker to document my contact with Shelly and her mother, I wrote a letter in which I tried to capture some of the dilemmas Shelly faced and to offer my thoughts about what we could do to help her:

Excerpts from My Correspondence to Shelly's Caseworker

Dear Ms. Kegan,

Although I know Shelly does not agree, I feel that most of her problems stem from her being isolated and continuing to participate in an emotionally and, on at least one occasion, physically abusive relationship with her boyfriend. Although it has gotten easier for us to speak about the situation, it is still very difficult for Shelly because she is very much in love with this young man and now has a child with him. Adding to the strain of our conversation is the reality that no one in Shelly's family likes or gets along with her boyfriend because of their feelings about how they have seen him treat her in the past and how they perceive him treating her now. Consequently, Shelly ends up feeling very alone in the relationship and her hopes for it to be different. I know that it has helped our discussions that I have tried hard not to be judgmental of her boyfriend as a person and limited my responses to my feelings about his behaviors and actions, as well as what kind of responsibilities in life I see him ready to take on—and how I perceive those to be different from Shelly's and her current needs from a partner.

I believe it is Shelly's relationship with her own mother (and support from her father and other family members) past and present that allows her to be such a good mother to Ariel. I believe Shelly's relationship with her boyfriend colors her judgment at times and keeps her from being present for Ariel in the best way she knows how and wants to be. It is my understanding that this is what resulted in Shelly's mother, with much reservation and angst, filing a 51A [a child abuse report] and seeking support and services from DSS [the Department of Social Services]. The rest of Shelly's family, in a meeting in which Shelly was present, told her they also felt such action was necessary. I also supported that decision.

Unfortunately Shelly's visits with her boyfriend resulted in Ariel being exposed to a physical environment that was unsafe and inappropriate for a baby. I believe this *situation* and those *circumstances—not* Shelly—were documented and found unfit for a baby subsequent to the DSS investigation. In our conversations Shelly acknowledged that she would find it unacceptable if a baby-sitter, for example, exposed Ariel to some of the experiences and practices that Shelly herself was involved in when spending time with her boyfriend. In fact, Shelly has said that she would find it totally unacceptable if, in the future, a boyfriend treated Ariel in the same way that Shelly's boyfriend often treats her— although she has said that if that were ever to happen to her daughter she might not interfere because she knows what it feels like to be in that position.

Sadly, in my experience, when a person is 17, 18, or older, any attempt to directly intervene in destructive and unhealthy relationships is futile at best and can in many instances make the situation worse. In my experience parents, siblings, friends, advocates, and counselors are better off supporting that person's participation in therapy, women's services, and continuing to provide an alternative to abuse in the form of safe, loving, and caring relationships. However, a situation in which a person's involvement in an unhealthy relationship puts a child or infant at risk is unacceptable and some kind of intervention or action is warranted, and in many cases mandated by law. It is this kind of problem that Shelly's mother and family were faced with and responded to. It was *not* their lack of faith in Shelly's role as a parent or her love for her daughter. Shelly's family—especially her mother—believe that outside of her *present* relationship with her boyfriend Shelly is a capable and good mother to Ariel.

At this juncture in Shelly's life, I feel strongly that making her choose between her boyfriend—the father of her child—and her baby is a grave mistake. Ultimately, in such a scenario, I think it is Ariel who would stand the most to lose. Ariel and Shelly need any and all healthy contact between them supported and encouraged. Placing restrictions or conditions on contact between Shelly and her baby that she cannot meet is not in mother or daughter's best interest. If the environment created when Shelly is with her boyfriend and Ariel cannot be improved and/or Shelly cannot make sound judgments about what is safe for Ariel in those situations, DSS should advocate that temporary custody continue to be granted to Shelly's mother. To me that seems the most logical and compassionate stance.

Sincerely,

Jonathan Diamond

cc: Shelly West
    Julie West

Following the DSS investigation, temporary custody of Ariel was granted to Shelly's mother. During that time Julie, Shelly, and Ariel continued to live together in Julie's house. With her mother's support, it took Shelly 6 months to have custody of her daughter returned to her. She also honored her agreement with her mother to stay in school and walked across the podium at her graduation with her baby in her arms. To Shelly's delight the local newspaper did a story on her and Ariel and her experience as a student mother. After graduation Shelly remained in an off-again/on-again relationship with Brandon for several years. They tried living together, but that didn't work out. Eventually, she left him for good. Shelly is now in school at the community college where her mother teaches. She recently took her mother's course, which was a bonding experience for them both, and now is planning on pursuing an advanced degree.

Therapists in the Nursery

Therapists often use pregnancy and birth as metaphors for therapy. The analytic dialogue or therapy relationship are seen as "fertile ground" for creating new meaning in people's lives. We refer to thoughtful pauses in the conversation as "pregnant pauses" because of the infinite possibilities the discourse holds for its participants. However, in my therapy with Shelly this metaphor took on a more literal meaning.

As mentioned in my letter to Shelly's social worker, my support for Shelly's decision to keep her baby had a positive effect on our relationship and the outcome of the therapy. In one sense, this development, not unlike Shelly's pregnancy, was unplanned. Supporting Shelly in her choice just seemed like the right thing to do. In another sense, how I chose to demonstrate that support was a more mindful process.

As a consequence of the adverse circumstances she faced, Shelly received a lot of input from people, some solicited, some not, about what she should do about her pregnancy. Relatives, friends, guidance counselors, her mother, all with Shelly's best interest at heart, asked her to consider having an abortion. Shelly took their advice under consideration but still felt strongly about keeping the baby.

It was difficult for me to resist the temptation to join the chorus of advice givers. I was concerned about the consequences of Shelly's decision to bring a child into her life at this time. However, I recall feeling that I hadn't earned the *author*ity to comment on such a deeply personal and intimate aspect of her story yet (remember, Shelly told me she was pregnant in our first session). There were many people in Shelly's life offering her counsel whose relationships were stronger, had more history, and were more influential than mine. Consequently, I decided that the best way to distinguish my voice was by keeping silent and providing Shelly a quiet space to sit with her own thoughts on the subject.

Another feeling I had was simply that if a young woman could stand her ground in the face of all this pressure and still feel as strongly as Shelly did about keeping her child, that was, in all likelihood, what was going to happen. This led me to think that if I had any chance of safeguarding a future for our therapy relationship—something I felt she needed now more than ever—I wouldn't help my cause any by participating in what felt to Shelly like a public referendum on her life and a unanimous vote against her decision.

I did ask if the feeling of isolation she was currently experiencing had any effect on her desire to have a baby. Did she think that having a child would give her a companion to love and who would love her back no matter what? She replied that she worried about becoming even more isolated if she chose to keep her baby because it might make so many people angry with her. When Shelly asked what I thought about her becoming a mother, I was honest with her. I told her that after 10 years of being in a relationship with the same person I was ready to start a family myself and yet I felt unprepared even after all this planning. I said I could only imagine what the financial and emotional burdens of the experience would feel like to two teenagers. I also expressed some worry about how much her life would change if she ended up raising the child on her own, but I told her these concerns would not change my support for whatever choice she made.

There were other themes I could have explored with Shelly: among these were issues that many of us were worried she wasn't thinking about—unconscious plots and storylines—that might have been influencing her decision. Did she think that she and her boyfriend would start up again and get along happily if they had a child together? Was this an attempt to heal any scars left over from her parents divorce (i.e., to mend a broken home and get her family back)?

The answers may all have been yes, and some of the ideas these questions raise are not foreign to any of us who have had similar childhood experiences and started families of our own. What's more, the reality is that grandchildren often do mend old hurts and cutoffs between people, and it was part of the effect that Ariel's birth had on Shelly's family. However, the exploration of these themes, some of which were introduced by Shelly herself during the course of the therapy before Ariel's arrival, didn't influence Shelly's resolve one way or another. So instead, I asked her what she needed from me during this time while she contemplated her choices. This, in fact, ended up being very little.

However, once Shelly made her decision and she and her mother were working together on preparing their home for the new family member, Shelly began using therapy to explore both her excitement and her fears— "terror" was the word she used—about becoming a mother. How would she know what to do? What if there was something wrong with her baby? She had nightmares about all the things that could go wrong. None of them came to fruition, and she gave birth to a healthy baby girl.

After Ariel was born, Shelly took a brief leave from therapy. Shortly after she started up again, she asked me if my wife and I had decided to start a family of our own yet. I told her that we were in fact going to have a baby. She smiled and said that she had a feeling this was the case. She offered to pass on anything about the experience that might be helpful to me. I accepted Shelly's offer.

During this time she was bringing her mother and/or Ariel to one session and attending the next on her own. As a consequence, I was able to witness many tender moments of laughter and joy between Shelly, Ariel, and Julie as they discovered what life together would be like. I also developed a deeper appreciation of the monumental changes a being this little can bring to family life and relationships. I looked forward each session to seeing and hearing what Ariel was up to so that I could brace myself for some of the developments that were in store for me with my own infant and family. I also listened intently to Shelly's list of things she wished she'd had in her possession when she brought Ariel home. There were also those things which she'd purchased or had asked for because she assumed they were essential, and then found that they never made it out of the packaging.

During one session, as I sat diligently writing the names of the products Shelly rattled off, I remember thinking that there was a third set of items Shelly hadn't mentioned: "things she'd acquired or been given that she never thought she'd need or use but were surprisingly helpful." I think therapy probably fell under that category.

Seeding the Clouds

I want to stress again that while the story of Shelly's therapy, especially the ending, has a certain symmetry to it, the work itself was not always smooth. Brandon, for example, was a very troubled young man but he was not the devil incarnate. Besides being Ariel's father, which meant Shelly's attachment to him would always be significant, he made several genuine attempts, with the help of his own family, to clean up his act and be a more responsible partner for Shelly and a better father for Ariel. Unfortunately, none of these efforts worked. During periods when Brandon was trying to straighten out his life, relations between Shelly, her mother, and Brandon were very problematic. When Shelly's relationship with her father was added to this already complex mix, therapy became nearly impossible.

It was a mistake on my part not paying more attention to Shelly's relationship with her father, Steve. Had I done so, I might have had more of an impact on this aspect of Shelly's life than I did. At a minimum, I could have avoided repeating the pattern that Shelly and her mother had established of buffering Steve from the worst of the bad news about Shelly's life and then expecting him to respond with an open heart in a crisis. Even if Steve had decided he wasn't able to do more than he was doing, at least it would have put the responsibility for changing his relationship with his daughter back onto him where it mostly belonged.

Adolescence is a challenging time for fathers and daughters under the best of circumstances. In girls' odyssey out of childhood, their bodies, emotions, and psyches undergo dramatic changes. These create awkwardness and tension in the relationships with their fathers that many men are not prepared for. Emergent sexual feelings, menstruation, dating, and intense mood swings are just some of the changes that occur during this phase of life. In many cases, the new pressures replace a comfortable sense of familiarity that existed between parent and child. Add substance abuse, pregnancy, and quick tempers into the equation, plus a number of other problems Steve and Shelly experienced in their relationship, and it isn't hard to understand why father and daughter had become estranged.

I found myself caught in this relational matrix when I received an angry call from Shelly's father. Steve was upset that he hadn't been asked to participate in the meeting with Shelly at my office prior to Shelly's mother filing the 51A. He also said that until he found out about the meeting he had no idea that Shelly was still in therapy and requested "weekly updates" on our sessions. Following our conversation, Shelly's father declined all my invitations to meet with us. Subsequently, I tried to reach out to him in a letter:

Excerpts from My Correspondence to Shelly's Father

Dear Steve,

I feel it was remiss on my part not to have at least cautioned Shelly to think about how her decision to not have you there would impact on her relationship with you—regardless of how the two of you were getting along at the time—or how it might make you feel. I take responsibility for this oversight, and although having this conversation may not have changed the outcome of the events it may have resulted in the feelings surrounding them being different. Again it was pragmatics that informed the decision (made in response to a crisis), and it was not my intention to make you feel excluded or left out.

As I shared with Shelly, at this point in her therapy I feel yours and her relationship is the area of her life that is most in need of tending to. Shelly is by her own and her mother's reports getting along better with her mother and her brothers at home, making more informed decisions about her health, setting up and keeping her appointments to apply for public support to help her with the baby, and pursuing employment. Currently, the most glaring absence in her life is the cutoff between the two of you. I now know how upsetting this state of affairs is to you and have known for some time how much it concerns Shelly even when she tries not to let on how much it hurts her. I do not think it matters how, or with whom, the two of you sit down to have this conversation with but feel it would be sad if this did not happen sooner than later. I also shared these opinions with Shelly following my conversation with you last week.

Steve, I am going to say something that may be hard for you

to hear and hope I am not overstepping my bounds by doing so. However, based on our brief phone contact and your note my sense is that you are a person who does not "pull any punches," so to speak, in your interactions with others and prefer to have people treat you the same way. I believe that some of the distance between you and Shelly stems from the perception Shelly has that she needs to buffer or protect you from some of the unsettling and upsetting truths and events of her life. It is clear that she knows you love her and care about her, but feels when faced with upsetting news about her life you retreat from the relationship until she is able to find some way to present things in a fashion you find acceptable, or the trouble has passed. Obviously, that has been a more daunting task for her lately.

Despite the contrite tone I took in my letter to Shelly's father, I also, in this communication, tried to respond to what I considered some dangerous undercurrents in the family's thinking regarding the possible causes of Shelly's substance abuse and other troubles. One of the more potentially damaging ideas was that Shelly may have gotten herself pregnant as a way to distance herself from Julie's lesbianism and to announce her heterosexuality with authority. Another was that Julie's being gay was having an adverse effect both on Shelly's judgment and behavior and also on Julie's ability to supervise Shelly.

As a result, following her divorce, Julie's behavior as a mother was assessed by different standards than her ex-husband's. For example, at a time when most parents are encouraged to model healthy loving relationships for their children, Julie's ability to "protect" her children was judged more by her ability "to act with discretion" and keep her personal relationships out of the home. In fact, rather than viewing Julie's having found a new mate as a positive development for both herself and her family, it was seen by many members of her family as something that could cause harm to the children.

Ironically, this is one predicament Julie and Shelly shared and were able to discuss in therapy. Although the circumstances were very different, both mother and daughter understood how painful it is to have a relationship in exile (i.e., to feel pressure to keep something or someone that means so much to you separate and cut off from the rest of your life). What made this particularly difficult for both mother and daughter is that these situations transpired at times when each woman ought to have been discovering ways to integrate—not exclude—intimate relationships into family life. In fact, from a relational perspective, rather than being seen as a distancing move, Shelly's choice of boyfriend can be interpreted as an act of loyalty to and identification with her mother.

Another popular misconception the family story about Julie's lesbianism fed was linked to the issue of whether a parent's sexual orientation has any bearing on her or his child's choices or predisposition to homosexuality or heterosexuality. The popular myth is that it does (i.e., that gay parents inevitably raise gay children). Research refutes this myth. One unfortunate outcome of this thinking is that people start to believe they can control or influence another person's sexual desires and choices.

Adolescents and adults need guidance and support, not myths and stereotypes, to help them cope with internalized forms of oppression and the confusing and contradictory feelings they generate. My intention, in my correspondence to Shelly's father, was not only to counter and discourage this kind of thinking but to introduce a more positive story about the influence of Julie's "coming out" on Shelly and her brothers, stories in which Shelly and her mother could take pride.

I was also trying to underscore that I do not regard fathers (or any parent) as peripheral to their child's life. Living or dead, married or divorced, loving or hating, distant or close, these relationships are sacred to people and, regardless of their status, helping clients come to terms with their feelings about them is paramount. These absences and presences are always in the room when we consult with clients. Encouraging people to show up for them is more important than telling people what to do about them.

Steve never responded to my letter, although I heard from Shelly at the time that he was still very upset. Currently, I do not know what, if anything, has changed between father and daughter. Obviously, a great deal has changed in Shelly's life. The thing about such a letter is that people can return to the ideas shared in it if and when they're ready. It is, in my metaphoric shorthand, a way of seeding the clouds.

(W)RITES OF PASSAGE: ADOLESCENCE AND THE FORMATION OF AN ALCOHOLIC OR RECOVERING IDENTITY

> *Newcomer:* How long do I have to keep going to these
> meetings?
> *Old-timer:* Only until you want to.
> —*LIFELINES*[3]

The phrase "once an alcoholic always an alcoholic" is one of the mantras of AA, and its members and other recovering persons take this slogan seriously, nurturing their recovering identities indefinitely over a lifetime. The medical community echoes the same sentiment, telling patients there is no cure for addiction but that it can be effectively "managed" in remission if a person commits to an ongoing regime of abstinence, therapy, self-help, and medication when necessary.

This kind of commitment is too much to ask of most teenagers. When I am asked to meet with an adolescent with a substance abuse problem, or speak with the parents, I make known my reluctance to label a teenager's condition alcoholism or addiction right away. This puts both child and parent more at ease. If people know up front how conservative I am in my use of these classifications, it makes them more open to hearing what I have to say, especially if I think their situation is serious. Therapy with substance-abusing teens, and with adolescents in general, often has a "drive-thru" feeling to it. Even within the context of a long-term relationship, I find myself stealing moments away from other conversations in order to introduce the topic of drugs and alcohol in a young person's session. Over time I try and build on these moments, stringing several together till they add up to an actual conversation. If I am patient and wait until clients invite me to speak to their experience— offering me what I like to think of as a spiritual entry point into this aspect of their life—eventually a genuine dialogue about the nature of their relationship with chemicals unfolds. The key is not ignoring what ails them or appearing too eager to get to my own agenda.

Judy was a 17-year-old young woman who was referred to me after she was arrested for buying pot. Her parents felt her problems stemmed from her drug use and said until she straightened her act out they no longer wanted anything to do with her. Judy said she abused drugs because she was depressed. Judy never missed an appointment and stayed for the entire hour. However, while in my office she said very little. She didn't want to talk about her depression or her drug abuse. One day Judy showed up with a brown paper bag in her hand which she held in her lap during the session. When I asked her what was in the bag she blushed and said face cream. She told me that she had terrible acne but that people couldn't tell because she did such a good job of covering it up with makeup.

I asked if I could see the face cream. She handed it to me. I held up the container to the light and examined it closely. "It's a beautiful jar," I said admiringly. "It smells nice too," I added. Judy looked at me in a funny way and laughed, as if the sight of a man taking such interest in a cosmetic item wasn't something you saw everyday. "You spent a lot of money on this. Does it work?" I asked. "Most of the time, unless it's really bad," she replied. "And if it doesn't?" I asked. "If it doesn't," said

Judy, "my mother and I get into a huge fight because I refuse to go to school. When I was younger I was teased mercilessly by the other children in school. If I have a really bad outbreak, I won't even leave the house." I thought about the shame Judy must experience during those bouts with her skin and appearance and said to her, "Let me share with you my only personal association with makeup," and proceeded to tell her the following story from my own mother's youth:

> "When my mother was your age she and her sisters used to get their hair done together. My mother lived in New York City. So every Saturday she and her sisters would march off to this one particular boutique on West 72nd Street in Manhattan. The store receptionist had an arrangement with the owner to sell her own line of cosmetics, which she made from scratch in her garage. These and other beauty products were displayed on a counter at the front of the store. If customers couldn't find what they wanted at the counter, and the receptionist wasn't at her station, they would ask the owner for help. The owner would look for the product and if she couldn't find it she would yell for her assistant in a voice that Mom described as a deafening nasal shrill, like the sound of the brakes on a subway train, 'ESTEE!!' [I used my heaviest New York accent to impersonate the shopkeeper's shrieking voice for Judy]. Then this very demure young woman whose other duties included sweeping hair and stocking shelves would come from the back of the store to continue the search. Mother said they always felt mortified for this poor girl when the store owner shouted her name like that. However, they stopped feeling sorry for her a long time ago, because Estee did quite alright for herself. My mother still can't look at an advertisement for Estee Lauder's cosmetics without hearing that shrill voice calling out her name. But, as Mom is quick to point out, 'The only place they shout her name like that now is on Wall Street.' "

Judy thought it was a riot that that shy store clerk had become the founder of the Estee Lauder cosmetics empire. I don't know what sense Judy made of my telling her this story. I do know that from that moment on the connection between us was a much stronger one. When one is providing therapy to substance-abusing teens, the importance of relating to the whole person and not just the addiction narrative can't be emphasized enough. In addition to strengthening the therapeutic relationship, it's good practice for adolescents to share intimate aspects of their lives not facilitated by or related to their drug use. Judy's disclosure of the shame she felt about her acne, and our playful exchange about the face cream which she covers it up with, opened the door to a more in-depth discussion of the shame she experiences because of her father's drinking. One of those "stolen moments" described earlier took place during this conversation.

Judy said that often when she came home in the evenings her father was sitting passed out at the kitchen table. One time his head was resting on his hand, which held a smoldering cigarette. Judy smelled something burning and realized her father's hair was starting to catch fire without him knowing it. Judy put out the flames and helped her mother carry him to bed. She said this type of incident happened all the time, but her dad never remembered anything he did when drinking and all her mother would say about it is that her father was working too hard and it was a miracle he didn't burn the whole house down, given all the stress Judy's problems were causing him. I asked Judy if she felt she ever used drugs or alcohol to "cover up" the shame her father's alcoholism caused her. This led to Judy disclosing more about her own drinking habits and pot smoking and the feelings that propelled them.

If the disease model and other approaches to substance abuse problems don't nest well with this population's experience of addiction and recovery, what does? I like to think of substance-abusing teens' journeys through recovery as rites of passage that help them shed self-destructive behaviors and replace them with acts of self-love and pride. My using my mother's voice to channel my message to Judy—about not letting feelings of shame or embarrassment about any aspect of herself hold her back—was intentional. Enveloping Judy in a story about the kind of women's culture and power she admired and identified with helped her feel more cared for. It also countered many of the messages of shame and worthlessness she received about herself and her appearance from her family and the larger culture.

I was first introduced to this way of thinking about therapy and recovery by Michael White and David Epston (1990, 1991). White and Epston apply the *rites of passage* metaphor developed by van Gennep (1908/1960) to substance abuse problems and therapy. This concept draws on ideas from cultural anthropology.

van Gennep proposed that all cultures use rites of passage—a triadic experience he labels *separation, liminality,* and *reincorporation*—as a means of facilitating transitions in social life from one status and/or identity to another:

At the separation stage, persons are detached from familiar role/statuses and locations and enter an unfamiliar social world in which most of the taken-for-granted ways of going about life are suspended—a liminal space. This liminal space, which constitutes the second stage of a rite of passage, is "betwixt and between" known worlds and is characterized by experiences of disorganization and confusion, by a spirit of exploration, and a heightened sense of possibility. (White & Epston, 1991, pp. 12–13)

Therapists, say White and Epston, can best gauge the extent of their participation in the liminal phase of a person's story by the degree to which they lose track of time and are unable to estimate the length of a therapy session, as well as by the degree to which their own thoughts and experience merge with their client's and the two individuals develop a sense of oneness, mutuality, and positive regard for one another.

Reincorporation, the last stage in van Gennep's triadic framework, writes White, "brings closure to the ritual passage and assists persons to relocate themselves in the social order of their world, but at a different position" (1991, pp. 12–13). It is through reincorporation, White summarizes, that new possibilities can be realized and people can bring their own—or their community's—hopes and dreams to fruition.

Ironically, many drugs used by young people, such as heroin, mescaline, and cocaine, are often shrouded in mystery and ceremony—rituals that in many ways mirror the rites of passage mapped out by van Gennep. However, when evaluating these experiences it is important to distinguish between ritualism and consumerism. In Native American culture, for example, drugs were used in the context of meaningful rites where the elders in a tribe bore witness to a significant event in the life of a younger member, such as a youth's observance of an important religious custom or successful negotiation of a challenging spiritual quest. In this country and other Western societies, colonialism, genocide, and later industrialization have ripped this process apart, separating native people from their environment and laying the foundation for many of the existential crises and phenomena we all suffer that often crystallize into addiction—powerlessness, isolation, alienation, materialism, consumerism, etc. As a consequence, market forces, not "vision quests," are what drives most drug use and the culture surrounding it found in our communities today.

Every culture has rituals that move adolescents from their status as children to adults, fully functioning as members of the tribe. In this book, and its reading of AA's steps and traditions, I am proposing a "(w)rite of passage" metaphor for therapy and recovery. Regardless of what we call it, adolescence is a period of time when issues of identity and identification are very intense for young people. Most teens harbor strong feelings about wanting to belong and fit in with others. Therapists can use their adolescent clients' innate curiosity about groups, as well as their need to create ritual and structure in their lives, to perk their interest in AA and other 12-step programs. For example, I find that it's not always necessary for teens to let go of chemicals altogether in order to benefit from AA or NA. The choice to identify with and begin to participate in a recovering "clan" or community is a powerful decision, one that many substance-abusing adolescents can benefit from.

In addition, adolescents have a strong sense of justice and fairness. Issues of their own and others' *rights* are just as sacrosanct as the need for ceremony and *rites*. AA, with its emphasis on making amends and concentrating on one's own problems rather than taking someone else's "inventory," offers teens what feels like an impartial source of unbiased wisdom to help them mediate their relationships. In this way, young persons are able to expose themselves to the healing power of a community of recovering people without having to buy into a long-term program of sobriety and abstinence they may not be mature enough, or ready, to take on.

Many adolescents struggling with a substance abuse problem are also grieving for the loss of the mothering and/or fathering they needed because of a parent's addiction. Alcohol and drugs offer these young persons a symbolic identification or connection to their missing parent. AA or Alateen meetings can provide adolescents ways to ritualize and honor their feelings for an alcoholic mother or father, and their need for nurturance, without turning to substances themselves.

Shelly was, as a result of her pregnancy, having to grow up quickly and come to terms with some problems in her life she might otherwise have been able to postpone dealing with until she finished high school. While I recommended that Shelly attend some AA meetings in order to provide her with a forum to explore her substance abuse, I also thought she would be more likely to meet women there who had given birth to children at a very young age in the midst of adverse circumstances. Although she was able to draw on her mother's experience (who was 19 when she had her first child), having role models closer to her own age who had overcome these kinds of challenges and accomplished many of their life's goals seemed important. At my urging, Shelly tried a few NA meetings; however, she didn't find them particularly useful and so stopped going. While she said she admired the people there, she felt her problems weren't as severe as theirs and that she no longer had a problem with drugs and alcohol.

I intentionally did not use Shelly's involvement with social services or the courts as leverage to require her participation at AA or NA. My thinking at the time was that asking Shelly to attend meetings against her will might have caused her halfhearted feelings about 12-step programs to sour altogether, thus exhausting an important resource she might need at another juncture in her life. This is always a judgment call on my part, and every person's situation is different; however, I do not recommend forcing people to stick with strategies that are not working for them. The reason is that if people find themselves in more desperate circumstances at a later date and it's suggested they try going to AA or NA, they will be less likely to respond that they already tried that once and it didn't help.

Unlike Shelly, Katie (the young woman whose narrative opened this chapter) wrapped herself up in the identity of a recovering alcoholic. Katie voluntarily checked herself into a 30-day treatment center for drug and alcohol abuse. When she returned home she moved out of her parents' house and into a sober apartment with several other women, found an AA sponsor, and attended four meetings a week while pursuing a degree in women's studies at a nearby college. During that time she used therapy and support groups to work through her feelings about the sexual abuse by her uncle. This culminated in Katie telling her mother and father about the abuse and, with her parents' support, deciding to press charges against him.

Three years after her inpatient stay, Katie said that she had sworn off drugs for good but wasn't sure she was a "true alcoholic." She was not convinced that it would be unwise for her to drink again:

> "I have no desire to drink today, but so many things have changed in my life I'm not comfortable saying what I will or won't be doing ten years from now. What I do know is that I want to go to grad school so it's definitely best that I stay away from alcohol for now. AA is like family. Between work and school I'm not able to get to as many meetings as I used to, but staying connected to my sober friends and the program is still very important to me."

In one sense, Katie's position is not entirely incongruous with AA's philosophy of taking life one day at a time. More importantly, she now has the tools she needs to see her way through a crisis should she get into trouble with alcohol or drugs again in the future.

Another client, a 15-year-old boy named Jeremy, used meetings as an outlet for his anger and rage. Jeremy was thrown out of private boarding school and asked to leave a residential treatment program because of his violent behavior and destruction of property when drinking. Jeremy knew his drinking problem was serious but didn't think he was an alcoholic. He pleaded with his parents to get him some help, but after his expulsion from the group home, AA was the only place left to turn.

Jeremy liked the people he met at AA. He liked the fact that they didn't pressure him to decide whether he was an addict and just accepted him for who he was. However, Jeremy hated the actual meetings themselves because, as he put it, "I can't stand any structured group that tells people what to do." In a wonderful paradox, Jeremy used his disdain for meetings as the motivating force for his participation. He went "because it pisses me off so much that I love to hate it." Jeremy's anger at the program seemed to diffuse a great deal of his resentment and frustration at home. His parents reported that as long as Jeremy attended meetings he was a much easier person to get along with. Jeremy said one of the things he appreciated most about AA was that no matter how upset he became at meetings he wasn't the angriest person in the room.

All three of the foregoing vignettes underscore young people's need for space to explore the world and experiment with their addiction narratives and recovering identities, while knowing they have permission to return home again, so to speak, in the event things don't work out. Shelly respected NA from a distance but continued the sort of organic recovery she'd begun on her own during her pregnancy; Katie threw herself into recovery with reckless abandon and continued to feel nurtured by AA and the relationships she'd made there even as she began to outgrow her recovering identity; and Jeremy brought to AA the same loving/hate that characterized all his attachments. For Jeremy, recovery was the first time in his life he was able to be with others without reigning in his emotions or being told his anger was too intense to be around.

There are no hard or fast rules for therapy with teenagers. But when people ask me what is the most important quality therapists must possess to work with adolescents, I tell them *therapists must have an affinity for working with this population*. The client and therapist alike must be enjoying therapy and having fun. As I've said, creativity, ingenuity, and humor are an important part of this phase of development in the lives of these young clients and ought to be reflected in the therapy. This includes the therapist possessing an ability to identify with the joys and pains of adolescence, and a high tolerance for challenging and rebellious behavior. More than any other group, adolescents require therapists to be spontaneous and prepared for the unexpected. It is incredibly demanding and exhausting but usually extremely rewarding work. As a rule, clinicians are either drawn to it or avoid it like the plague. Rarely are people indifferent to this work.

I also make a point of telling therapists who work with teens to try and resist the temptation to bring adolescents to an adult level of functioning in order to do therapy. Too often we try to push young people through delicate stages of development too quickly because it makes it easier or more comfortable for us to work with them. In such cases, we're doing a great disservice to our clients. Meet adolescents where they're at, and allow younger children their feelings. Young children and adolescents need the experience of working through feelings of anger, rage, despair, powerlessness, dependency, and other emotions within the context of a safe, caring, and holding relationship. Often therapy provides them the only opportunity to do this important and necessary work. Because so much of what happens outside of the structured therapy space is where the real healing and mending takes place (this is particularly true of work in a clinical milieu), therapists need to be creative—walk together, use art, music, letter writing, make tattoos with vegetable dye, shoot baskets, and the like.

WORKING WITH INVOLUNTARY AUTHORS

I'm all for rational enjoyment, and so forth, but I think a fellow makes himself conspicuous when he throws soft-boiled eggs at the electric fan.
—P. G. WODEHOUSE

I often find myself telling my adolescent clients that the object of recovery is not learning how to be a "good" boy or girl and stop raising hell and causing so much trouble. Rather, the trick is to learn how to cause trouble and raise hell without using drugs and alcohol. This is good advice for many adults as well, who often feel that when people ask them to get sober what they are really wanting them to do is stop being such a bother (i.e., to be seen but not heard from). In therapy with addicts and alcoholics, it is important to remember that it's their consumption of spirits that's the problem, not their spirit.

Winnicott (1965) said that where there is delinquency, or what he called an "anti-social tendency," there is hope. These behaviors are children's attempts at self-cure. Alcohol and drugs allow people to externalize rage—to, as Buber said, personify it.

While many individuals with substance abuse problems are referred directly by the courts, most adolescents that seek therapy are, more or less, given an offer they can't refuse. However, there are some special considerations when therapists are working with clients sent by the courts or another institution. Again, many of these principles carry over to work with any client pressured by family, teachers, or friends to seek help.

In mandated work our legitimacy does not come from our clients' invitations but from the state or the courts. Consequently, it is important to maintain a constant vigil for ways of providing such clients with opportunities to take ownership of the work and form more meaningful connections to the therapy.

In the late 1980s, I ran a court diversion program for adolescents. I found that after the rules and limits had been carefully established (and tested relentlessly!) it was very important to allow each group to develop its own unique rituals, routines, and culture. In one particular group this meant reading the daily *Dear Abby* column during members' "check-ins" at the beginning of meetings, except instead of reading Abby's replies to the letters the group members formulated their own. The same group organized a trail hike and picnic at a scenic lookout for their last meeting.

Perhaps the most important principle that helped us realize our goals in that program was the idea that mandated groups could be *fun* and did not have to be punitive in nature in order to be effective. When doing this sort of work, I'm always looking for ways to speak *with* authority, not *from* authority.

Family involvement was an important aspect of the program, but because of court restrictions we could not require parents' participation in these monthly multifamily groups. The meetings were held in the evenings, and attendance was poor until we sent a letter requesting people to bring a favorite dish and join us in a potluck supper. In the same correspondence we also assigned homework. We asked people to bring the story of how their family came to this county and why they chose to settle in this particular town. The message the letter gave recipients—with its request for food and their stories—was that they had something to offer us. We were also trying to communicate that their family's story was not the sum total of their child's legal and substance abuse problems.

When we are providing therapy to adolescents, there are other ways to use AA and the culture of recovery to expand teenagers' thinking about addiction without asking them to make commitments to AA or sobriety that they're not ready for. In these court groups I always arranged to take participants on a field trip to a treatment center, or I sent them there with their families for a "look-see." This was an effort to remove as much fear about hospitals and rehab centers as possible and to demystify the recovery process. Nowadays, if I make this suggestion in a family session, I always tell adolescents to look in the trunk of the car and check the backseat to make sure their bags are not packed. This is a lighthearted way of addressing a teen's anxiety and fears about being shipped off for "brainwashing."

Cultural Considerations

Programs and therapy can't compete with the high a child gets from drugs. You cannot detox patients and then send them back into deprivation and poverty and expect them to stay free of drugs. Agencies collaborating with inner-city families suffering addiction or substance abuse problems must have an informed analysis of the effects and workings of racism and poverty as well as a firm grasp and understanding of the dynamics and etiology of addiction. Most importantly, these programs must have a joint-action plan with the community to combat these problems.

Hospitals need to make their facilities—often the newest, safest, and best-kept physical structures and facilities in the neighborhood—available to the community. They can serve as a haven or safe gathering place for youth programs, recognition ceremonies, and public memorial services to mourn the loss of family members and friends to drugs, AIDS, and other illnesses. These facilities can also be used as sites for festivals, celebrations, and marketplaces (e.g., art fairs, craft sales, and workshops).

Therapists and their agencies must maintain an active presence in the schools and neighborhoods of the people who use their services, as well as designing programs that are available and accessible to clients in their homes. Developing connections with and offering to serve on church, school, and housing boards as well as involvement in local political action groups are other necessities. A clinical position of neutrality in the context of communities under siege from racism, drugs, alcohol, and decay is not an option for therapists or agencies.

These issues of community involvement are not only relevant for therapists working in the inner city. During the time I was leading the court diversion groups in the 1980s, one of my jobs at the same agency was to reach out to children and teachers in elementary and junior high classes in an effort to publicize the therapy groups we offered to this age group at the clinic and in the schools. To generate discussion and referrals, I invited children to write about a problem they'd experienced in their lives. I'd ask them to say as much as they were comfortable saying about "what happened, who they reached out to, and the eventual outcome." I explained that this was both a way of developing compassion for others who might be having difficulty asking for help in the face of an emotional hardship, and a way of exploring what it would take for any of us to ask for help with a problem of our own. In addition to sharing something about themselves, students were also given the opportunity to ask for an individual appointment with a counselor or to express their interest in a group.

The following excerpt, by an 11-year-old girl named Sarah, is an example of the sort of writing generated by these discussions:

Excerpt from Sarah's Letter

Not to long ago, my parents got into a huge fight. My father was seriously drunk and my mother was angry because he spent his check on beer and cigarettes and other junk when we really needed the money. They started throwing things and yelling and soon there was glass everywhere and the kitchen was trashed. My brother and I were upstairs until I couldn't handle it anymore and took us to a neighbor's house. We spent the night and the next day went home forgetting anything happened, like always. Nothing good came out of it.

Sarah's letter was not unusual. I found these groups and classrooms—situated in the public schools of a small, unremarkable New England town—filled with similar stories which children desperately wanted to tell and talk about.

In addition to demonstrating her need to speak about her experience, Sarah's writing illustrates the thick wall of family denial many children run into when trying to make sense of their pain and trauma within the context of an alcoholic home. While not every child with a substance abuse problem grows up in a situation like Sarah's, these are training grounds where children learn how to use drugs and alcohol to cope with painful feelings and experiences.

The Making of a Family Therapist

In his book *Dead Reckoning: A Therapist Confronts His Own Grief* (1997), author and family therapist David Treadway described one of many painful encounters with his mother's alcoholism:

I remember one night in my living room at 22 West Cedar Street when I was about sixteen. I was there with some friends. We were drinking beer. Mom was drinking bourbon.

At first we all had a good time. She was being very funny and teasing us about how we were managing our "hyperactive hormones" and stuff like that. My friends thought she was a riot. As the night wore on she began to slur her words and not make any sense. Everyone started getting embarrassed because she was clearly drunk. She wouldn't stop talking and even began flirting with one of my friends. I was so ashamed of her.

Finally she announced that she was tired and that she was going to take a nap. She lay down on the floor in front of everybody, cradled her head in her arms and promptly passed out. My friends started teasing me about my Mom's difficulty holding her booze. I couldn't stand it. I had to get her out of there. No matter how drunk she was I didn't want my friends making fun of her. I remember yanking her up off the floor by her arm like she was a bag full of wet sails. She was a small woman, only 5 feet 2 inches. It wasn't hard to get her up. I put her arm over my shoulder and my arm around her waist. Her head flopped onto my chest.

My friends were stone silent. They were all looking away. I dragged her out of there. It was probably the last time I ever held my mother in my arms. (pp. 161–162)

Parents who withdraw from parenting and emotionally abandon their children in these ways leave children (like David and Sarah) in roles of responsibility they're not ready for. This leads to a pseudomaturity in many adolescents that gets them into dangerous situations or results in their making decisions or agreeing to do things they're not ready for, such as having sex with older boyfriends or experimenting with drugs. They may also take over responsibility for the functioning of the household and the raising of younger siblings before they're old enough. To facilitate proper development, children need to live in child-centered homes. When an alcoholic parent is actively drinking, his or her children live in an alcohol-centered, not a child-centered, home.*

In therapy, children often express feelings of responsibility for parental drinking. This often stems from parents' outbursts when angry: "If you weren't so difficult and stopped doing things that upset me, I

*In the following discussion, I am indebted to Robert Ackerman (1986) for his research on alcoholic families and his clear formulation of these ideas on children's emotional development.

wouldn't drink so much." Also, a child may feel that if Mom or Dad "really loved me she (or he) wouldn't drink so much." Conversely, children may be angry at the nonalcoholic parent and blame him or her for the other parent's drinking: "If Mom didn't hassle Dad so much, he wouldn't drink." Children may also worry that a parent may get hurt or die from drinking (by falling asleep with a lit cigarette, falling down, driving, etc.). Or, in situations where children feel that when drunk their parents are more permissive, generous, fun, or affectionate, they may want their parents to drink, but then feel guilty for feeling that way.

Once children are old enough to understand that others frown upon their parents' drinking, they begin to internalize an intense sense of shame and embarrassment about it. The child's sense of shame is amplified when the parent tells the child not to tell anyone or discuss the drinking with anyone outside the home. When the nonalcoholic parent tries to cover up the drinking or pretend it doesn't happen, the message becomes reified and the shame grows—"Mom's drinking must be so terrible we can't tell anyone." For younger children who don't understand that unusual behavior is the result of drunkenness, when other family members cover up or pretend in this fashion the consequences can be even more serious. In this situation the child may start to feel that she or he is crazy.

The dance of development that takes place between parents and children from the earliest stages of life to the launching of a child from home is crucial, but, as Robert Ackerman (1986) observes, for children of alcoholics because of their parents' impairment there is no partner. They dance alone.

There are a number of altruistic reasons for improving and increasing the sorts of services and therapy that we offer these children and their families. Nevertheless, we as therapists, in particular, and our professional communities, in general, would greatly benefit from taking such steps as well. My own experience and anecdotal research tells me that for every child of an alcoholic that follows down the road to addiction, another one readies her- or himself to join the next generation of therapists.

CHAPTER 11

Narrating Our Own Stories
Therapists in Recovery

The motif that keeps coming back to me, again and again and again, is that this is all about being human. This is absolutely all about being human. Jon, you pose a question about to what extent do the issues that we encounter as recovering therapists differ from generic issues that any therapist would encounter? I think, fundamentally, they don't. I think, fundamentally, the question is: How [do] . . . therapist[s] reconcile their humanity with their role as . . . therapist[s]? And the special challenge and the special opportunity and the special, I think, advantage that we encounter as being therapists in recovery is that we are forced to address that issue very directly and very explicitly.

You know, I've long felt that when we go around the rooms and we say, "My name is Roget, and I'm an alcoholic," or "I'm a sex addict," or "I'm a compulsive gambler," or "I'm an overeater," or whatever the hell it is, that the magic of that, the power of that is that we're saying, "My name is Roget, and I'm a limited, mortal human being. This is my acknowledgement of that." So when we're in a twelve-step meeting with clients, and we identify with these phrases, we are affirming, "Yup, I am another Bozo on the bus." You and I have a certain formal relationship that positions me in relation to you as an ally, hopefully a capable ally. But the bottom line, and the centerpiece of the relationship, is that we're both human beings.

—ROGET LOCKARD

Roget is a treasured friend of mine. At different times in my life he has served as sage, consultant, colleague, and therapist—sometimes all four at once. Consequently, it's hard for me to think of him being in pain or imagine him compromised in any other way personally or professionally. However, pain is not a synonym for injury. Pain is our psyche's way of preparing us to grow. This chapter is about our experiences as therapists in recovery. But, like the rest of the book, it is not a typical text in that it does not offer a specific approach or set of guidelines. The information is revealed in the storytelling. Roget shared the following anecdote about a difficult time he experienced in his recovery and its impact on his practice:

Four years ago we had a house fire and a number of other painful things in my life all seemed to converge at once, and I became very depressed. That launched for me a period of about two years when I struggled with more self-doubt than I can ever remember. Including when I hit bottom with my alcoholism. For awhile, I used to say that it was the hardest period that I was able to show up for. Imagining that maybe other times were harder, but because of my drinking I wasn't able to show up for them. But as this period stretched out I just decided, "No, this is just plain the hardest time that I've had in my life." The centerpiece of it for me was a deep, core experience of, I don't know. I don't know how to fix this. I don't know how to restore myself so I feel viable and adequate. Those were the key words to me.

And so, for about two years, my personal experience of viability and adequacy was really tentative and often substantially lacking. Kind of, you know, moth-eaten, full of holes. And, in the meantime, I had a living to make, and clinical responsibilities to fulfill. Boy, I don't know how to explain what I did. It felt really important to find some middle ground between being authentic with my clients and not pretending to a sense of adequacy that was unsupported within me—and, at the same time, representing myself as a capable ally, in their work. And I must say that there were rare moments, almost crisis moments, catastrophic moments is the word that occurs to me, when that bottom line seemed to be iffy. Am I a capable ally? Jesus, I'm not sure. You know.

And I have to tell you, one of the peculiar things is the universe exquisitely conformed itself to my capability. That first summer of the house fire, I was shattered, and not at all aware of how shattered I was. And since I opened a practice, I've never had such a slow summer. I asked myself "Where have all the clients gone?" And there was no clear, obvious explanation. It did not appear like clients were fleeing, but people weren't calling to replace the routine attrition—the things that would open up by vacation or people graduating or terminating or whatever just didn't get filled. And I remember there was one period in the summer when I looked over my schedule for the coming weeks, and I said, "Oh my Jesus, I'm almost exactly five hundred dollars short of what I would typically be making in a week and need to be making to pay the bills." And then a day or two later, I went to the supermarket, and while I was in the check out line I purchased a lottery ticket. To my astonishment it turned out that ticket was worth five hundred dollars. Now that helped a lot. I mean, of course, the five hundred dollars helped, but even more deeply, what helped was kind of this affirmation: "The reason you don't have clients is because you're not supposed to have clients. Because you've got all the clients you can handle. In the meantime, you're going to be taken care of; we're not going to let you starve."[1]

*   *   *

In my work with the Kelly family* a "breakthrough" moment in the therapy occurred when the mother, Cynthia, agreed to go to Al-Anon. I'd been patient yet persistent about some of the changes I thought might result from her willingness to try meetings. I explained that in my experience families in which any member of the family gets involved in a 12-step program increases any other family member's chances of getting sober or overcoming a substance abuse problem exponentially.

One session, Cynthia agreed to go to Al-Anon and asked my advice about where to start. I eagerly offered my suggestions about meetings in her area I thought might appeal to her, as well as some that met at times she'd said were convenient for her but I knew less about. One thing that is important for therapists to appreciate is that even after a conversation like this one it may take a while for clients to act on their intentions.[2]

That's why I was both delighted and horrified when I ran into Cynthia at what we both thought was an Al-Anon meeting, but one look around the room told me this wasn't an Al-Anon meeting, but an AA meeting. The meeting itself was being held in the gathering space of the local sobriety club rather than a church basement or hospital conference as is customary. As a result, the smoke in the room was so thick you could barely make out the people mulling about and sitting in chairs prior to the meeting's start. The majority of folks present were older men, all of whom looked as though they'd been drinking longer than either Cynthia or I had been alive. I recognized a few younger people with tattoos and leather jackets as members of a sober bikers' club in the area. They were cloistered together in the hollow of a bay window

---

*The story of my work with the Kelly family can be found in Chapter 9.

where they could keep a better eye on their motorcycles parked outside. Standing in the middle of this scene was Cynthia, my client, looking more than a bit out of place.

Cynthia looked at me and shouted above the din, "Jon, it doesn't look like there's an Al-Anon meeting happening here tonight." She sounded anxious and fearful, but the disappointment in her voice came through as well. With the number of AA and Al-Anon meetings that take place on any given night, it's amazing, I thought, that scheduling miscues don't happen more often. Regardless, I knew what it took for Cynthia to get there that night and couldn't believe that the meeting wasn't happening as planned on the one evening she'd decided to go. After a pause that felt like 30 minutes but was probably closer to 3 seconds, I said, "No, it doesn't, but if you have some extra time I know where there is another meeting that hasn't started yet and is only 20 minutes from here. You can follow me there if you like." She agreed, and we were out the door and on our way.

Driving in my car, I had plenty of time to think about how I felt about attending a meeting at which one of my clients was present. I remember thinking at the time that it would make a good journal article, except now it had quickly snowballed into a book chapter or short story on my feelings about taking clients to meetings! An exchange with my supervisor several months prior kept swirling around in my head. He said Cynthia had a flirtatious energy with me in sessions, which I had noticed as well. What's more, I told him the attraction was mutual. She was a charismatic and energetic person, and although she didn't have a striking outer beauty she had a radiant personality that seemed to light up a room when she entered it. My supervisor and I had been talking about what a stark contrast her dynamism was to her husband's equally powerful but more somber and cynical presence. When I expressed concern about any potential harm these feelings might have on the therapy, my supervisor said he saw the attraction between us as a positive development—that such feelings, acknowledged or not, were an important part of every therapy relationship. In his view, one I have since adopted as my own, the absence of such feelings in the consulting room is more cause for alarm, as it indicates a lack of chemistry between the parties. My supervisor made the case that the absence of this kind of passion in a marriage is one of the reasons clients come to therapy in the first place, and he added that Cynthia continued bringing her family to therapy in the hope that she and her husband might rekindle it in theirs.

However, our conversations about the issues that feelings of attraction between therapist and client raise took place in the context of the consulting room, not an Al-Anon meeting. The management of both sexual tension in the therapy relationship and outside-the-office contact of any sort require that therapists have a strong and unwavering sense of boundaries.

Great, I thought to myself, what would my supervisor have to say about what was transpiring now? Would he see it as a positive development? And if this was just more grist for the therapy mill, adding to the "idealized transference" between Cynthia and myself, what if our "date" was a bust, would she still want to keep dragging her family to therapy? It was one thing to decide not to stay at the meeting in town, but how would she feel about driving 30 minutes out of her way (I could already tell from the exit signs on the highway that I had underestimated the travel time) for a meeting she found to be no help at all? Obviously, I thought of giving her directions so she could go by herself, but the meeting was located in a church rectory in a building that was very hard to find. As I hadn't been there myself in quite a while, I wasn't confident I could give adequate instructions.

Images of my client going from feeling totally out of place at one meeting, because of a mistake on my part, to becoming totally lost trying to find another contributed to the dilemma I found myself muddling through. I also debated showing Cynthia to the group and then leaving. However, as she already knew I'd planned on going to a meeting that evening, I worried that it would be obvious that my not staying was because of her, which might shame her into feeling there was something wrong or inappropriate about her having gone in the first place. I wasn't too lost in these thoughts to recognize that my obsessing about these things was a sign that at least one of us needed to get to a meeting that night.

The good thing about the extra driving time was that by the time we arrived I was much calmer. As Cynthia and I got out of our cars and walked downstairs to the meeting, I remembered I was often telling clients that in my experience Al-Anon always managed to leave situations involving alcoholism better than it found them. So, regardless of anything else that transpired as a result of our unexpected field trip, I knew I could count on that much. By the time we took our seats, my anxiety had almost subsided completely. Then I looked up and saw my elder brother sitting at a table in the front of the room ready to chair the meeting. He saw me right away, came over to where we were sitting, gave me a bear hug, and said, "Hi, Bro." With an enthusiasm and curiosity usually reserved for the eyeing of a passing celebrity, Cynthia exclaimed,

"This is your brother!" I introduced the two, and then my brother went back to his seat to start the meeting.

It's customary in AA and Al-Anon for the chairperson to "qualify" briefly before introducing the speaker, step, or topic for the evening. This is an opportunity for people to say something about themselves and how they found their way into these rooms. So, as my brother read the meeting's preamble to the group, I had a chance to ponder what other aspects of my personal life might be revealed to my client in the minutes to come. However, much to my relief, part of the chair's responsibilities at this group was to ask if there were any newcomers present and, if so, to suggest they attend a beginners' meeting about to take place in an adjoining room. Cynthia, who hadn't expressed any nervousness until then, turned to me and asked if I thought she should join that gathering. In a voice that caught the attention of everyone sitting on our side of the room I said, "Yes!"

I looked for Cynthia after the meeting, thinking she might need to talk about her experience and say good-bye. When I found her she was surrounded by half a dozen people from the newcomers' group. They were having a boisterous conversation, their sentences punctuated by laughter. Cynthia acknowledged my presence with a quick wave and barely noticed my departure. All of a sudden I found myself feeling very small and insignificant. On the one hand, I imagine some of my disappointment stemmed from my having wanted, in some part of my unconscious, for this to be a real date. More poignant for me, though, was my realizing how much I needed clients to need and rely upon me in tough situations. I don't know which was more upsetting: this discovery or finding out that, more often than not, like Cynthia, they could get along just fine without me. I made a commitment then that the next time I put myself through so many machinations over being with my brother and someone's mother at a 12-step meeting, it would be our own mother.

I had taken clients to meetings many times prior to my experience with Cynthia, but these were primarily adolescents who were going with me as part of a planned activity, and often in the context of a therapy group. Whatever other feelings or fantasies Cynthia had about our excursion (I certainly wasn't going to ask her about them at the time), she seemed genuinely appreciative. At the next family session she said, "What you did the other evening meant a lot. The fact that you were willing to go so far out of your way to show me the other meeting showed how much you care about us and that this isn't just a job to you." She added that because these were clearly problems that I had to deal with in my own family, she felt more comfortable in therapy. Obviously, I wasn't telling her to try things I hadn't gone through myself.

I was more inexperienced then, and the Kellys were one of the first families I'd seen in therapy. But if I had it to do over, I would change very little about what happened. The most notable exception is that when I saw Cynthia at the sobriety club I might have told her that I believe in every kind of coincidence except "just coincidence" and I might have suggested we both stay for the AA meeting and share what we heard or learned there at our next session. Another difference is that now I would have talked ahead of time with a client about the possibility of our running into one another at a meeting if I thought there were any chance of that happening. Also, had Cynthia been an individual client of mine, or in couples therapy exclusively, it would have muddied things up a bit more and might have changed my response at the time or how I discussed it with her in subsequent sessions.

However, it's also possible that were I seeing Jim and Cynthia now, I would turn to Jim in our next meeting and in my impish way share my discomfort about the "extra session" offered Cynthia. I would explain that because of my inability to reconcile these feelings, he and I had better go to an AA meeting together—in order to balance the ledger, so to speak. Regardless of a clinician's personal style, any interactions with clients outside of sessions ought to be explored. In Jim and Cynthia's case, for example, standard practice would be for me to ask Jim if Cynthia had mentioned our experience at the Al-Anon meeting—then to inquire why not, if not.

These are not uncommon predicaments for therapists in recovery, or any clinician for that matter. I shared this particular story to highlight some of the boundary overlaps and countertranference/transference issues unique to addictions therapy that will be explored in this chapter. For those of us in practice who are in recovery ourselves or are healing from past childhood trauma, as so many of us seem to be, these dilemmas can be painful and complicated. We may find ourselves paralyzed with fear when confronted by a bullying alcoholic parent, or disassociated and confused when witnessing parts of a client's story whose traumatic experiences closely resemble our own.

My experience with Cynthia reminds me of Roget Lockard's comments about being human. Therapy is between two human beings in a room, and neither of them has all the answers:

> That's just so much an informing perspective for me, the idea that the vagaries of human relationship are not susceptible to our formal pref-

erences; that people are going to like each other or not like each other, and things like that, based on the chemistry of it all—the convergence of incalculable variables. And so, while our work as therapists is informed by certain principles and senses of responsibility, we also have to accommodate the chaos of human existence.

Now, one of the things I've noticed is that this is distinctly unwelcome news to certain clients. Very alarming. Very disturbing. I'm remembering one client in particular; a very touching moment where this young woman came to a meeting specifically because I was speaking. It was an anniversary meeting, the anniversary meeting of the Saturday night meeting, so it was huge. Hundreds of people there. And at one point during my story, she literally fled the room in tears—never to return. Of course I asked her about this in our next session, and she explained that her reaction had come at a point in my story when I alluded to a time in my later progression where I would have a hard time holding onto a coffee cup—even with both hands. And I made a gesture of my hands trembling. And that did it. She . . . that picture of me being that vulnerable, that human, that compromised, was poignant in a way for her in a way that she found intolerable.

At the same time, as I think about who she was and what her issues were, it was, like, perfect. It was no mistake that she was there to encounter that experience. She was in the process of becoming a therapist herself. She's a very talented, intelligent woman and will make a skilled therapist. And there's no doubt in my mind that she will be very helpful. And yet she was at that point utterly dedicated to the idea that no one should ever find out who she really is, including, conspicuously, for example, her husband, family, supervisor, co-workers, etc., etc.—never mind clients.

So, you know, it was no mistake no misfortune that that incident happened; it raised issues for her that were poignant both with respect to her personal work, and her perspective as a therapist in training. And at the same time, I don't know—it was interesting for me. Like I said before, I feel that in my actual day-to-day experience, I feel oriented most of the time. I rarely feel, "Gee, how am I going to handle this situation with this client?"—this situation of both of us being at the same AA meeting. But this is not because I have thought this through and formulated like a policies and procedures manual, or something, which makes me a little uncomfortable. I mean, it's sort of an obvious and appropriate thing for any clinician to, it would seem to me, to have thought this through systematically. And I can't really claim that I've done that. I'm afraid over the years—especially when I worked in the "high-volume" field of detox treatment, which is where I started out—I just improvised ways of dealing with these issues in very extemporaneous ways, and these ways have worked well enough so that I haven't challenged myself to think about the subject in a rigorous or systematic way. So when I think about it now, at your prompting, Jon, I'm rather disappointed in myself.[3]

I like the juxtaposition of my story with Roget's (including his remarks about his own "existential emergency" that introduced this chapter) because one represents the panic of a fledgling therapist with 2 years in Al-Anon who thought he was supposed to have all the answers, and the other the panic of a senior therapist, more than 20 years sober, who knows he's *not* supposed to have all the answers. Admittedly, though, it has been a bit disconcerting to discover that this sort of self-doubt is not limited to the start of a person's career.

I also appreciate Roget's candor about not having looked at these issues in a formal way. I don't think most of us have, and that was one of the reasons for my writing this book. I wanted to pose some difficult questions. I am not interested in vilifying or valorizing therapists because their work with addicts and alcoholics is or is not informed by a 12-step program. I just think that therapists who have had such experiences offer an interesting perspective, one that has not been investigated with much rigor. I want to begin a dialogue in which questions are considered about the way our own work in recovery touches our client's lives and the way our work with them in therapy has something to offer all of us, not just clinicians who work with addiction. And this inquiry is a timely one, as nowadays both therapists and clients are entering these meeting rooms in large numbers.

HEALING HEALERS: THERAPISTS IN AA AND AL-ANON*

> Psychoanalysis was not so formal then. I paid Miss [Anna] Freud $7 a month, and we met almost every day. My analysis which gave me self awareness, led me not to fear being myself. We didn't use all those pseudoscientific terms then—defense mechanisms and the like—so the process of self-awareness, painful at times, emerged in a liberating atmosphere.
>
> —ERIK H. ERIKSON

Erikson was talking about the unfettered experience of being a patient, but many of us find that being a therapist is a liberating experience as

---

*I prefer the sentiment captured in the expression "healing healers" over the term "wounded" in spite of the former term's somewhat awkward phrasing.

well—that what we get back from seeing people in therapy is more than we put into it, even when we give a lot. Oftentimes, I have the impression that as therapists we're supposed to hide our reverie—or worse, feel shame for having it. Somehow the process of helping people heal, while sublime for clients, is supposed to be somber for practitioners. We are not supposed to take any pleasure in our work with other people's pain and suffering. We can take pride in our skills, but the therapy itself is serious business. How can our enjoyment and pleasure be justified? Better to emphasize the frustration, the pain, the travails than to reveal the joy of helping people overcome adversity.

When Michael Elkin jokes that therapists are the only people in need of 25 or 35 hours of therapy a week, he's not far off the mark. But that's not just a sign of our pathology or the tremendous amount of therapy we need ourselves. For most of us, it's what we choose to do. What better reward for this work could there be than having some aspect of our own experience in need of healing revealed through our work with a client? Isn't this part of what draws us to this craft? It's certainly not the money or the fame. We enjoy life's dramas, the intensity, and the intimate moments of engagement with people—the aliveness. It's what men and women athletes mean when they talk about all the hard work, grueling hours, personal sacrifice and commitment not mattering—they do it for the "love of the game."

Nevertheless, therapist burnout is real. But if we can only bring one set of emotions into the room, if "the analytic attitude," borrowing Schafer's (1983) expression, has no place for the zeal and personhood of the therapist, then of course people will find themselves breaking more easily under the demands of the work.

How do we find authentic ways to sit and bear witness to people's narratives when so many of the gaps and missing pieces in our clients' stories mirror our own? The following pages present three distinct voices of therapists in recovery who are muddling through these sorts of questions and challenges in their practices—quandaries we all struggle with.

Denise: "There But for the Grace of God Go I"

Denise's involvement in recovery programs preceded her decision to start her therapy practice. She received her MSW degree in the late 1970s, and moved in the 1980s to the area in which she lives now. At that point, she went into administrative social work and then clinical social work: "I moved out of the policy stuff but stayed in the kinds of clinical and casework practice that avoided going really deep into my own process." Denise's encounter with a client during a home visit gave her the courage to get sober and begin her recovery.

Denise's Story

Sometime after I left school I was working for a private nonprofit family agency. I was actually recruited into that job, away from a very secure State job by the executive director of a large children's clinic, who felt that I was a very ethical and principled worker, and said she'd like me to run this particular program. I protested in the interview that, you know, while I was flattered that she was recruiting me, I really didn't have much clinical experience. That I was largely a policy and administrative type. And her response was, "That's OK. We really need someone to stabilize our operations administratively in this area. We know that you can work very well independently. You do the administrative work, and we will teach you how to be a clinician." And they made good on their word. They gave me a very good supervisor who had a lot of time, a super warm, caring person who helped me. Developmentally, it was a very important time for me.

There was always, however, a piece of my story I couldn't bring into supervision. I was still actively drinking. Even at the time it struck me as ironic that I could sit in a room and talk about countertransference with clients and all kinds of stuff about my personal life, but there was this whole piece about me, my alcoholism, that didn't enter the room.

I had used alcohol for, at that point, probably 16, 17 years. And it had had an escalating pattern of dependency. It had started out abusively but the dependency built. And I would say in the last four or five years of my drinking I knew it was a problem. I just didn't know how to stop. And I tried tricks, you know. Bargaining. And I would say, "OK, when I come home from work today and I stop at the red light where the street, the bifurcation in the street if I'm not sort of predestined to drink today, then my car will, when I start up at the light, my car will go home. If I'm predestined to drink, when I start up my car will go to the package store." It was a very primitive sort of bargaining going on. And I even had some perspective on that. But again, being an alcoholic, I couldn't stop. No matter what tricks I played.

So it was in that phase of time where I knew it was a problem. I had somatic symptoms that, in retrospect, were highly related to alcoholism. I had lots of joint pain. I had pain in my lower abdomen which, when I would speak to doctors about it and say, "What is here?" And they'd say, "The liver." And I would say, "Uh-huh." And I would take in that piece of reality but I wouldn't say anything more.

I was actively surveying in those days. I was basically asking the environment to tell me to stop drinking. I wanted an external control. I used to ask nurses at my health plan, "So, how much is too much alcohol?" And, there was one nurse who said, "Well, why do you ask?" And I said, "Well, I have a few glasses of wine every evening." She said, "Well, the latest research indicates that that's good for you. In fact, people should drink a moderate amount of wine," blah, blah, blah. And so then I would take that as permission to keep doing what I was doing, but I would also be pissed off. Because I really realized I was looking for someone to say, "Stop." Of course I was answering three instead of five or eight. I was a person who probably could have been aided by a DUI. Because there wasn't anything in the environment that stopped me. I didn't stay away from the car though, I drove drunk a lot of times. But I always got away with it. Always got home. I didn't weave on the road or do anything to attract a lot of attention. I was a very overly controlled, tightly wrapped person who just drove straight ahead and put the brake on at the appropriate time. So it was in that context that I got hired to work for the child and family clinic.

Bottom happened when I was coming home from a home visit. In the context of this particular home study my task was to make a clinical evaluation of a married couple to see if they were appropriate to parent a child not born to them. And was it a good time for them? And there were, without going into a lot of detail about suspicions I had about this couple, there were gaps in their job history and their house wasn't quite built. It just seemed like they were almost 40 years old, and there were just sort of missing pieces in their life. Absences that might be explained by something like drinking.

I remember asking the husband, you know, because he acknowledged earlier, much earlier, he had had a lot of barroom involvement and drinking problems. But he denied any current problems. As I did the house tour, which is a routine inspection, part of the licensing, of the home, the wife took me off and showed me the house. The husband went elsewhere. I think he went to the garage. Then the husband came back and walked me out to the car to say good-bye. As he walked me out, I clearly smelled gin. I knew he had some kind of hard liquor on his breath, but I wanted to make certain, so I moved closely to him, so I knew what I was smelling. Then I knew it was gin!

Anyway, I got home. And on my way home, it was sort of biblical. I mean I didn't get struck off my horse or anything. But I had an epiphany of sorts. My hands were on the steering wheel and I'm driving, going, "How can you slow this guy down in his desire to have children?" How can I confront him and do follow-up work about what was going on. "Why were you drinking at two in the afternoon? If you don't have alcohol issues, couldn't you wait until after I left?" It was so sneaky. You know, I mean, I knew I had to do some sort of confrontation. I knew I had to talk to the agency about this. And what that did for me is it finally broke through my own denial.

I'd been teetering on the edge of that reality, the reality of myself as an alcoholic, for a few years. But it was in the context of knowing that I needed to confront this guy about his alcohol that I sort of felt that there but for the grace of God go I. You know, I could be the woman at home sneaking a drink in the middle of a home study because I want a baby. And somebody comes in and judges me because I smell like gin. And here I am, a mother of three sons I'm actively raising who were biological kids so I didn't have to talk to anybody about my appropriateness as a parent. And so I really remember shaking. My hands were on the steering wheel. And I sort of vowed that, the next day, as I followed up with this case, I would also call my HMO and refer myself for alcohol services. Which I did.

Fortunately, I was assigned to a woman who knew what she was doing. As we sat down, she said, "Why are you here?" and looked at what I had filled out on the intake, in the waiting room. "Oh, two things," she said, "your relationship with your mother and your possible drinking problem. I assume your mother can wait, I want to know about your drinking." And so we went through that whole dance of how much, and how it fit in to the whole picture of my life. And she basically at the end of the first session made me a deal. She would be my therapist. And she would try to stay involved as long as she could within that system, to support me. But that I had to be in a peer support group. And I remember saying, "You mean AA? That God group?" And so she clarified that that's what she meant.

And I feel very grateful for this. I'm not a person who would have gone to AA at all voluntarily. I wouldn't have gone unless my, as they say in AA, my ass was on fire. And I didn't feel like it was on fire. I just felt like I wanted to do something about this overuse of alcohol. And had she not lowered the boom on me I may not have gotten sober. When I came back the next week and reported that I had looked around at a lot of meetings but I couldn't make it there, she said, "OK, don't make another appointment to come back then." She took that hard a stance. And for someone like me, I think it was the ticket. It was the thing that turned the corner, for me.

Initially I told her, "I'm in the field. I can't do that." And she replied, "Well, shop around and talk to people." She wasn't very concrete about how one might check out how to be discretely at a meeting. She left that entirely up to me. In retrospect, I think she wanted me to think of myself as an addict or an alcoholic first and a therapist second. Because she wasn't too concerned about whether I ran into someone I knew. However, I could have used more guidance, as going to my first meeting was terrifying. I had a panic attack in the car on the way, but I wanted so badly to go back and talk with her, I could see that she was going to be helpful. She was a very straight-ahead no bullshit person. Even in my denial, I've always been a pretty intuitive person. I knew there were certain things that I needed for myself. So I wasn't going to do anything to stand in the way of therapy with that person.

So I found in the *When and Where Book,** a meeting in the city. It was in a building where my children used to go for an afterschool program. In the basement. I went in. On the way over, I remember chest pains and problems breathing. And I tried to, you know, normalize my breathing. And then I asked myself, "What am I worried about?" And I was worried that I would bump into someone I knew. And then I thought, "Well, that's ridiculous because we'll both be ashamed." I tried to use that kind of logic to get myself through it.

When I walked in the door, indeed, that scenario occurred. A man who I had known for years was there. He was the father of a girl who was friendly with one of my kids. We knew that he was a bad alcoholic. He had one of those raucous personalities, a real scoundrel. He had a really dramatic story, the kind that when you hear you can point to and say, "I am not an alcoholic, now he's an alcoholic!" He went and put his head on a railroad track and waited for the train to come—the whole classic thing. So, when I saw him there, I thought, "Oh, my gosh. I guess there's different kinds of alcoholics."

He came up to me and said, "So, Denise, fancy seeing you here. I never figured that anybody who lives on your side of town would wind up here." Fortunately, I knew enough about my entitlement to be there. I had moved through a lot of fear to get there. So I just turned on him and I said, "Fuck you so-and-so. I deserve to be here too. Don't give me that classist shit." And it took him aback, shall we say. And he thought about it, and then approached me and gave me a big hug and said, "Of course you deserve to be here. Would you sit next to me and let

---

*This is a directory of AA meetings printed by local and regional AA Intergroups. These groups and their offices can be located in the phone book.

me show you the ropes?" So it stopped him in his tracks. Because, you know, it's so hard to get there. And that was eleven years ago. May. Exactly eleven years ago.

Melanie: "I Feel Like If I Drink, I'll Kill Myself with It"

Melanie is a psychologist with a diverse caseload and 9 years of sobriety in AA. She was seeing clients and going to Al-Anon meetings for 6 years prior to getting sober herself. Although she has a reputation for doing good work with persons in recovery, she prefers not to limit her practice to therapy with alcoholics, addicts, and their partners because she believes it gets in the way of her own recovery. Here she shares her insight about how her suicidal feelings helped her come to terms with her alcoholism.

Melanie's Story

Growing up I was not aware of addiction in the way that I am now. I was a scared kid who had this shameful father. I was living in fear on a daily basis, and I was taught that it was "us and them." We were poor too, not as poor as people who don't have food, but I've been buying my own clothes since I was in junior high, decided I wanted to go to the dentist and paid for that. My father was an angry drunk; you didn't want to be around him when he was drinking, and so I learned to manage intense anger and conflict as a matter of survival. I needed these skills to protect myself, keep myself safe, as well as my brothers and sisters. I guess you could say my training as a therapist started very early.

I'd been going to Al-Anon meetings for 6 years. My marriage had broken up and I was drinking the way I always drink, which was not a lot. When I first drank, I drank to get drunk, I just didn't drink often. To me, that was one of the ways you would measure whether you're an alcoholic. So I didn't drink like my dad did, however I had all these rules around drinking; I stopped drinking vodka because I got mean like my dad did, and I didn't drink when I was angry, and I didn't drink when I was sad, and I didn't drink when I was around certain people. These are things that I paid attention to: while I'm feeling so-and-so, I'm not going to drink, while I'm going to be around so-and-so I guess I won't drink tonight, that kind of thing.

Here's the guts of my story. I had a birthday party for my partner. It was October 23, 1989, and I drank, and I ate chocolate for dessert—and I was playing around with not eating sugar, not eating chocolate. What had happened earlier in the day is that I'd gotten really angry at my partner. I don't even remember exactly what it was but I had gotten really angry and then took her out to dinner. I drank for a couple of hours, then I started feeling suicidal. I told my partner and I cried and cried and I decided that I probably shouldn't drink, and I probably shouldn't eat chocolate.

I started going to OA, because I figured I had a serious problem with sugar. For nine months I went to OA and off and on through that nine months, I longed to drink. I felt like there was a death, like I was grieving, but I didn't drink. I might not have even drank twelve times a year; some years I might not have even had anything to drink more than three times. But what happened to me when I drank, and what I was able to see through this nine months, was that I felt much more comfortable in my skin when I drank. Sort of able to just be okay.

A couple of times when I drank, like when I was getting dinner ready for my kids, I would have a glass of wine, and it was the best. The kids could fight, things could not be timed right and I felt like I had everything in full control. The other times when I didn't drink (I found this out in retrospect) I was a dry drunk. The kitchen counter showed it. You know, I almost broke my hand once by slamming it on the table. I was really out of control.

So, nine months later we're on vacation. My grandson had just been born two weeks prior and I was at the birth. It was normal and the baby was healthy. So there I was sitting there on vacation, and this wave of feeling came over me and all I could think about is how much I wanted to drink, and then I felt suicidal. I told my partner about it and she said, "Do you want to go to the meeting? There's one in town this morning." And I said, "Sure." So I went. She'd been telling me off and on, because I had so many rules about my drinking, that I might have a problem. As she's a recovering alcoholic, she'd ask if I ever related to any part of her recovery or if her story made it more difficult for me to see my drinking as a problem. Also, during this period, I was getting really angry in Al-Anon. I just felt like I wanted to do outrageous things and shake these polite people up. Polite and sweet and nice is how I was in the world (though it wasn't necessarily how I was at home). I think I was seeing a lot of myself and I was just not happy about what I was seeing.

So I started going to AA and shared, "I'm here because I felt like killing myself and I felt like drinking." I was a therapist, and we were there on a two-week vacation. The kids came down for their birthdays in the middle. All our kids came. About four days before they arrived I was sitting in the vacation house, which had a cathedral ceiling with an open balcony. While sitting down in the living room, looking up at the balcony, all of a sudden there I found myself spontaneously trying to figure out how I could hang myself from it. That really scared me. So I talked about it in the meeting, which I never could have done at meetings back home. I have since talked about it some years later. I just didn't know what was going on; it was just so weird, I felt like I was emotionally falling apart.

Now, mind you, I was going about the business of doing my day, and nobody would have known that I was feeling this way. And I haven't felt that way since. But I just kept going to meetings, and I kept saying, "I don't know if I'm an alcoholic but I know that I'm miserable. And I know that I feel like if I drink I'll kill myself with it." I realized that a lot of my thoughts about drinking, over the previous years when I wasn't drinking and I would want to drink, would be about dying, just isolating, and drinking. It wasn't working for me anymore, anyway. Then I started realizing all the things I did when I was drinking that I never would have done sober. The only times I ever stole anything were when I was drinking. It was as a teenager, but I was pretty squeaky clean because I didn't want to be like my dad. So that's what happened. That's what got me into AA. I was scared of dying actually. Because I knew there wasn't any real reason for me to want to die. It didn't make sense, and it all seemed tied into the drinking.

Oh, it was very hard for me to feel like I belonged in AA, even though I could identify with a lot of what people felt when they would tell their story. For me it was 25 years—at least 25 years—of drinking, but it wasn't a physical addiction. There was certainly something emotional, and my body would respond to only one sip of alcohol. It is a progressive disease. I mean, I drank two glasses of wine once when I went out with my kids for dinner, and I needed help getting out of the place and I used to be able to drink *much* more. On my honeymoon, I remember ordering triple vodkas. I went through a six-month period drinking nothing else. Triple shots of vodka. I weighed about ninety pounds. I could do that and still be standing and remember the whole night. Towards the end, I couldn't handle two glasses of wine. It's amazing how that works.

Being a therapist and in recovery myself, it's like mud, sometimes. It feels like mud, which is probably a reflection of the work I have yet to do. That's where I'm feeling pushed right now. There's work I need to do—ACOA and healing from childhood trauma. The meeting I really like is often attended by some of my clients. The other day, at the meeting, I scoped the room out really well to see if any clients of mine were there before I shared. It isn't that what I shared was awful, but there are people who wouldn't want to know that I had embarrassed myself, that I was out of control in a family situation. There are people who would get pretty freaked out about that, but they weren't there that week. I guess that's what it's like. I feel like my life's available. It's too available sometimes.

Rachel: "Straddling Two Worlds"

A psychiatrist devoted to her patients and with 15 years of recovery in Al-Anon, Rachel said she discovered the healing possibilities of community in these groups and that they helped her organize what felt like a totally unmanageable life.

Rachel's Story

My childhood was like the movie *Ordinary People*. My parents were not demonstrative people but, like the couple in that film, they tore each other to pieces with words and glances. What was going on inside, what we were feeling never mattered as long as everything looked perfect on the outside. My parents coped with this situation by staying high on prescription medication and alcohol. In every family photograph mother has a glass of wine in her hand and father is holding up a tumbler of scotch. The children all overachieved. We lived to make them proud but nothing was ever good enough. That didn't keep us from trying though. We won awards for academics, athletics, and all received scholarships to elite schools and colleges. Everyone except my younger brother. He had some learning problems but mostly he just wasn't like the rest of us. It made him very depressed. He was also asthmatic. Not having all the clubs, activities, and games to keep him busy and get him out of the house meant he suffered more of my parent's sarcasm and scorn than the other children. One day he went out to the garage put a hose on the tailpipe of my father's Porsche and asphyxiated himself. He timed it so both our parents were home and would find him. I don't think he intended to die—I think he was just trying to get their attention. Because of the asthma his organs weren't as strong as the rest of ours and had a lower tolerance for toxins.

My father was a surgeon. I remember his disappointment when I chose psychiatry as my specialty. He said it was for people who couldn't hack it in real medicine. He said the fact that my brother had committed suicide made it even more pathetic. That even if my training helped me understand why he did it that it wouldn't bring him back. "If you want to save lives why don't you go into surgery or emergency medicine where at least you're working on the living."

After med school I was intent on keeping what happened to

my brother from happening to anyone else. After my residency and a few tours of duty at a state hospital with very chronic people, I took a position at a high-powered teaching hospital. I worked longer and harder than anyone else on the faculty. My patients came before anything or anyone else. This contributed to my marriage ending but even the divorce didn't slow me down. The pace was starting to catch up to me. I used to bite all my nails down to the cuticles, I chain-smoked at home so know one would see me, I was becoming a nervous wreck. But I didn't feel like I could stop. People were depending on me. I was publishing articles, serving on committees, writing recommendations, but most of all I didn't feel like I could abandon my patients. I felt I was the only one who could help them. If I took someone on I told them I would never stop fighting to get them healthy or give up on them. All I asked in return is that no matter how bad things got they not quit on me. They all understood what I meant. My commitment and dedication was not without its rewards. Many people I worked with got better. Many did not, but for years no one ever made a serious suicide attempt while in my care. I took great pride in that.

Eventually my streak came to an end. A patient of mine came into the ER—she'd cut both her wrists along the veins, it was very serious. Just as there are two kinds of canoeists, those who have tipped and those who haven't tipped yet, if you do this work long enough inevitably something like this is going to happen no matter how careful you are or who you are. I was devastated. I had a breakdown of sorts. I was missing deadlines, meetings and became very angry with staff if patients acted out in my office. When residents and colleagues started complaining to the department chair about my treatment of them I knew I had to do something.

I went into therapy with an analyst who had been a visiting faculty member in our department at one time. He helped me grieve, for the first time, what happened to my brother and stand up to my father when I went home. Throughout all this, however, I never stopped working. If anything I worked harder just to prove to people that even though I was in therapy I hadn't lost any of my skills or competence. My blood pressure was off the charts, I was smoking at work now as well, and I thought I was going to die. I was terrified. It wasn't that I wanted to kill myself or anything like that, I just couldn't stop working so hard. I had no social life outside of the hospital, no relationships, and because of the tension between my father and me at the time very little contact with my family. I was also aware of my growing dependency on wine to help me sleep at night.

That's what it took for me to get myself to Al-Anon. I'd

been sending patients and their families there for years. Because of my experience with both my parent's alcoholism I considered myself a kind of "enlightened doctor." For years I'd had literature and meeting schedules in the waiting area of the office where I keep a small private practice, separate from the institutional setting where I work. The people in these rooms saved my life. For the first time in my life I felt part of a community of loving and caring people. Although I'd been helping people with their problems and relationships for years, I didn't know how to connect with others myself. I knew how to "network" to advance my professional career, but until I started using this program I couldn't manage my own life. It taught me how to focus on others without abandoning myself.

I still care about my work and my patients as much as ever, I just have an easier time letting go now and accepting that even if I've done my best work—"fought the good fight"—there are some people I can't help or who may not be ready to get better. I also quit smoking and cut down on my drinking. People at work noticed the change in me as well and just assumed it was from the therapy. And, as they were partly right, I just left it at that.

It's hard. The circles that I've been moving in, professionally, in the last nine or ten years have been pretty conservative ones. And that's challenged me a lot as a human being. In the institution I work in people are openly scornful of 12-step work and recovery, and extremely conservative psychodynamically oriented psychotherapists. When people do talk about 12-step it's talked about as "those programs, they're wonderful for very character disordered people." And I sit there and these people don't know I'm in recovery. I've made the choice not to talk about that in this particular setting. It was a political decision on my part about what was best for my career and a very conscious one that may not be the best one for me personally. I feel like I'm straddling these two worlds.

Al-Anon profoundly changed the way I think about therapy and work with patients. Unfortunately, I often feel in my practice and at the hospital that what I'm doing with clients—the way I use myself around 12-step—I have to be somewhat secretive about.

MANAGING MULTIPLE CONNECTIONS: WHEN THERAPIST AND CLIENT ARE BOTH IN RECOVERY

In her book *An Unquiet Mind*, Kay Redfield Jamison discussed her ambivalence about telling the story of her lifelong struggle with manic depression:

I have had many concerns about writing a book that so explicitly describes my own attacks of mania, depression, and psychosis, as well as acknowledging the need for ongoing medication. . . . I have no idea what the long-term effects of discussing such issues so openly will be on my personal and professional life, but, whatever the consequences, they are bound to be better than continuing to be silent. I am tired of hiding, tired of misspent and knotted energies, tired of the hypocrisy, and tired of acting as though I have something to hide. One is what one is, and the dishonesty of hiding behind a degree, or a title, or any manner and collection of words, is still exactly that: dishonest. (1995, p. 7)

Like Denise, Melanie, and Rachel's stories, Kay Jamison's words inspire me. I need to hear accounts of therapists' lives who, after mending their own wounded spirits and relationships, find that working with others whose narratives have been similarly broken reminds them (the therapists) of the gift they've been given. It is not that I endorse the potential boundary violations of some impulsive acts of self-revelation, but I do not think it would be reckless on our part as therapists to be more transparent with one another in consultation and supervision about the ways our clients' traumatic memories and addiction narratives resonate for us. In fact, I imagine it would have the opposite effect, making it less necessary for clinicians to burden the people they see in therapy with their own grief because it's one of the few places they have to remember or recall these experiences. In this way, when a therapist decided to share certain painful aspects of her own experience with a client—or some other details about her life—she could be more confident that it was her client's needs that were foremost on her mind at the time and not her own.

These gaps in therapists' conversations with one another undermine the messages we try to give clients about the need to break their silence and tell their stories. In cases of trauma and addiction, acknowledgment of an individual's experience by a larger witness group or community of people authorizes the person's story in a way that therapy alone cannot. These experiences can then be taken back to others who may feel isolated and trapped in the same kind of dilemmas and suffering. This is as true for therapists as it is for clients.

I also appreciate that for Denise, Melanie, and Rachel recovery is a work in progress. I admire their struggle with the contradictions inherent in their experiences as therapists and alcoholics in AA, or as members of another 12-step group and community. Balancing the needs of their own recovery with their clients' needs and managing multiple roles often results in their feeling lost and confused. The trajectory of their clients' recovery and healing is not always on track with their own. The two experiences often feel out of sync with one another, and at these times the process can feel chaotic and unruly.

Dialogues about overlaps, multiple roles, and boundaries between therapists and clients aren't new to the therapy community, nor are they unique to therapists in AA or Al-Anon or to therapy with persons in recovery. Feminist therapists have been discussing similar issues for years. In feminist circles the discussion revolves around the concepts of mutuality, power, and authority. I also think that therapists who are members of a minority group or some other marginalized community, such as alcoholics, have also had to deal with these issues. That if, for example, a gay or lesbian therapist in a small town ruled out working with members of the gay and lesbian community because of overlaps with her clients, she would quickly starve. This is a situation where the realities posed by sexual orientation and identity as a member of an oppressed group transcend clinical orientation. In such a scenario it is virtually impossible not to see people in other contexts, some of them very intimate ones (e.g., dances, political meetings, and parent groups). If the therapist is in recovery himself, his world gets that much smaller.

These overlaps do not mean that only certain kinds of therapy and clinical theory apply or can be practiced in these situations; rather, they must be adapted to a different set of circumstances. Another tendency is to see these situations as less desirable or "making do," especially if analytic work is being undertaken. This is not the case. In fact, just the opposite is true. These situations require that therapists stretch their models and ways of working with clients. They challenge us to create theories that fit the needs of our communities rather than shaping our communities to fit our theories.

The most important consideration when it comes to managing boundary issues with clients is the therapist's understanding of and use of her own power. Power can't be wielded the same way in 12-step programs as it is in therapy. Nor is it languaged the same way. We have seen how in AA and other 12-step programs power is closer to the feminist concept of "power in relation to" rather than "power over" someone, and yet there are important differences.

In 12-step programs, issues of power tend to revolve around people's struggle with the concepts of acceptance and surrender and the relinquishing of control to a Higher Power in the presence of fellow sufferers. These programs take a very clear stance against abuses of power. However, the responsible use of power in relationships in the sense it's conceived of in therapy, does not come up in AA very often. That's because in AA no one is authorized to use power in this fashion.[4] In AA, members talk to newcomers "not in a spirit of power but in a spirit of humility and weakness" (*AA Comes of Age*, 1985, p. 279).

As therapists, we cannot have mutuality in relationships with clients without first acknowledging the inherent imbalance of power there, by virtue of our different roles. We have to be explicit about that and fastidious about what that means in terms of self-disclosure. In classical analytic theory these boundaries are more rigid and any overlap is seen as a transgression. There's a joke in analytic circles that transference has the half-life of plutonium. The point being that if there's any maternal transference, there's always maternal transference. And it doesn't mutate. It doesn't transform. You don't have dual relationships with clients, ever.[5] You have your termination, and you don't see people again after that in any other way—even as a client. In actuality, I do not know too many therapists, even analytically informed colleagues, who are this strict in their practice.

Some clinicians who teach will see clients who were students. People find therapists through their work in the way Rachel described finding her analyst. A cherished colleague asks me to see her best friend's child who is in trouble and who has already seen a number of therapists. Could this be a rescue fantasy on my colleague's part? She is a talented therapist who knows me well and is familiar with my way of working. If she says she thinks the therapy would work and be helpful to this person, I want to trust her instincts. But what if it doesn't, or what if the problems this adolescent client brings up causes me to seriously question the parenting or judgment of her mother, my colleague's best friend? We make decisions like these all the time. There is no textbook that tells us what to do in such situations. Training and experience inform us, but mostly we rely on intuition. We do what feels right, after weighing the pros and cons, and applying whatever logic we can bring to bear.

I find I use my intuition in managing the overlaps that happen between myself and my clients in a 12-step group. Each decision is specific to the individual. With every new therapy I find myself asking: How am I using myself differently with each person? Who am I to this person? And what is the meaning of her seeing me in this context? So I'm always thinking about both planes. I'm also trying to be a member of the 12-step community as it exists in the area where I live. Those things often clash for me. I often have a difficult time reconciling the two processes. When, for instance, I'm thinking of referring a client to a particular Al-Anon meeting where I often go, sometimes it's fine, sometimes it's not fine. I don't always make the right decision.

The Therapist's Use of Self in Psychotherapy with Persons in Recovery

The practices that therapists employ when reflecting on "transference" in trauma and addiction therapies are different from those of more traditional psychotherapies. The anxiety and safety issues of addiction and trauma require addiction therapists to bring the "real" therapeutic relationship into the conversation sooner than more conventionally trained therapists might. In the case of addiction, therapists may need to offer clients reassurance and be more active and open with people in order to minimize their clients' anxiety. In psychoanalytic terms this means refraining from encouraging a transference to unfold completely—into a "transference neurosis"—and collaborating more closely with the client on developing self-protective interpersonal skills and a sense of connection to a safe and supportive recovering community.[6]

This is a stance which therapists and analysts are gravitating toward more and more in their work with all clients: in the analytic dialogue the discussion is about "being in the now"; therapists at the Stone Center in Wellesley, Massachusetts talk about the use of "empathy" and "mutuality" in the therapy relationship; and narrative family therapists are developing storylines about "two-way accounts of therapy" and "taking-it-back practices." The terms we have been discussing here involve allowing for more of the vagaries of human relationships in therapy. These practices are first and foremost expressions of an ethical commitment. They are about acknowledging our own humanity in the work and bringing it into the therapy relationship with more conscious intent.

In work with addictions, this requires moving away from what White (1997; borrowing Sharon Welch's expression) calls an "ethic of control" and bringing to the therapy process an "ethic of collaboration" and concern.[7] To accomplish this, therapists need to be familiar with their own narrative center of gravity. In other words, how do their own hopes, dreams, imagination, vicissitudes, and preferences in life inform their work with the people they see in the therapy setting.

Having this information about themselves doesn't obligate therapists to share it. The argument for more transparency in the therapy relationship is not an either/or proposition. These newer approaches to therapy are meant to expand, not narrow, the clinical dialogue. Replacing the old analytic primers with a new set of rules or "how to" books does not represent an advancement in the field. There are many situations where it continues to be advantageous for therapists to remain opaque in the therapy relationship. This stance helps therapists keep the focus of the work on their clients, buffers clients from therapists' own biases and concerns, and helps therapists avoid reassuring clients in order to foster the emergence of people's anxieties and other symptoms (in the case of addictions, this practice keeps therapists from rescuing clients from the experience of hitting bottom).

Mitchell (1993) asks us to consider the hopes of the obsessional patient (which we can here translate to mean the alcoholic) at the beginning of treatment. Alcoholics are not interested in giving up their life's work of controlling everything that happens in their own experience and that of those around them. In fact, they are likely to be hoping that therapy will help bolster their skills at control. Therapists' hopes, Mitchell observes, are likely to be very different—more oriented toward enabling their client to live life in a different and richer fashion, which becomes possible only when clients relax their efforts to omnipotently control their experience. We are not able to say, "Look, I understand you are hoping I will help you become better at controlling your drinking and the other relationships and concerns in your life, but I can help you give that all up and find a much fuller and more meaningful life." If the therapist did say something like that, the client would likely leave, and rightfully so. According to Mitchell (1993), "To sign up under those conditions would be to commit to a conversion process, not analysis. So instead the analyst says, 'Let us begin an inquiry into your experience, and we will see what we find' " (p. 225).

Where does that leave therapists working with people in recovery or suffering from alcoholism? In the case of addictions, we *are* asking the client to sign up for a conversion process. We often tell them that, under the current circumstances, for therapy to have any lasting effect, or to facilitate any positive change whatsoever, they need to get sober. This *is* what needs to happen.

My aim in presenting this material is to help therapists come up with ways of using their own experiences and their relationships with clients to effect this kind of transformation. An important part of this process is allowing people to arrive at the fact of their addiction in their own time and way. Or, if we do need to present news that is shocking or jarring to our clients, to do so in a way that is respectful. It's a paradox. We need to *both* safeguard the hope that a person will eventually choose to get sober *and* accept the real possibility that, despite our own—and often our clients'—best efforts, it may not be in their stars to do so.

Therapists in recovery who have made the decision to get sober with the help of a Higher Power may understand this dilemma better than any. At the same time, it may be more difficult for them to sit with people in this quandary without transposing their own experience onto their clients. Provided these experiences are offered up to people to use as they see fit, and not imposed on them, I think therapists with a conscious spiritual orientation in their work and lives are advantaged, *not* disadvantaged, in their work with alcoholics and people in recovery.

A conversation about the spiritual life of therapists and how this shapes the therapy relationship will follow. Prior to that I want to present several other themes related to the therapist's use of self, and the question of therapy for therapists in recovery.

Accompanying Clients to Meetings

Clients in AA who know their therapist is in recovery also may expect more sharing and self-disclosure from their therapist. The transition from the atmosphere of camaraderie and fellowship at meetings to the quiet intimacy of a therapy office can sometimes disappoint clients. It's certainly okay not to gratify clients in this way if it does not suit your personal style. If you opt not to do so, you just need to make sure clients understand that this is a reflection of your own boundaries and sensibilities; if it's part of your overall theoretical approach to the work, you should provide clients with a clear rationale for it.

Honoring a client's request to accompany her or him to a 12-step meeting is often thought of as "breaking the therapy frame" (that is, engaging in behavior that results in the therapist stepping outside his or her professional role). The discussion then revolves around the pros and cons of such action and whether it's in the client's best interest. Regardless of how one feels about this practice, conversations about accompanying clients to 12-step meetings are clinical discussions and the activity itself is a treatment event, not a social outing. (Furthermore, in the case of addiction, such meetings are certainly less outside the treatment frame than clients' weddings, graduations, and other social events that therapists often attend.) I also find disconcerting the way these conversations become organized around issues of credentialism in which providers are divided into two types: the para- or nonprofessionals who engage in this sort of activity, and the "real" professionals who for reasons of therapeutic integrity do not.

Traditionally, the case for us as therapists taking a more professionally distant role in therapy is to allow clients to project onto us their anxieties and insecurities. Accompanying people to 12-step meetings is another way of allowing ourselves to be used by clients. We are in a very real, not just symbolic, way safeguarding our clients' future. In the case of people we are seeing on an inpatient basis it can also help facilitate their transition from the more sheltered existence of hospital life to the community. We are—again in a literal, not just metaphorical, sense—lending our belief in the strength and courage of other human beings to those clients until their faith in themselves is restored or mended. This is what psychodynamically oriented therapists refer to as "borrowing the therapist's ego."

Some may argue that therapists who accompany clients to 12-step meetings are taking on a parental role or standing in for their "super-egos" and that such a practice is too intrusive into people's personal lives. However, in some instances, because of the intense level of danger drugs and alcohol pose, taking a more active and directive role in clients' lives is not only necessary but imperative (this is often especially true in therapy with children and adolescents).

Clearly this practice has some disadvantages and, despite the case I'm making for it here, in my own work I tend to be more conservative. In many cases accompanying clients to meetings, or seeing a person in any other context outside of the consulting room, can be disruptive to the treatment relationship, especially in therapy with trauma survivors where boundary issues are paramount. The feelings of other clients or potential clients who may also be present at the group also need to be considered. What makes sense for one person may not for another, and therapists ought to be prepared to discuss people's reactions and feelings to seeing them with another client in this context. (The more consistent such attendance is with a therapist's practice, the less this will be an issue.)

However, even if accompanying clients to meetings isn't standard operating procedure for you as a therapist, that shouldn't keep you from considering it. I recommend making that decision on a case-by-case basis, as one would the decision to attend a client's wedding or commitment ceremony. Consider each case individually. Witnessing and participating in rituals that acknowledge people's transition from one phase of life to another or the incorporation of a new aspect of their identity are powerful ways of supporting clients. Discussions with clients in response to a request to accompany them to a 12-step meeting, honored or not, provide opportunities to expand the therapy conversation in rich and interesting ways.

Sharing 12-Step Meetings with Clients

For the therapist in recovery, sharing a meeting with a client is more complicated than just accompanying a client to a meeting. As Melanie said, it can lead to the feeling that one's life is too available. Choosing to do certain kinds of therapy or address certain problems with a person may require putting that client's needs at a meeting before one's own. This is not about "getting it right," "having one's life all together," or "becoming a perfect being." It's a gesture. It means one's identity as a therapist and a person in recovery is more integrated.

Obviously if you are a therapist in relatively early recovery, this may not be possible, and there are crisis times when you cannot afford to do this regardless of how much sobriety or recovery you have. As a general rule, therapists need to tread cautiously when walking the borders where professional and recovering identities meet. My sense is that it is easier for the "analytic attitude" to run roughshod over a sober mind or recovering heart than vice versa. Therapists should examine whether they are using their identity as professionals to avoid taking risks at meetings. As one colleague observed—it doesn't necessarily have to:

> One of the things I've realized is that I'm . . . what would you call it? I'm sort of an honorary member in good standing in SLAA [Sex and Love Addicts Anonymous]. You know, certainly with a history to justify my seat there. I don't go to the meetings with any regularity at all. I usually go just to introduce people to the meetings, make it easier for them to go. But one of the things I've realized is that if I were asked to speak at one of those meetings, I wouldn't. And I wouldn't, because of clients. And I just have a deep inner sense that for me to tell my qualifying story at SLAA would be excessively provocative for them. And that's true. But I have a sneaking suspicion that there is a way to tell my story where that doesn't have to be true. This is, you know, this is a work in progress, internally, for me.

It is difficult to make decisions about what to share about one's recovery at a 12-step meeting or in a therapy session, especially when people ask specific questions about these experiences. Attend first to what and how your client presents. Those clients who present as fragmented and who are obviously having a difficult time containing their anger may find it hard to use information about a therapist's recovery constructively. Those clients who are struggling with the discovery of a parent's alcoholism may not need or want to know that their therapist is a recovering alcoholic. News of their therapist's vulnerabilities and flaws may be unwelcome even if the eventual discovery of this information might be therapeutic; as we saw (earlier in this chapter) with Roget Lockard's client, a therapist herself, who came to hear him speak at an AA meeting and fled the room during his description of his alcoholic tremors. Of course, this sort of information has a way of surfacing at the most inopportune moments in the therapy, especially in a small community. The trick is to transform these moments or crises into healing ones.

Again it is not the achievement of perfection that is required but the intent. For example, saying to a client "I am sorry you had to find out about my being a recovering alcoholic that way—how awful!" or "I hadn't shared this information with you because I didn't think you needed to be burdened with it while you were trying to figure out what to do about your relationship with your alcoholic father" is different than "I think you should know that I'm an alcoholic too, so that you understand that all drinkers are not the same." Obviously, the latter is a very simplistic illustration, but the point is that telling people something for their own good, whether in therapy or life, usually is not for their own good but is driven by another agenda.

Rachel discussed a specific encounter with a client that generated a number of questions about the sorts of dilemmas that recovering therapists face when sharing or considering sharing meetings with clients, as well as offering some solutions:

Rachel's Dilemma

I'm having a real dilemma right now. I'm working a new 12-step program that is probably the newest 12-step program on the scene—Debtors Anonymous [DA]—which looks at one's relationship to money, debt, time, depravation, and abundance—the whole ball of wax. It's really an amazing program, and it's in its infancy. Right now there are only two meetings in the area, and usually there are no more than four or five people at a meeting. It has the power, I imagine, that early AA once did for its members, or that any program does that's in its infancy. Everybody is pulling everybody else along for their own survival. It really feels like there's just a tremendous amount of service going on and phone calling and intimacy. It's very powerful. There's no mainstream acceptance. It's not chic. There's a tremendous amount of shame and stigma, and all the people in the room are in some other program. Some of them have not disclosed to the people in the programs that they're in that they're using DA. It seems to me that money—issues around money—even more than sex and incest and all kinds of things that have hit the psychotherapy community, are particularly shame-laden for people.

So, what's interesting for me is that, since I'm in very early recovery in this program it feels like I'm just starting to peel away the layers of the onion and getting to some core stuff for me. And now I have a client who's asking me, who's begging me, for information about where to go to deal with compulsive spending, debting. "Is there a support group, is there anything that you can share with me about this?" she asked. In all other situations when I'm talking to people about OA, Al-Anon, or AA, whether I go to those meetings or whether I'm simply drawing on my own experience, if I self-disclose, if I don't, I feel very comfortable, very grounded, about what I share with people.

This time I was flabbergasted. She's now asked me twice. I deferred her the first time and we went on to something else. The second time I said, "I need to do some thinking about that." I bought some time for myself so I could think about what it would it mean for me to have her be sitting in these meetings with me, on Tuesday or Friday night, with three other people. Where I'm at my most lost and vulnerable and most out there, could I do that? And, I'm very selfishly thinking about myself. Am I willing to give these meetings away? This is what it feels like. And then I'm thinking about this particular person, who she is in terms of her history and her character and her other addictions and other recovery programs—all of who she is, and all of who I am to her.

Maybe I'm letting myself off the hook here, because I'm also thinking about the way in which she is desperately moving from program to program, and therapy modality. You know shamans, and astral projection. I don't mean to make a joke about this. This is real for her. She's really searching, and my feeling is, "Would it be different?" I keep asking myself if I felt like this was somebody for whom this was the primary core issue, where she would go and hook up with this program and take off with it, if it would be life transforming for her to be in these meetings. I feel as though, if this were the case, somehow we could work with that, that it would be okay. Yet, I feel like what would happen is she would drop in and drop out again. I think that's very true, but is that a justification for not sharing what I know with her? That's when these issues were really hitting me right between the eyes.

I also thought about if I didn't say anything, and she found out anyway and saw me at a meeting. Because she can ask around. She's a resourceful person. If she were to show up at a meeting, and then I was there, and she asked, "Why didn't you share this with me?" What would that do to the relationship and the trust between us? I wondered if I were to just come clean with her and share my dilemma with her, what would that do to the relationship? I'm often really transparent with people, and that's what I do if I'm in a dilemma or stuck place with them, but around this, because it's so early in the recovery process for me I found I wasn't willing to do this. It felt too unworked and unclear to me.

What finally freed me up was something someone in the program said to me who is also a therapist: That if my client had to choose between being in therapy with me and going to meetings, she should go to the meetings. That the therapy relationship, as he put it, "Needs to be eligible to be relinquished." That in this instance it wasn't about what I was thinking or should propose—because I know, without being grandiose, that I could hold her in therapy and wasn't sure these meetings could—but about what I was willing to have happen.

What I ended up saying to this woman was, "Look, candidly, the reason that I've needed to study this for a couple of weeks is because I am involved in my own recovery work around that issue, and this work is of fairly recent vintage. And I needed to . . . I've needed and wanted to give some real delivery of thought to the question of how to interact with you around this. For one thing, because I don't want you to be looking at me as the person with all the answers, when I just got here myself. And secondly, there's this very small community that I want to tell you about. But it's a very small community. And we need to talk about how can we negotiate this in a way that is respectful of both of our interests without making this work either difficult or perhaps impossible? Let's collaborate."

This is, by the way, not the kind of conversation I feel I can have with every client. It has to be with someone who can maintain her boundaries in a certain kind of way. There is another person I'm seeing who if we negotiated, for example, separate meetings, she would want to come to the meetings that I'm at. She would push the limits. She's already found out where I live and other things about me that make me uncomfortable. In her case, asking her to do that would be negligent on my part because I'd be putting her in the position of taking on something that she's not ready or capable of.

One thing that was hanging me up was that I feel as a member of a 12-step program, anytime, anywhere someone reaches out, I have a responsibility to be there. And I feel that around DA very, very powerfully. And then the same colleague corrected me. He reminded me that the tradition actually says "I want the hand of AA to be there." It's not "I have to be there," but that's how I interpreted it and how it gets paraphrased.

Progress, Not Perfection

Therapists need to bring lots of compassion to these interactions, both for themselves and their clients. Clinicians trying to negotiate these boundaries with clients are a lot like the early pioneers in AA Rachel referred to above. There are few, if any, role models in the field to follow, or guidelines in the literature to refer to. Although the newness and small size of DA made Rachel's an especially difficult situation, she did a good job of mapping out many of the machinations therapists in recovery undergo when they consider the consequence of attending the same meeting as a client or referring clients to 12-step programs. In some instances, encounters with clients at meetings can be informative and therapeutic; at other times, therapists need to carefully negotiate boundaries with clients to try to ensure they do not attend the same meeting.

What's most desirable is not always possible. Roget Lockard talked about the dilemmas he faced as a therapist in the fellowship because of his work at a treatment facility:

> Working in the detox as the entry point for my being a treatment person in the field of addictions, and a person in recovery myself, absolutely required that I come to terms with being at meetings with clients. It was literally not an option. I would have to drive a couple of states away to be absolutely confident that I would be at a meeting where there were no clients. And in the years that I still worked in a detox setting, and even for several years after, I would notice from time to time at, for example, an AA meeting that more than half the people in the room either were present clients or former clients. So, you know, I just had to come to terms with that context, because I didn't have an alternative. (personal communication, June 1998)

Roget's circumstances are unique to therapists in the recovery field, but not unusual ones for them to encounter. Many therapists with similar vocational histories find it challenging to protect their own and their clients' anonymity at meetings. Melanie described her relationship with a client in recovery who became very anxious when she discovered that Melanie was a recovering alcoholic:

> "She used to get concerned about whether I was still sober, if she'd had a little break from therapy, or if she hadn't checked in with me in a while, even though we were meeting every week. I know it used to make me uncomfortable when she'd do that. I used to feel like I needed to have a certain kind of program. I needed to go to a certain number of meetings. I don't do that now. I decide what I want to do, and where I want to go, and how many. And if she asks me now, I'm more secure."

Worried about her client having to manage this anxiety on her own at a time when her client's sobriety and their therapy relationship were especially fragile, Melanie worked out a way for her client to check in with her between sessions. The need for this kind of reassurance, more prominent during the beginning phases of therapy, eventually subsided, and the two simply discussed the client's concerns at their next session. Melanie also discussed the dilemma presented when another client aggressively challenged her recovery and what she was doing to take care of herself:

> "There was one woman who definitely needed to be more into recovery; she's the kind of person who would say to me, 'Why should I be going to so many meetings when you're an alcoholic and you don't even get to half that many?' I think if anyone said that to me, at this stage of the game, I would say that my feeling about anyone going to meetings is that they need to use the program more when they need it. They need to use it in a way that works for them, and when I have a crisis going on, I go to more meetings. That's just how I do it, so if that's what was going on for a client I would say, 'What I'm seeing is that there are some things that aren't working well for you, and this is an avenue that I would encourage you to pursue.' Just like I would."

While some of the details of this discussion are particular to work with addictions, the questions they raise are not. How to manage personal information about the therapist whether it's inadvertently discovered by clients or intentionally disclosed by the therapist is a challenge that every clinician faces. It is also a challenge with which therapists who see recovering therapists in their own practices must grapple.

Therapy with Recovering Therapists

Just as some therapists who are new to trauma work will discover their personal trauma histories through their work with survivors, therapists will often come face to face with their own addictions through their work with clients' alcohol and drug problems.

What therapists in recovery need most from their own therapy is respect for their need to be clients. Many of us in this work grew up in alcoholic homes in which we were given too much responsibility as children. Whether caring for siblings, running between adults in the family in an effort to diffuse conflicts, or tending to the emotional and physical needs of the nondrinking and/or the alcoholic parent(s) when they were children, these persons do not need to have the experience of being "parentified" in their own therapy.

We should not assume that because a therapist knows how to take care of clients she knows how to take care of herself. This is often welcome or comforting news to a therapist who worries that tending to a crisis in her own life—giving herself permission to "fall apart"—will result in her practice becoming unraveled or her clients being deprived of the care they need. Further, it's not important whether a therapist "knows" what she needs to do to take better care of herself or just needs to "follow her own advice." What's healing is hearing the same words and ideas she shares with clients expressed to her within the context of a caring and empathic relationship.

More than any other people we see in our practice, working with a person who is also a therapist is going to have us questioning our own experiences. Consequently, it's important to have our own consultation and supports in place prior to taking on this work. It is also a good idea to encourage therapists we see in therapy to do the same. Ensuring that people have adequate clinical supervision in their practice is the best way of preventing the therapy relationship from being transformed into a supervisory one. I do not mean to give the impression that these are strict boundaries that should never be crossed. All clients need to discuss their work in therapy, and this is no different for therapists. For us therapists, our own therapy is always our best training. Some supervisory relationships evolve into clinical ones, and those therapists who were once clients will often seek out a former therapist for clinical mentoring (although this scenario may well be a complex one). Having the two processes in place conjointly simply allows us to be more creative and play more in supervision and therapy. It also ensures that regardless of what's going on in our therapy, our clinical work is being held and tended to in whatever ways both our clients and we are in need of at that time.

Seeking ongoing consultation when seeing therapists in our practices is just as important and is a good way to keep our envy and competitive emotions in check. It's important that we be capable of taking joy in all our clients' work and success, to appreciate what they do better than us, and still be present in the ways they need us to be for them. As Pearlman and Saakvitne (1995) counsel, for persons providing supervision or consultation to therapists, regardless of the context, remember that supervision of trauma and addiction is always a consultation about a relationship, not a client.

As careful as we need to be about all recovering persons we see in our practice not using therapy as a substitute for going to meetings, this is even more essential in work with the recovering therapist. Is the person hiding behind her identity as a clinician in order to avoid her alcoholism? If the answer is yes, we might ask her the following question. As she has started to feel more adequate and competent as a professional, does she feel that she's supposed to be "over her problems" or no longer needs these kinds of supports to remain sober?

The specific issues will be different for therapists depending on the stage of their career. Rachel, for example, experienced some shame about her recovery issues. An accomplished and experienced clinician, her recovery felt like the one thing holding her back or keeping her from advancing to the upper echelon of her field. Other therapists who are very comfortable in their identity both as senior clinicians and as people in recovery may feel pressured to always "have it together"—not in the way that a novice or student might, out of a sense of insecurity or inadequacy, but from the stress of being held up as cultural icons of sorts and as heroes or pioneers by the larger professional and recovering communities. Publishing and touring the lecture and workshop circuit can be very exciting and stimulating work that nourishes a healthy ego, but it doesn't do much for the soul. We need to feed both.

Therapist Relapse

From the standpoint of addiction, there is no more vulnerable or dangerous space alcoholics can occupy than the one they find themselves in immediately *after* they've taken that first drink. It seems ridiculous to point out that drinking is an extremely dangerous activity for an alcoholic. However, alcoholics *will* drink. It's what they do. If sober alcoholics are going to avoid drinking, their "moment of truth" transpires well before they actually pick up a glass of alcohol. Once they have a drink in their hands it is usually a forgone conclusion that they're going to consume it. The crucial question then shifts from what they can do to avoid drinking to what they're going to do about it once they are drinking.

Therapists in recovery who work with alcoholics and other addicts are no less vulnerable to relapse than oncologists are immune to cancer. However, in addition to whatever action the recovering therapist or her sponsor feels is necessary to get her recovery back on track, a therapist's slip has implications for her practice which she must consider as well:

Denise's Relapse Story

For me, my relapse has such educational value about recovery. And fortunately I was awake enough to notice what the lesson was.

I had not consumed alcohol since about four or five years into attending AA. And I was going to meetings. I was working my program, and I was working as a clinician exceptionally hard. My husband and I had a lot of financial responsibility in those days. We were supporting seven people and paying a mortgage and just working very, very hard, both of us. I think I had two or three jobs, you know, including the private practice. And raising kids and carpooling and stuff. So it was a stressful time. I hadn't really developed all the stress management skills I needed. And I was really unaware of all the different aspects and sort of permutations of codependency in work and in my personal life.

So there was one Sunday afternoon when I was at home, a sort of gray day. My husband was out doing some lawn work. So he was available to talk to and the Rolodex with all of my hundred AA names was sitting where it always does.

Up until the relapse, I would fumble through the Rolodex. I would take calls from other people who needed me. I would call on the people when I felt good, or when I wanted to socialize. But actually, my social life was so full outside of AA that I didn't really use those names for a lot of socialization stuff in the way that some folks do, and I didn't call anyone when I was hurting either.

If I called anybody in the program I called after the fact to review what I had done about feeling so bad—sort of show and tell—rather than in the midst of the crisis. I hadn't used those names in the Rolodex that way, up until that time, so I wasn't really fully mutual with my fellow AAs. I was still the therapist who should figure it out and then tell people about it.

Then on this afternoon, I felt very empty and depressed, this real existential funk. I'd never felt that way for more than a moment, but that day it lasted hours. I was cooking something for our dinner, and prior to that day, I had never really had any difficulty with abusing the cooking wine that sat on the spice shelf. Occasionally we'd have a chicken dish or something we'd splash some cooking wine on. But it was not a drinkable wine. It was from the grocery store—you know, salty. It was just there, almost as an herb or spice. But this day I was feeling desperate. So instead of exercising any other options or making any other connections with people, I just very quickly, while in the midst of cooking, picked up this cooking wine and guzzled down a couple of swigs. It tasted awful. I didn't get any high out of it. There was no euphoria, it didn't work in any way to make me feel better. It was done totally compulsively.

Probably ten minutes later, I was still cooking, chopping vegetables, my husband came in and he could read me, he could tell that I looked very strange. He confronted me about what was

going on. I said, "Nothing, nothing." I was extremely defensive.
He asked again. This is another thing I feel very grateful for,
people in my life who have along the way helped me to keep
looking in the mirror without harming or shaming me. My
husband persisted. Apparently, I looked out of it or whatever. . . .
I meant to ask him how I looked. But he knew to pursue
questioning what was going on with me, and he did pursue it,
and he listened. Finally he said, "Do you ever feel like drinking
when you feel like this?" I just said I felt very empty and sad and
couldn't name what was going on. "Do you ever feel like
drinking?" he asked. I said, "Yes."

And then he paused a moment and asked, "Do you ever
drink when you feel like this?" I avoided him and went into the
bathroom and closed the door. I thought, "Shit. What do I do
now?" I had a choice of lying or not lying. I guess I had been in
the program too long to lie. At least for me, I didn't think that it
was wise to try to cover over what had happened. Even though it
was just this brief moment with no apparent intoxication. So I
came out of the bathroom and I said, "I'm sorry. I did drink.
Yeah, not only do I feel like it, but I did. Look at this," and I
got the bottle out. He just very calmly asked, "So, what do you
think you're going to do about that?" This is the value of going
to a lot of meetings because you get programmed into knowing
what you should do in certain circumstances. I said, "I'm going
to go to a meeting and talk about it." "When are you going to
do that?" he asked. "Tonight," I said. And I went to a meeting
that night.

One of the first people I ran into at that meeting was the
same man who four years earlier had given me the hard time and
then come around. He was there, and I very instinctively went
over and grabbed him and said, "I need to talk with you." I told
him the story. And he was very non-shaming and non-facetious,
and gave me a lot of good advice. He said, "You know, you're a
person who hasn't had a relapse experience. This is a time where
you need to do 90 in 90.* You also need to get to know some
different people in the program, people who can tell you how to
come back in without shaming yourself out into another relapse.
You probably don't hang out with people who go in and out?"
he asked. "No, I don't," I replied. "Well, you need to do that
now," he said. He mentioned some first names of some people
that I might approach. To humble myself to them and say, you

---

*This refers to AA's recommendation that newcomers and others struggling to remain so-
ber make an effort to attend 90 meetings in 90 days.

know, "I just picked up, can you tell me about your experience?" That was very sound advice, I thought. He helped me to get more deeply into the program and my process.

So I listened to this fellow's advice. Part of me wanted to still compartmentalize, to do my recovery from the relapse in some group that was for therapists or helping professionals only. But, for some reason, I didn't explore that. Instead, I listened to another part of my mind that said, "Stop covering your tracks. Denise, just be in the world." So I went to the Looney Nooner, which is like a big downtown coffee shop a hundred—a hundred plus people. I was on the 90 in 90 track, and this must have been about the second or third day back from my cooking wine.

I sat at the table instead of sitting on the periphery. I did what they told me in the program. I sat up at the table and as the discussion moved around to me instead of just identifying and saying, "I pass," I said, "Hi, I'm Denise. I'm an alcoholic and I'm coming back in from a slip." All the voices said, "Welcome back Denise, keep coming," as the voices say in the room. As I looked up from the table, I guess I had been talking with my head down, I surveyed the room and I saw client, client, active client, former client. Maybe four people who I had some involvement with as a therapist, and I said to myself, "Oh shit," because I realized the implications of that. Here I had used this venue to acknowledge what was current for me and maybe that wasn't the best thing to do. It necessitated my approaching each person, at least my active clients, to explore their experience of the meeting. I took it up with them in therapy at the beginning of the session. "What was it like to see me there?" I asked.

They may have been caretaking me or setting aside what they heard there in their own denial about who I was, because it didn't fit their idealized picture of me. I don't have any way of assessing what their experience was. But what they did tell me was that it was very powerful to hear me acknowledging my drinking in an open way. Two people said, "That's what's different about you as a therapist. I would never go to see a therapist—if I was working on an active addiction—I wouldn't go to a therapist who wasn't in the soup herself."

I realize I didn't go out on a magnum or a case of beer, but I was pretty clear about why I considered it to be a relapse, and acknowledged it to my husband, acknowledged it to others, and kept doing intensive work in AA. It was because of the extreme compulsivity of it. It frightened me that there was almost no pause between the morose feeling that overtook me and the solution that involved taking the cap off the bottle and chugalugging. So it wasn't the amount. The volume wasn't relevant to me. And my only regret, of course, is that I didn't get high out of it. You have to humble yourself so much when you come back in after a relapse that I would have liked to have had a high.

That sums it up right there. It was the compulsive nature of the act. It was how alcohol owned me, how it spoke to me as the ultimate solution. Just the level of hold, the level of claim that alcohol as a solution had on me, and the compulsivity of the decision making is what caused it to stand out for me. This was especially true in face of the fact that there were so many people I could have talked to, friends who would have loved and supported me and helped me do what I needed to do. That I had so many options and still chose to drink for affective regulation of my feelings told me not to minimize it. For me, I needed to treat it as a slip or a relapse, and I would tell a client that too.

When I was going to all of these cajillion AA meetings, I recognized that all and all I've been blessed because the trajectory of my recovery—what's promoted further, deeper healing—and my therapy practice were interwoven. What I learned from the relapse is that it was my codependency, my failure to self-care, and my desire to take care of everyone in the entire world (except for me) that led to my desperation, and resulted in my drinking the cooking wine. That was an important insight—one I followed up on by doing work in Co-Dependents Anonymous [CoDA] and Al-Anon.

Shame

The idea Denise received from her friend in AA about needing to seek out other people who had recently relapsed or slipped, in order to generate some strategies of her own and combat the shame and embarrassment, was sound advice. A poignant Buddhist story drives this point home: A 3-year-old boy dies, and his mother can't accept it. She walks around the village with his corpse in her arms. Finally the villagers send her to the Buddha. He listens, then assigns her a task. He tells her to visit every house in the village and bring back a mustard seed from every house that has not known death. Obviously, the woman comes back empty-handed. When a client is having difficulty accepting a slip and moving on or expressing shame at having drunk, I often share this story with her. I then tell her to visit every AA meeting in town and to bring back a penny from every alcoholic who has not known relapse.

The feelings of shame a person experiences after a slip are often amplified for professional health-care providers by what I call the "fallen-angel syndrome." Physicians, nurses, psychotherapists, and other healers are archetypal figures in our culture who symbolize authority and nurturance. Consequently, when they stumble or falter their actions are often viewed as acts of betrayal and abandonment of the people they've committed their lives to protecting and serving.

Denise talked about not using a specialized group of professionals in recovery in response to her relapse, because she wanted to "just be in the world." But there are support groups that model themselves on AA and that are tailored to the specific needs of health-care providers. These are good resources for therapists and other clinicians to consider when responding to a slip or getting sober for the first time.

I encourage therapists that I see in my practice to think of a relapse in the same way as they would think of a death in the family or some other personal emergency. I recommend they stop taking new referrals until they've had a chance to regroup, and to take as much time off as they need to get to more meetings. When deciding whether or not to tell clients about their own relapse, therapists need to consider the possibility of clients who are also in the fellowship finding out about the slip on their own or from someone other than their therapist. Also, just as some individuals we've been working with for years know when all in our world is not well, clients do not have to have been informed directly in order to sense the effect a change or shift as significant as a relapse may have on the therapist's experience of herself. The decision to tell clients ought to be talked over with a supervisor, a consultant, and peers. As with any personal crisis, what is shared and how much is shared with any given client will depend on the relationship the therapist has with that particular individual. In the case of ongoing abuse, the therapist will need to suspend her practice entirely until some long-term sobriety is achieved again.

AA's ninth step encourages alcoholics to make amends to people they've hurt with their drinking "except where to do so would cause more harm." This can also serve as a guideline. Ultimately, what therapists choose to share with both clients and colleagues comes down to the needs and personal preference of the individual therapist. Regardless of the venue used to acknowledge the experience, the most important qualities that a recovering therapist who has relapsed needs a larger "outside-witness group" to share are compassion, love, respect, and humility.

Despite the positive feedback she received from clients about her slip, Denise said, "If anything like that ever happened again, I would do things differently. I would not want to subject my clients or my relationships with them to so much of my relapse history." She went on to say that she would find meetings with a lower profile or in another location, further from her practice, where she could share her experiences.

The Language of Psychotherapy and Recovery

Some final remarks on the vast topic of the therapist's use of self and the language I use to describe these experiences. I have said on a number of occasions throughout this book that I find the terms "transference" and "countertransference" unsatisfactory to describe the kinds of spells and relational states that are conjured up for us and the people we see in therapy. However, I find much of what certain analysts have to say about these topics inspiring. Earlier, I've proposed alternative terms—hybrids of literary theory and psychotherapy—such as "countertrans-pondence," but these are less than adequate as well.

Many therapists express concerns which I share that the use of these terms leads to our privileging, in our conversations with people, the "micro-world of therapy" over the "macro-contexts of people's lives."[8] These cautionary messages are in response to the idea that to be effective, the therapy relationship needs to be sealed off from realities and problems of ordinary life or removed from the experiences of peoples' everyday lives. Classical theory has done little to dispel this myth with its warnings of "contaminant properties" outside the analysis. However, this is not an accurate reflection of contemporary psychoanalytic theory and the therapies informed by them. What these ideas tell us is that therapy is not about being with people in another world; rather, it's about being in the world with people in a particular way.

Authenticity in the analyst, says Mitchell, has less to do with saying everything than with the genuineness of what is actually said; what is unique about therapy and psychoanalysis is that the two processes "demand a curiosity about one's feelings on the part of both participants especially a curiosity about the moments when one feels a virtual lack of curiosity" (1993, p. 146). The outcome is not a less authentic experience than we would have outside of therapy but one with a different emphasis.

I have a client who knitted a wool comforter (or throw) for my couch. She worked on it during AA meetings and at family functions that she started attending for the first time since making the decision to get sober. Periodically, she would bring the comforter to sessions to lay out its colors and patterns against the color scheme in my office. She said that knitting it helped her feel more connected to me and her therapy, and provided her a sense of safety when she needed to take risks in the world. How do you find a language or theory of therapy that captures that?

I thrive on the dreams, predilections, hopes, fears, and therapeutic needs of my clients and their situation at hand. It is particularly gratifying when you watch someone use your relationship with them to transform something about their life or themselves. There is no greater satisfaction for me than that. It's about more than therapy—it's seeing that you do have a wonderful effect on another person.

THE SPIRITUAL LIFE OF THERAPISTS

> Those of us who have come to make regular use of prayer
> would no more do without it than we would refuse air,
> food, or sunshine. And for the same reason. When we
> refuse air, light, or food the body suffers. And when we
> turn away from meditation and prayer, we likewise deprive
> our minds, our emotions, and our intuitions of vitally
> needed support. As the body can fail its purpose for lack of
> nourishment, so can the soul.
> —THE TWELVE AND TWELVE

When I started out I was pretty circumspect about including spirituality in the therapeutic conversation. And I just found that the preponderance of time it was a refreshment. It was welcomed. And the times when it wasn't it was still a useful line of conversation to open up—to explore. And it may not go much of anywhere if the person doesn't have a spiritual perspective but they usually do. And, once that is factored into the conversation there's an exponential enhancement of what happens. It authorizes a level of intimacy that makes sense. It shifts people away from fixing the problem when you have that bigger way of working.

—ROGET LOCKARD

I bring Spirituality up a lot in the context of trauma and sexual abuse, particularly exploring what contributed to a person's resilience. Even if they didn't call it a Higher Power or spirituality when they were children, where did their sense of being held or connection to the world—the sense of a protective presence in their life or the universe—come from? I think it not only opens up and enriches things, it gives you new language that is freeing. It diffuses a lot of the transference and breaks up the intensity of that dyadic team working on fixing things. Suddenly you have a triad. And at times, especially when bearing witness or talking about things that are unspeakable, that's a great relief to people.

—DENISE

People's spiritual beliefs are interesting and really hard for me to talk about. I'm beginning to read some Buddhist teachings, and what I read is sort of like what I've always believed—at least what I've believed since I was about 24, when my mom died: That whatever happens in my life is there to provide meaning for me, it's there to teach me a lesson. And so, I use that. I don't talk about this very much, but I use that in how I might invite a client to explore their feelings when their coping mechanisms are strained or silent around a tragic loss or other trauma. I guess I use it more for myself. I use my own faith and beliefs to help me to detach from what's going on with my clients. I used to dream about clients. I used to be, you know, really thinking, "What am I going to do to help this person?" Or "What am I doing wrong?" Not that I still don't think about these things. But, more often than not, I realize their life is their path or their journey, and they have to follow it.

—MELANIE

I often invoke the presence of God for myself when I get into a place where I feel stuck with a client. Or, if I have a personally strong reaction to my own transference to them. I use imagery. I imagine their higher power and mine together, and us being held together in therapy, in that process. I do that much more explicitly. Even in sessions, I find myself doing that. Sometimes I feel like—or ask to be—a channel in a session for our Higher Power. And I do that so much more often than I ever used to do. It's really very present for me in the work. And I don't talk about it, necessarily, unless somebody brings it up.

—RACHEL

*   *   *

Prayer and meditation have been part of AA and 12-step culture since its inception in 1935. While not the only factor in AA's dismissal, until recently, by the "helping professions," it was the primary one. Some of the history behind these rifts and the evolution of AA's spiritual practices were presented in Chapter 4. I have also tried in this book, when presenting the stories of the people I see in therapy, to be as transparent as possible about the ways the 12-step programs' spiritual steps and clients' interpretations of them—"the God stuff"—

informs my thinking and practice. The remaining passages of this chapter relate more specifically to how the therapist's spiritual beliefs and sense of the sacred (i.e., the clinician's conception of God or a Higher Power) affects the therapy relationship.

While 12-step programs clearly influenced each therapist's sense of faith and spirituality, Melanie talked about the influence Buddhist readings have had on her thinking as of late. Conferences and workshops on meditation and other Buddhist spiritual practices have been part of the New Age psychology landscape for years. Recently news of these practices have been cropping up in more mainstream forums, and one can hear the whirring of the next *Networker* feature readying to hit the presses with a picture of the Dalai Lama and the headline "Leader in Exile or Psychotherapist in Residence?"

References to Buddhism abound in psychoanalytic and family therapy journals, literature, and professional conferences. Initially the promise of this approach was its offering a potential crossroad where psychotherapy and Western medicine could finally meet. Innovator Jon Kabat-Zinn (1994) adapted Buddhist practices and principles in his pioneering work with hospital patients and other people combating stress, high blood pressure, and chronic pain. Now third-party payment for workshops consisting of rooms full of people in hospital auditoriums being guided through relaxing imagery, breathing exercises, and Zen meditation is becoming standard practice, and the types of referrals and problems for which such exercises and meditation are "prescribed" include posttraumatic stress disorder, addictions, anxiety, attention-deficit/hyperactivity disorder, and certain forms of depression.

For therapists, meditation offers gentle ways of helping us stay present for clients, letting go of our own stress, and restoring our spirits after years of absorbing people's stories of trauma and pain. The attraction Buddhist meditation holds for therapists and clients is an obvious one. Its attention to people's experiences of suffering and happiness and its emphasis on staying in the moment and being present make it particularly well suited to the psychotherapy process.

In addition, the concepts of "acceptance" and "letting go" are cornerstones of the philosophies underlying the spiritual beliefs of both Buddhism and 12-step culture, and the two worlds nest very comfortably with one another. There are many therapists who have been steeped in these spiritual ways and have used them in their relationships with people for years. However, because of the more accepting atmosphere in general about spirituality that exists today, the road is being paved for these practices to impact the psychotherapy culture and theory on a much larger scale.

These perspectives can also make us more available to assist clients who are in despair about their disconnection from their own spiritual and religious practices, even when these traditions are not where their therapists find their own sense of the sacred. Denise talked about her work with one client who had fallen away from the Catholic church, and then returned to his faith by virtue of what happened in a conversation between them about spirituality:

> "There was a man—a recovering alcoholic—who said to me he really objected to the subject, to my raising it, when it first came up. He objected to my saying, 'I think that you're being too controlling in your own head, keeping yourself away from the sacraments. Because you are an adulterer. It was eighteen years ago and you're still punishing yourself. You're doing it all yourself. You're running your own show. Here's another manifestation of your alcoholic mind. You never asked anybody, you never went to Father so-and-so up there at Blessed Sacrament and asked him what he thought about your coming back into the fold. You're doing it all on your own. You're doing your own program.' And he hated that. He absolutely hated that I suggested it. And I told him, 'You've got to have another voice in here sometimes, other voices that can help you decide how much shame, how much flagellation is appropriate. And when is there acceptance? When can anybody come back into the community? I'm not a Catholic, so maybe I'm treading on ground where I shouldn't be, but I suggest you bring some other voices in on this.'
>
> "And, by God, he came back the next session, and said he had gone to Easter services with his kids. He's a divorced man. He's getting involved in his children's lives again. And he's going back to church and going to start taking communion."

AA emphasizes that it's not the symbol system you use but the way you use it that counts. I don't share the one Denise's client used, but he certainly made it count.

What Religion Were You Raised in, and What Are You Now?

In her book *Amazing Grace*, Kathleen Norris (1998) writes about being invited to chair a panel at a literary gathering, at which she says she naively suggested the topic: "What Religion Were You Raised in, and What Religion Are You Now?" Norris quotes Samuel Taylor Coleridge who said, "An undevout poet is an impossibility" as a way of explaining her desire to learn more about her spiritual roots. Just becoming aware of the way religion is unfolding in her own life, she thought it would be interesting to hear from other writers on the subject. She was not prepared for the high emotion her question generated. Some were angry at her for raising the subject of religion at a writer's conference. Others took her aside to say that while the subject was of great interest to them, it was too personal (or too painful) to talk about in public. According to Norris, "Several writers declared themselves, in no uncertain terms, to be 'In the religion of Whitman,' having happily substituted literature for religion in their lives" (p. 78).

When I first heard Norris' account, I found myself having the same reaction as the latter group of writers. I shared the secular sensibilities these authors had about their profession. As a psychotherapist, I'd lived with a similar separation for years, keeping, as Norris writes, "religion in a box labeled "past" and, in my case, psychotherapy in one labeled "present." Like Norris, this neat division has ceased to hold for me. Because of my work with people in recovery, I find myself exposed to a variety of spiritual practices and have begun to doubt that the split between psychotherapy and religion need be as severe as I have made it.

Also, regardless of whether or how a therapist has thought about the role of spirituality or faith in her work, the act of showing up for her practice can bring the issue front and center. It's hard showing up day after day for our client's problems if we do not know what's in our hearts or what we believe in. Overcoming a family history of alcoholism or their own addiction presents clients with impossible choices. It requires sacrifices that seem to have no meaning other than to test people's faith—both the client's and the therapist's.

A recent week in my own practice illustrates the point. I go into it very aware that the anniversary of my father's death is fast approaching. The holidays seem tougher than usual. It's been two years this month. The trail of tears starts on his birthday, November 6th, and seems to stretch right through Thanksgiving, Christmas, to his memorial day, December 27th. We are expecting our second child. Three years ago with his body ravaged by cancer the big question was would my father live to see his first grandchild? He did. This time around it's not an issue.

On Tuesday, I arrive at my office for my nine o'clock appointment and find my client is not there. She is a recovering alcoholic, with 6 months of sobriety. I've only met with her a couple of times, but she seems very motivated. She's pregnant, but she's had three miscarriages before. This time she's made it to the second trimester, and she and her husband are full of joy. When I finally talk to her, she says she tried to call me. She'd had a miscarriage and lost her baby. She sounds devastated and asks if I can see her later in the week. On Wednesday I receive a message from a client whose family I've been seeing for the past five years. He's an ex-army medic, employed as a nurse, who works all kinds of crazy shifts. He depends on his wife, a cancer survivor, to keep him, their three children (ages 13, 11, and 4) and his home in some kind of order. His first wife was an alcoholic who abandoned their two children when they were little. Several weeks ago he missed an appointment that his wife had scheduled; it was the third or fourth session he'd missed in a row. I tried to get hold of him without any luck. His message said his wife was out of remission from her cancer and that she had died suddenly several days ago. He asked if I would please come to the service and call him. Now I have to cancel all my Friday appointments, including one with a mother who just lost her child, so I can be present for three children who just lost their mother. It's the second time that the two older kids have been left by the woman that they call Mom. In the midst of the frenzy of phone calls and scheduling changes required to attend the funeral, Robin, another client, tells me she did not make it to the Al-Anon meeting I suggested she attend. Actually, she made it to the meeting but couldn't get herself in the door. It turns out the last time she went to the church where this particular group meets, she was attending her mother's memorial service. Her mother had died two years ago that month. She said she would try again next week, but again, this time she couldn't go in. She just sat in her car and wept.

I tell her that two years is a heartbeat.

The point is that many of the so-called emotional crises that people seek our help with—alcoholism, drug addiction, divorce, trauma—and the challenges they pose for therapists might be more appropriately labeled "spiritual emergencies." In this book I've emphasized clients', not therapists', stories. However, in a book about how we sustain ourselves when faced with problems and situations that seem to defy our best skills and technical know-how, or that are so despairing they cause us to question everything we thought we believed in, the lines get blurry.

At an interreligious conference of Buddhist and Christian monastics held at a Trappist monastery, a reporter asked the Dalai Lama what he would say to Americans who want to become Buddhists. "Don't bother," he said. "Learn from Buddhism, if that is good for you. But do it as a Christian, a Jew, or whatever you are. And be a good friend to us." This is good advice for therapists as well. In order to be "a good friend" to our clients, to be present for them in the spiritual emergencies and crises they face, we need to know what experiences and beliefs inform our own skepticism and faith—what Kathleen Norris (1998) calls our "religious inheritance." For some of us, unpacking our religious inheritance may feel like a necessary chore, while for others, it may represent an epiphany, a turning point in our career or our lives. In either case, when it comes to treating addiction, knowing where our own spiritual center of gravity rests and utilizing our clients' spiritual resources in therapy is an essential part of our work.

The Promises for Professionals

Spirituality isn't just about mending our lives, it's about surviving them. My client, Cara,* is telling me about having felt suicidal and even having had a plan to go through with it. She said she felt all her affairs were in order and that she had made her peace with all the important relationships in her life, but the reason she didn't take her life was because she couldn't find a way to say good-bye to me.

The events that precipitated all this took place when Cara returned home for a weekend to help care for her aging mother. It was her first visit home in years. Her mother still lived in the house where Cara was raised and the neighborhood where she'd been sexually abused by her friend's father as well as another man she'd trusted. I commented to Cara that the contrast between the two experiences was striking: the intense sense of isolation and disconnection she experienced during her visit home, on the one hand, and her reluctance to leave the safety and security of our relationship, on the other. Thus, for Cara, thoughts of suicide were, in a sense, part of her quest for continuity (i.e., her effort to experience someone or something more permanent in her world that wouldn't abandon her). Cara felt such relief as she listened to this interpretation that she knew it held a profound truth for her.

I too felt relieved. However, I also remember asking myself, what am I supposed to do with my feelings about the suicidal plans Cara made and chose not to see to their conclusion? I was very anxious. Sometimes holding onto the choice to end their own life is all some people have left, and you can't take that away from them. That doesn't mean I would not take steps to prevent such clients from taking their life, but when we work with people in their most despairing and hopeless places this tension is not going to go away because of a contract for

---

*Cara's story introduced in Chapter 7, is discussed extensively in Chapter 8.

safety or psychiatric risk assessment. We can take steps to minimize the danger and our liability, but we can't plan for every contingency. During these times we rely on our intuition, experience, and training, but sometimes it isn't enough.

Somehow during my entire conversation with Cara about her suicidal feelings, I managed to avoid any further discussion of the intense dependency, reliance, and trust she'd invested in our relationship or the huge sense of responsibility that came with that trust. We didn't duck the issue completely because Cara was clearly expressing how much our relationship meant to her. She was also telling me how scary it was for her to express her vulnerability and allow herself to have faith in another human being, especially a man, again. Either way, sometimes in these situations all we have to hold onto is our faith and trust in our own and our client's Higher Power.

When people ask me after an experience like this if things are going to be okay, oftentimes this faith is all I have to offer them. When people ask where my faith comes from, how I know it won't abandon me or let me down, I answer honestly—I don't. I just prefer the way my days feel and life unfolds when I act as if it won't. I prefer to choose the problems and disappointments I face by believing, rather than the way life feels when I go through it without that belief.

This hasn't always been the case. Most of us who have had our spirits broken the way Cara has, falter. We stop believing in ourselves or anything else. When I identify at 12-step meetings I often feel like saying, "Hi, my name is Jonathan, and I'm a recovering professional"—that my life as a therapist sometimes poses as much of a challenge as any trauma I faced in my childhood. David Treadway (1989) wrote that sometimes being in therapy is what people do to avoid change, and sometimes being a therapist is a way to avoid ourselves—that, "we all have our moments of hiding out in the therapist's chair" (p. 199). A grandson tells his Jewish grandmother his great news, "Grandma, I'm going to become a doctor of social work!" His grandmother replies, "That's wonderful! So tell me, what kind of disease is social work?" In some ways, clinical training is like a disease. Many of us need to consider the possibility that we won't complete our own recoveries until we have recovered from being therapists.

My encounter with Cynthia at the 12-step meeting is a good example of how my professional identity and my need to be in control can get in my own way. There was a lesson in all the worry and anxiety I experienced running around trying to control every aspect of the situation for her. I needed to realize that the cosmos had a plan for Cynthia as well, and that once she found Al-Anon she didn't need me to keep smoothing the way for her, or removing all potential obstacles in order for her to get where she was going. We all have trouble understanding sometimes that wherever we are is where we need to be. We are not accustomed to thinking, as Julia Cameron (1992) says, that God's will for us and our truest dreams for ourselves may coincide.

Things happen that affirm my faith—sometimes the lessons are not subtle and the signs hard to ignore. Earlier this year a colleague asked me to present some of this work to a gathering of social workers at Cambridge Hospital. When the date for the training arrived, I was frantically trying to catch up on one of my many missed deadlines for this book and so had very little time to prepare for the talk. Consequently, I wrote the entire presentation out ahead of time and uncharacteristically decided to read the paper verbatim. For some reason when I came to reading some samples of client letters I decided to share one that I'd never used in a presentation before. The letter I read was Larry's correspondence to marijuana (This correspondence and Larry's story can be found in Chapter 3). I then shared some of the things we had learned about addiction and recovery.

Cambridge is on the other side of the state from the town where I work and live. On the way home on the Massachusetts Turnpike I stopped to check my answering service. The only new message on it was from Larry, whom I hadn't heard from in 7 or 8 years. It was very brief. "Hi, Jonathan," he said. "It's Larry. I wanted to let you know that today is my 10th anniversary. I've been sober 10 years to the day. Congratulations, you do good work! Hope you're well." I returned Larry's call to "take back to him" how excited I was to receive his call, as well as how much his news meant to me and lifted my spirits. I also told him how I'd been reading his letter and sharing parts of his story with others at the same time that he was leaving word of his milestone on my answering tape. I'm not suggesting that Larry's message was a sign from God or the work of angels. For me, it was the type of ordinary occurrence or coincidence (i.e., an everyday miracle) that keep me hopeful and passionate about what I do. The real miracle is Larry's 10 years of sobriety.

These reflections on spirituality are not part of a cosmic road map or instruction manual to enlighten therapists in their work with addicts. They're simply a collection of my own and other people's thoughts on our use of faith, prayer, and meditation in therapy with persons in recovery. I use them to help me take better care of myself (and my clients) whenever I feel lost in some of the more daunting places to which this work leads us.

I have a wooden chest next to my chair that sits on the floor between clients and me. It serves as part coffee table, part file cabinet, and its paint has a distressed look which makes it hard to tell just how old the piece is. With its purple tint of varying hues children find it magical looking. Its best feature is the 18 tiny drawers that make up its facade and give it the feel of an oversized jewelry box. I use them to keep letters, poems, cards, and thank-you notes that clients have given me or asked me to hold in safekeeping for them. Its drawers store people's fears, resentments, worries, hopes, and dreams. Because of the assortment of geodes, shells, and other treasured objects that rest on its surface, some people call it my "puja" or "worship table," while others, because of its contents, refer to it as my "God box."*

It helps me when meeting with the people I see in therapy to have something in the room that reminds me that these relationships and the work we perform are sacred. I think it's good for all of us to have symbols like this in our work spaces. It doesn't have to be an altar or shrine. It might be a picture, a photograph, or a candle that rests on a windowsill, something hallowed yet whimsical so we don't take ourselves and the process too seriously. No matter how elaborate or contemplative the arrangements on my chest/table become, it's still a place to put my tea mug. "Why is it that angels can fly?" a client asks. "Why?" I query. "Because they take themselves lightly."

---

*In AA, many sponsors suggest their sponsees use what they call a "God jar" for similar purposes. The idea is for people to use the container as a prop to help them turn their anxieties about events in their lives over which they have no control to the care of God or their Higher Power.

Commonly Asked Questions by Therapists
in Recovery Who See Addicts, Alcoholics,
and Other Recovering Persons in Their Practices

What do you answer during an interview if a client asks you about your own drinking or drug habits or personal experience with recovery?

Some recovering alcoholics inquire about a therapist's background and personal experience with sobriety issues because they want to work specifically with someone who is in recovery and using AA him- or herself. Responding to these kinds of inquiries about our experience is no different than any other situation we encounter with people. On the one hand, this is only one facet of the work and therapy relationship. We do not have to be experts in every aspect of people's lives or know their story "from the inside out" in order to be a capable ally to them. On the other, people have a right to want these credentials in their therapist (or potential one), and there are more than enough competent clinicians who have them so that if that's what they're looking for they should have no problem finding an excellent therapist with whom to work.

When a sober alcoholic or anyone else asks me specifically about my own recovery and personal experience with addiction, I explain that I have an intimate knowledge of the pain alcoholism can cause individuals and their families. I disclose that I have spent many years as a student of Al-Anon. However, as for my own drug and alcohol dependence, I cannot represent myself as having "been down those mean streets" myself. Consequently, I will understand if it is their desire to work with someone who has. If so, I offer to help them find such a person. Usually, even recovering addicts find this a sufficient response. Most clients are seeking reassurance that you have some frame of reference for understanding their plight and are familiar with the language and customs of AA or other 12-step groups. I also think therapists who haven't any personal experience with addiction in their life or their practice—I personally haven't met any but trust they exist—yet demonstrate a willingness to learn from their clients and seek consultation will find that they make satisfactory candidates as well.

The issue is more complicated for therapists who are also members of AA. If a clinician already has a reputation in the community as a person in recovery, then this is often why a person has chosen him or her as a therapist in the first place. If this is not the case, and even if it is, therapists should be cautious about how much of their own recovery they disclose to people. Don't assume that the boundaries and guidelines used to govern people's interactions in 12-step meetings are adequate or even applicable to the consultation room. It is, for example, not fair to disclose one's recovering identity to clients and then expect clients to respect one's (the therapist's) anonymity. In many instances this will be experienced as akin to being asked to keep "secret" the fact of a parent's or other family member's addiction, and is an unfair burden to place on clients. Situations like these highlight why it's always a good idea for recovering therapists to have knowledgeable and reliable clinical supervision in place in addition to whatever recovery work or therapy they pursue for themselves.

Is alcoholism and addiction best treated by specialists only?

Like the popular gangster line—"Who wants to know?"—the answer depends on who's doing the asking. It's a widely held misconception that addiction experts don't get fooled by clients who are actively abusing substances. In fact the more of this kind of work you do, statistically speaking, the higher the probability of that happening. It's true you may have more cases with a successful outcome too, but all the experience and training in the world is not going to serve as an immunization shot that inoculates clinicians from being taken for a ride, so to speak, by a person's denial. So, if someone is making a referral because she expects you to set that client straight—literally—and not be taken in by his denial system and the other problems and hardships he faces, disappointment is likely.

Experience can make a difference in determining how we therapists respond to being misled or deceived by someone in the throws of addiction. However, even in these places we are all susceptible to becoming too involved or letting our own story interfere with our judgment about what's right for a client. The only way to acquire this experience is to get practice doing the work. As far as client considerations are concerned, my bias is that working through these difficult places in the context of a safe, reliable, and ongoing therapy relationship is preferable to carving these problems out and "subcontracting" them to another clinician. No therapist need be an encyclopedia of information on recovery and addiction to be a capable ally to clients in this area. AA meetings, consultation, and other resources can provide this kind of support when necessary.

I feel this idea is often used as a way for clinicians to avoid looking at their own issues with addiction or perhaps because they see sobriety issues as outside the realm of therapy or, even worse, somehow beneath it. However, if a clinician genuinely feels, because of an awareness of her own experience or lack thereof, that she is not the best person with whom a client ought to be having these conversations, the responsible thing for her to do is to refer the case to someone else.

If you have a client suffering from addiction and another serious condition, which do you treat first?

The concept of dual diagnosis treatment is a ruse of sorts in that it tells us more about the way a specific professional community identifies a cluster of problems than what to do about them. Therapists, like others in the scientific, medical, and healing professions, are, what Evelyn Fox Keller calls "a colluding community of common language speakers." This is what we mean when we refer to therapy as a discipline and talk about developing standard procedures and professional practices. No matter what linguistic or material conventions we follow or forge together, each of us still has to apply them to our clients' stories in a process that allows for our own sort of muddling through and makes sense to the people we're trying to help.

In the case of the "dual-diagnosis patient," if the person is actively using drugs or under the influence of alcohol, the patient should be strongly encouraged to go through a detox process first, and then to participate in AA or another 12-step program. But this only applies uniformly in "textbook" cases. As has often been demonstrated in this book, each person's situation is unique. The only principle I can universally apply is to start where clients are. Where do they want to begin? What ideas move them? What ideas are they willing to try?

I recommend AA even to clients with quite severe mental illnesses, based on the dramatic changes I have seen in such people who have found a group where they feel safe and to which they can commit.

At what point, because of a person's ongoing substance abuse, is it appropriate to end therapy?

This is another situation where the personal boundaries and sensibilities of the therapist take precedence over any set clinical formulas or 12-step principles. A client who consistently shows up to therapy under the influence of alcohol and drugs is giving a clear message he or she needs inpatient, not outpatient treatment. Obviously, there are guidelines that can help us make these decisions; however, within these parameters there are many judgment calls. Behaviors one clinician is willing to tolerate in the therapy relationship may be unacceptable to another. In general, I prefer the problems that stem from hanging in too long with clients rather than letting them go too soon. However, a therapist who is paralyzed with fear about the activities her client may be engaging in is not going to make a very useful ally and may need to end or postpone her work with that person because of this.

I find the best approach to these scenarios is to avoid getting into them in the first place. I require that someone who is still actively using chemicals—after a significant amount of time in therapy and 12-step group—participate in a treatment program as a condition of remaining in therapy. This frees me from having to "police" a client's drug or drinking habits. This is a common practice for psychiatrists who are monitoring a person's medication. All inpatient and most intensive outpatient programs require drug screening as a condition of enrollment. By establishing participation in a treatment program as a criterion for continuing in therapy, therapists put the onus of responsibility for making this decision back on their client. It also gives people who are not ready to get sober a way to leave therapy without severing the relationship—that is, to end treatment with the message that they're always welcome to return, along with a means of doing so should they have a change of heart.

The therapist who is in recovery herself is no less vulnerable to these dilemmas. She may, because of her own contertransference, find herself being more hardline, so to speak, with clients around their addiction issues, or overly empathic and tolerant. These are very appropriate issues for supervision.

Should therapists in recovery themselves sponsor people in AA and other 12-step programs?

There is not a correct answer to this question or one that applies to every clinician. You choose your problems, not your solutions. One therapist with many years in the program offered these reasons not to sponsor others:

> "I don't sponsor to take care of myself. It's too close to what I do for a living. I help people. I'm available for 12-step conversations, calls, so forth and so on. But I don't—for both of those reasons, and other clinical considerations—formally sponsor others. I find this avoids situations where both clients and I feel set up: 'Well, you sponsor him . . . how come not me?' "

On the other hand, there are important benefits that the sponsoring relationship offers therapists that they may not get from clients. Rachel, who clearly understands the concerns about boundaries, feels it's a question of balance:

> "If I had a full-time private practice, I couldn't sponsor. However, since I have a one-quarter caseload, it's very different. When I was first in the program I did a lot of sponsoring. And to me, it was totally mutual, the power differential was not there. Regardless of the kind of practice you have, whether you're a feminist therapist or whatever, they're giving you money. When sponsoring I got just as much from people as I gave. And the process of using the tools to be in the solution and not the problem is a very different process of how the energy of expenditure and the giving it back works and so forth."

My own preference—when actively involved in Al-Anon or any other 12-step group—is to find other ways of performing "service" at meetings. Sponsoring people is hard work and can often add to the particular kind of fatigue I experience from being a therapist. Sometimes, I have found it's a good idea for me to spend the time that I'm not practicing therapy taking care of myself in other ways, instead of looking for other ways to take care of people.

PART IV

No Conclusions

There is nothing so dangerous as an idea when it's the only one you have.

—EMILE CHARTIER

CHAPTER 12

A Less
Convenient Fiction

Robin: Suppose you fall down the stairs . . .
Morris: Get hit by a car.
Robin: Run up against some mean virus.
Morris: Or abuse your arteries.
Robin: And the hero doctor rushes in and saves your life,
   but maybe you don't notice who's been taking care of
   you all along. Life is community art—and artists are so
   good, so subtle, we got everybody thinking we are
   obsolete and unnecessary. . . . Each person is a piece of
   art, a masterpiece, ancient and modern.
                                   —ANDREA HAIRSTON

Like a painting, therapy, and other creative processes, a book is never finished—it simply stops in interesting places. Some of the places we'll be pausing here, in this book's final chapter, include some summary remarks on the language we use to describe alcoholism and addiction, methods of collapsing time when therapy with alcoholics and addicts needs to be brief, and some additional thoughts on letter writing and other narrative techniques in psychotherapy and recovery.

Every artist knows that psychiatry, psychology, and social work have no monopoly on the power to heal. Even the DSM-IV text and criteria editor, Michael First, MD, admits that "it is a convenient fiction to suppose the patients' problems can be broken down into discrete categories. We don't understand the etiology of mental illness, and lab findings are practically never found that are diagnostically useful" (American

Psychiatric Association, 1994, p. 26). From the standpoint of psychiatry and medicine, when it comes to understanding the etiology of alcoholism and addiction, the present book offers a less convenient fiction.*

Fiction, it is said, often reveals truths that reality obscures. In her play *Strange Attractors,* Andrea Hairston makes the case that poets and storytellers save more lives than do doctors or medical research. Consider this scene between the two characters Robin and Morris, who ask:

> How many times a year does a doctor actually save your life? How often is a truly big breakthrough in medicine discovered? How many times did you even go to a doctor in a year—most of us don't even have a relationship with a physician we see regularly. Compare that to the number of movies you saw this month—or last week. How much music do you listen to everyday? What about TV? How many images do you look at everyday or stories did you hear in the last twenty minutes? How often do you try and express yourself, fix your hair, buy clothes, or make a gesture?
>
> When we try and figure out who we are, what we want, and how we're going to get it—how do we know what's possible? What roles we can play in life? Where do we get a sense of what we can be ten years from now? How do we make plans? We fall in love, or have a passion for this or that—how do we come up with all that? Just from our own experiences, our innate nature, our own personal culture? (1997, unpublished script, pp. 32)

Jay Efran and his coauthors (Efran, Hefner, & Lukens, 1987) make the same point about the ways we've come to theorize and treat addiction. Current theories of addiction are not based on the outcomes of scientific research or critical experiments but are part of a backlash to 19th-century moralism that labeled people bad or evil as a result of their drinking and other social habits. Citing Blume's work (1983), these authors discuss how the "disease model"

> allowed for the diagnosis of clients based on common features, encouraged the establishment of treatment facilities instead of reliance on jails and psychiatric institutions, protected the civil rights of alcoholics and addicts as disabled persons, promoted health insurance coverage, and gave impetus to funding for research and training.

A Less Convenient Fiction: Poets and Writers Revisit the DSM-IV is the title of an anthology of poetry and prose I am coediting with Emma Morgan.

Thus, a large and beneficial program of action emerged from this way
of thinking and talking about addiction and drinking. (p. 44)

The authors point out that the disease model did not free us of
moral issues—it simply cloaked them in more antiseptic and modern-
sounding medical, psychiatric, psychological, and sociological jargon.
Moralism and addiction have not achieved anything like a satisfactory
divorce. Since problems and solutions are always found in language, *any*
approach to a problem reflects a value position. Morals are hidden in all
human enterprises, even those that purport to be value free. It's time to
give up the pretense that the answer to questions can be found purely in
science. Answers, these writers conclude, are always a function of the
questions we ask and the language we use, and always have moral implications.

In "Poetry Is Not a Luxury," Audre Lorde states that "poetry is the
way we help give name to the nameless so it can be thought" (1984,
p. 37). Meanwhile, for all its authority to name and label human experience, the language of medical science can only hope to approach this experience.

The issue is language. "Language," says poet Adrienne Rich, "is as
real, as tangible . . . as streets, pipelines, and telephone switchboards"
(1979, p. 247). A client gives us a poem that puts words to her pain and
takes our breath away. When the session ends, we hand it back to her
and write notes in a file that correspond to each itemized problem identified in her treatment plan with a corresponding DSM-IV code. Why is it
that a poem or a short story can capture so much of a person's experience but when it comes to informing ourselves about their condition and
the challenges they face we turn to the DSM-IV or another psychiatric
tomb? Audre Lorde deems poetry "a vital necessity of our existence. . . .
It forms the quality of light within which we predicate our hopes and
dreams toward survival and change, first made into language, then into
idea, then into more tangible action" (1984, p. 37). Within the light cast
by DSM-IV and other psychotherapy texts, what kind of dreams do we
predicate?

I began this book stating that I did not intend to grab onto the ris-
ing star of narrative therapy and postmodernism and would deploy a
number of lenses that would help the reader make a critical assessment
of these ideas. Over the course of the book's pages many strengths and
advantages as well as contradictions and concerns about narrative therapy were uncovered. Nevertheless, now, at the book's conclusion, one
point remains certain: narrative therapy, in all its incarnations, is gaining

in notoriety and fast becoming the "new wave" in psychotherapy. However, as suggested by philosopher Richard Rorty's celebrated phrase "facts are dead metaphors," every new idea for therapy is eventually replaced by still newer ones—laying the old one and our thoughts about it to rest.

Scientists and astronomers exploring our physical universe offer their own account of this process. When long ago, some distant stars burned out in our galaxy, the Milky Way, they shot countless carbon atoms into space, the same atoms from which all earth-bound, carbon-based life forms—including humans—derive. In other words, as these scientists and stargazers point out, we are all made of stardust. Perhaps, in our own way, this is the phenomenon we narrative therapists are invoking when we talk about people discovering the "sparkling facts" of their lives, and why we human beings seem to shine so when given the opportunity to tell and share our stories with one another.

SHORT STORIES: BRIEF PSYCHOTHERAPY
WITH RECOVERY ISSUES

What a ludicrous notion of emotional efficiency! Americans really believe that the past is past. They do not care to know that the past soaks the present like the light of a distant star.

—LEON WIESELTIER

Certain aspects of narrative therapy's growing popularity concern me. Some therapists wanting to be on the "cutting edge" may, for example, use letter writing, rituals, stories, and other components of the narrative approach to gain access to clients' experience of trauma and addiction, yet find themselves without the proper training to address the complexities of these problems. Asking persons to write about their experience without the binding of a caring and knowledgeable relationship to hold the pages of their stories together is frightening and not freeing.

In my experience brief treatment of addiction and trauma is always disadvantageous and not my preferred way of working with these concerns. However, when circumstances do not offer the therapist any choice, brief therapy can help people suffering with an addiction and sometimes help a lot. I like what the authors of the Milan approach (Boscolo et al., 1987; Cecchin, 1987), in particular, have to say about the way we use time to punctuate therapy sessions, as well as how change takes place, and the sense of randomness and unpredictability that surrounds it, when working in this fashion. Although I prefer to see people over time, I try—especially when working with families—not to become wedded to a set schedule and to remain flexible about the intervals between sessions. In this sense much of the work presented in this book, especially in Parts I and II, could be considered brief—not "time-sensitive"—therapy.

However, if, when working with someone in therapy, you need to collapse time, then introducing the idea of writing a letter, or a similar activity, can be useful sooner rather than later.

Drinking: Charlie's "Favorite Pasttime"

When Charlie came into my office he was bereft. He'd just been arrested for his third DUI (driving under the influence, i.e., of alcohol) and was going to lose his driver's license for 5 years. He talked about every man in his family being alcoholic: "Some kids played baseball with their dads—we drank with ours." Charlie and I met for a total of five sessions every other week. Charlie couldn't afford to meet more frequently as his insurance only covered these kinds of services if provided at an area health clinic. Charlie said he didn't want to return there as he didn't feel the other people were serious about getting help. Mostly it reminded him of the other two tours of duty he'd undergone at the clinic, he said, "when I thought my drinking was all a big joke." Charley knew he was going to have to go to inpatient treatment as part of the sentencing for his DUI, but he didn't feel like waiting that long to start getting some help for himself. He said he didn't know what he was going to do about his drinking, but he knew he had to do something. After our first meeting I suggested that he write a good-bye letter to alcohol. Here it is:

Charlie's "Good-Bye" Letter to Alcohol

Dear Alcohol,

When we first met all my friends knew you. We all felt that you changed our characters and made us people we wanted to be. You took away our fears and problems and made us feel everything was ok.

I felt that I had known you since I was a child, knowing your effect on people and not always caring for it. But they say when in Rome do as the Romans, so we became best friends.

First my neighbor and I would meet you in the field across

the street. We would get real silly and have a lot of fun. All our problems and worries were all forgotten. When we were with you nothing else mattered and nothing could hurt us.

Shortly after I would bring you to outdoor parties and that was the first time we would start our relationship with the law. The local police saw us together so often that they knew we were best friends. It was all fun and games back then. Playing cat and mouse with them but the game was just in the first inning and I was up to bat and swinging. By the second inning, fresh out of high school, I had rolled my parents' cars and got my first DUI in Vermont at age 18.

As far as friendships went I don't think I ever hurt anyone with my drinking. I was, for the most part, a funny harmless drunk. Although there were probably many people that I hurt including myself by making a fool of myself and just not remembering because of a grayout or blackout.

As far as blackouts go I did what any normal everyday fucked up individual would do and said, "Gee, I'll never drink that much again!" or better yet, "I got to stop drinking vodka and just stick to beer."

Well it's the bottom of the ninth and I struck out. I could write a book on our relationship, fit the good parts on a notepad and the bad parts in a novel. It's been good to know you and I'll remember the good times along with the bad. In conclusion: you learn something every day. Yesterday's gone and today has just begun,

See ya!

C.R.

AA often puts people's lives and experiences in a developmental context, looking, for example, at people's years in the program as corresponding to where they're at emotionally and developmentally. The jubilation experienced within the first months or year of sobriety—referred to by AA as the "pink cloud"—is compared to a child's love affair with the world experienced during the first year of life. Then, the "terrible 2's" come with the discovery of the limits of recovery and the word "no": "What do you mean I can't have my old job back? Do you have any idea what I've been through this year!" As people get further along in recovery these analogies break down, and they're never intended to be applied literally. They are metaphors for some of the experiences people encounter in recovery.

In addition, AA talks about taking things "a day at time" to help members combat their anxiety about the future, but also to help people stay present and not become overwhelmed by the amount of time the journey can take. There's a saying I've heard at many meetings: "If you walk 40 miles into the woods, you're going to have to walk 40 miles to get out of the woods." In other words, AA does not offer people a fast solution to addiction or a shortcut to recovery. Attendance at meetings and heeding some of the advice shared at them may lessen the amount of time it takes people to get sober, thereby diminishing their loneliness and pain, but the process involves a great deal of time and energy, especially at the beginning, as most things worthwhile do. Recovery requires ongoing attention and practice.

Initially Charlie was going to have his lawyer keep postponing his case as long as possible to put off going to treatment, but now he said he was looking forward to it. A week into his stay I received the following letter from him:

Charlie's Letter from Treatment

Dear Jonathan,

It's Tues. Morning 6:30 A.M.

I'm at the Alcohol Institute and a lot of the people are bored and think that it sucks here. They don't understand that in a couple of days you all get to know each other and it starts to become fun. I just know it'll be an easy 2 weeks of sobriety and I'm going to have fun here and make the best of it.

I'd just like to say that when I came to you I had to change my life and didn't know how. I'll have to admit I don't remember everything we talked about but I do know every time I left your office I felt like I accomplished something and I felt real good. You steered me in the right direction. Everybody, who knows what I'm going through, from friends to the people at the clinic, have been really supportive. I've been keeping myself busy in sobriety and don't have time to take a drink.

Thank you for all your help. I couldn't have done it without you. My life has changed for the better and I deserve this.

Thanx for everything,

Charlie

AA understands that people are not always available for help or ready to act on their convictions. When a suffering alcoholic turns down the hand of AA, members of the fellowship do not consider their efforts wasted. They call it "planting seeds." In therapy we also like to leave the problems people seek our help with better than we found them. In therapy letters can be ways of planting seeds. They are spiritual mulch.

SOME ADDITIONAL THOUGHTS ON THE USE
OF LETTER WRITING AND OTHER NARRATIVE
TECHNIQUES IN PSYCHOTHERAPY AND RECOVERY

> The newest computer can merely compound, at speed, the
> oldest problem in relations between human beings, and in
> the end the communicator will be comforted with the old
> problem, of what to say and how to say it.
> —EDWARD R. MURROW

I often tell clients to consider their letters and journal entries as a form of compost. Writing, like therapy, rakes our conscious minds, taking shallow thinking and turning it over. Even, for example, if an angry or emotional letter crafted in therapy is not sent, its contents can be stirred into the batter of the therapy conversation. Sometimes it makes no difference whether the words actually make it onto the paper or not. Just talking about the idea can enrich the discussion. Nothing is wasted.

Unfortunately, I cannot offer readers a recipe book or "how to" manual for performing this work or crafting letters to clients. To those readers who, despite all the disclaimers in the book's first part, held onto the hope of being provided with a blueprint for creating these kinds of documents, I understand (and share) your disappointment. However, there are some principles which can be gleaned from the stories presented in this volume which can guide therapists' pens and keyboards.

In my correspondence to clients I always strive for a conversational tone. Despite the numerous metaphors borrowed from literature, these letters are therapeutic communications, not literary creations. When writing them I don't have a list of items to include or themes that must be touched upon. No matter how similar clients' struggles with addiction may seem on the surface, no two individuals' problems are exactly alike and neither are the therapy relationships that accompany them. If every therapist responded to the same person's predicament in the form of a letter, I assume that each response would be entirely different and reflect the unique personality and point of view of its author. I do not think these techniques should be used in a uniform fashion or that there is some "pure" form of narrative therapy that needs to be adhered to in order for this method to be effective. There is no template.[1]

Nevertheless, while the decision to write a letter to a client is almost always a spontaneous act that reflects my connection to that person, or response to the specific circumstances he or she faces, the actual process of writing a letter is often more calculated. For instance, it might take me several drafts to find the right tone or style of address for a particular client or situation. In addition, although when writing a letter I always try to embrace an overall attitude of curiosity and inquisitiveness, I often have my own agenda and reasons for writing people. In general, I find few problems result from using a letter to influence people's actions or decisions in this fashion. Where I get into trouble is when I become too attached to the idea of a letter having a particular outcome. For example, while I used my letter of apology to Shelly's father (in Chapter 10) to raise some concerns I had about his and Shelly's relationship, I tried not to become too invested in his responding to these ideas in a certain way or changing his behavior as a result of my efforts.* This was an attitude I was also trying to role-model for Shelly and encouraged her to take when dealing with all the significant relationships in her life, but especially her father.

When I write a letter to a client I am very conscious of the fact that I am extending the therapy relationship beyond the walls of my office. Consequently, I try to model in my writing the same stance in relation to people's addictions and other problems that I strive for in my face-to-face consultations with them (i.e., an attitude of acceptance and compassion).

Specific kinds of letters may require more time and thought than others. An invitation to a client to examine her relationship to an addiction is obviously not going to be as involved as a summary of my relationship with a client, such as the document requested by Sylvia and Jeff (the couple in Chapter 5). When it takes more drafts or pages to find the right tone for a particular correspondence I can become frustrated. Sometimes, I worry that this is a sign of my having become "overinvolved" in a particular individual or family's story, or that I'm trying to exert too much control over a particular situation. Although that can be the case, more often than not these efforts are a reflection of my strong attachment to and concern for the people who have entrusted me with their most intimate thoughts and treasured relationships. I hope that the time I take mulling over my ideas or obsessing over the words I choose when describing people's experiences, regardless of their accuracy (or people's agreement with them), leaves the recipient of a letter feeling more held and cared for.

How do therapists incorporate these ideas and concepts into their practices? Should we trade in our MSWs and doctoral residencies for MFAs and writing retreats? While the latter might well be for other rea-

---

*Excerpts from this correspondence can be found on pages 251–252.

sons a more fulfilling (and tougher) career path, it is not necessary in order to effectively employ any of the practices advocated in this book (and certainly wasn't my route to a narrative approach). Clearly, some of these ideas may resonate with clients and therapists who enjoy writing in the same way people who enjoy a fascination with dreams may be drawn to various types of Jungian psychotherapy and thinking. But clinicians needn't possess exceptional writing skills to use these methods effectively.

A questioner at a presentation once said she could see how letter writing could be a useful addition to her practice. However, she asked what advice I had for people who didn't, in her words, have a gift for writing or the ability to draft such beautifully crafted letters to people. I explained that the reason I felt these productions advanced the goals of therapy and were experienced as helpful by my clients wasn't because of how they were written but that they were from me. (I also mentioned that when publishing or speaking I always try to circulate my best efforts; however, a letter doesn't have to make good "copy" or read like poetry in order to get the job done or have meaning to the person receiving it.) I told her that if I wrote one of my (what she called) "masterpieces" to one of her clients, it might seem insightful and clever at best, or shallow and objectifying at worst.

The timing of letters in therapy—when and how I actually introduce the idea in a session—varies from one situation to the next. The decision to write a letter myself is easier. If any documentation is required by me in the course of a person's therapy, I always prefer this genre. Regarding clients' letters, an invitation to craft a letter almost always involves a certain amount of humor and playfulness. In groups I offer samples of work created by other clients, like the illustrations shared in this book, to give people a sense of how others have used these ideas. Sometimes I just simply share my bias about therapy needing to find ways of allowing people to express what's important to them rather than putting them through a series of psychological tests and other mental gymnastics hoping to crack their soul's code. Also, I'm lazy. I'd much rather have a client write a letter that tells the story of her addiction than have to pull together a lengthy questionnaire or survey which I then have to score and interpret.

With people who are accustomed to keeping a journal or diary, these ideas are often viewed as a natural extension of practices they already consider an important aspect of their healing. For others, sometimes introducing the concept of keeping a journal about some of the themes that come up in therapy prior to asking them to write a letter can be helpful. In this way it's possible to introduce the idea of their using writing as a simple means of tracking thoughts, feelings, and experiences before suggesting a specific task. Still for others, especially teens and men, I might suggest they purchase a notebook to keep or record some exercises—"homework"—I may suggest they try between sessions. After they've acquired such a notebook, I recommend a "good-bye letter" to alcohol or drugs to inaugurate their book and get them started.

If people seem ambivalent about writing a letter, I'll share something of the origins of these practices and suggest we try one to see if we can learn something that's been escaping us about their predicament. These practices, I explain, are not tests. They are more of a collaborative effort, or partnership. Sometimes it helps to remind people what I shared with Karen (in Chapter 7) about every letter taking place at the moment in time in which it was written—that whatever they write is simply a snapshot or a photograph of where they're at with these concerns right now, today. It may change tomorrow, and it may not be the same as it was yesterday. All we're doing is exploring possibilities together.

THE POLITICAL IMPLICATIONS
OF WRITING IN THERAPY

> There's nothing to writing. All you do is sit down at the typewriter and open a vein.
> —RED SMITH

In her book *Talking Back: Thinking Feminist, Thinking Black,* bell hooks offers the following description of "writing autobiography" and her efforts at healing and self-discovery through writing:

To me, telling the story of my growing up years was intimately concerned with the longing to kill the self I was, without really having to die. I wanted to kill that self in writing. Once that self was gone—out of my life forever—I could more easily become the me of me. It was clearly the Gloria Jean[2] of my tormented and anguished childhood that I wanted to be rid of, the girl who was always wrong, always punished, always subjected to some humiliation or other, always crying, the girl who was to end up in a mental institution because she could not be anything but crazy, or so they told her. She was the girl who sat a hot iron on her arm pleading with them to leave her alone, the girl who wore her scar as a brand marking her madness. Even now I can hear the voices of my sisters saying "Mama make Gloria stop crying." By writing the autobiography, it was not just this Gloria I would be rid of, but the past that had a hold on me, that kept me from the present. I wanted not to forget the past but to break its hold. This death in writing was to be liberatory. (1989, p. 155)

This description recalls Sophie's thoughts about physical pain being preferable to spiritual death (Sophie was one of the women clients whose writing and therapy was presented in Chapter 7). Sophie's cutting and self-mutilation, driven by a loss of all feelings, was a desperate effort to feel again and to return from death to life. Both women's writing reveals a personal quest for identity and sense of self in the midst of a deathlike isolation and emptiness. Each author—Sophie through her poetry and letters, and hooks through autobiography—was trying to break the spell of this deathlike mode of being:[3]

In the end I did not feel as though I had killed the Gloria of my childhood. Instead I had rescued her. She was no longer the enemy within, the little girl who had to be annihilated for the woman to come into being. In writing about her, I reclaimed that part of myself I had long ago rejected, left uncared for, just as she had often felt alone and uncared for as a child. Remembering was a part of a cycle of reunion, a joining of fragments, "the bits and pieces of my heart" that the narrative made whole again. (hooks, 1989, p. 159)

These reflections by hooks emphasize the process of self-knowledge and authentication that personal writing affords. Claiming the freedom to grow as human beings was connected for hooks and Sophie with having the courage to be open, to be able to tell the truth of their life as they experienced it in writing: "To talk about one's life—that I could do. To write about it, to leave a trace—that was frightening" (hooks, 1989, p. 156); hooks's experience of the difference between writing and speech is not surprising. Writing can be more threatening than speech. With speech you can take the words back, but writing stays. It doesn't go away. It makes events seem more real.

Mary Olson (1995), citing Ellen Carter's (1994) research (a beautifully written thesis that looks at writing as a therapeutic act in women's lives), reminds us of the caution and forethought we need when asking people to write in therapy. For some, writing can be a disorganizing experience that conjures up fears of not being a good enough writer. For this reason, when I introduce the idea of writing a letter to a client I do it cautiously (usually after a therapeutic relationship has been established) and check in frequently with people about their experience. If the process is in any way unhelpful, we discontinue it.

Psychoanalytic feminists connect postmodern ideas about writing and therapy to our thinking about the unconscious linking psychic and social life. In this conceptualization of psychotherapy, says Cushman (1995), the unconscious is not an interior thing; rather, it is part of our social landscape that contains potential feelings, thoughts, and experiences unavailable to us because they lie outside of our "horizon of understanding."

In therapy and recovery this creative process can only happen in connection with others. For some, writing provides an opportunity for reflection and, says Mary Olson (1995), a path between our own experience and its articulation with others. Our interior voice is not a monologue but is in constant dialogue with the outside world. The sense of "being" human only comes into existence when we are engaged in a dialogue with people. The decision to delve into one's past may also serve as an avenue into one's future. We may be powerless to change the past but, as Stephanie Covington (1988) writes, "A new understanding of the past can give rise to new hope" (p. 157).

In the end of her writing-about-writing autobiography, hooks concludes:

> The longing to tell one's story and the process of telling is symbolically a gesture of longing to recover the past in such a way that one experiences both a sense of reunion and a sense of release. It was the longing for release that compelled the writing but concurrently it was the joy of reunion that enabled me to see that the act of writing . . . is a way to find again that aspect of self and experience that may no longer be an actual part of one's life but is a living memory shaping and informing the present. (1989, p. 158)

The work of hooks reads like poetry; she stir our emotions, as she struggles in a tough-minded fashion with the same issues taken up by other social scientists and theorists whose ideas about narrative, story, and therapy were presented in this book. However, hooks's writing does more. Her writing demonstrates not only what narrative ideas have to contribute to the process of psychotherapy but how the actual creation of narratives—the act of writing itself—can be a form of therapy, a story in which writing no longer serves as the midwife for therapy but is itself the defining moment and healing encounter in a person's life.

Myerhoff (1982b), when writing about the popularity and attention that the act of keeping a journal has gained in contemporary psychotherapy, found it most interesting that writing crosscut such a variety of theoretical approaches. Letters, maintaining journals in groups, and other forms of writing, says Myerhoff (all therapy techniques that owe their origins and much of their form to the women's movement), appear to transform experiences and emotions of derision and shame into gifts to be shared with others, who in turn are transformed and feel privileged to witness them. Letter writing is a powerful healing tool and much of its strength lies in its ability to transform painful and traumatic experiences into lasting moments of privilege and honor. As David Epston says, "The words in a letter don't fade and disappear the way conversation does; they endure through time and space, bearing witness to the work of therapy and immortalizing it" (1994, p. 31).

The letters and people's stories found in this book occupy a space between the spiritual and the therapeutic. I've long felt that the letters and other written productions collected over the years and presented in the foregoing chapters, like the characters in Pirandello's play, were searching—crying out—for an author to tell their story.

Muddling Through

Suffering ceases to be suffering in some way at the moment
it finds a meaning.

—VIKTOR FRANKL

In a piece he wrote for the *Family Therapy Networker*, Garrison Keillor
said that it is "an author's fate—to write the books and then go and live
them" (1991, p. 68). In this story, the narrator and main character, Al
Denny—a self-help guru and millionaire a hundred times over—confessed that he had nothing left to say about his area of expertise, as he
had said everything there was to say about the subject before he knew
anything about it. The destiny of this book and its author is not unlike
the protagonist in Keillor's story. Its ending, as the reader who has made
it this far will soon discover, is anticlimactic.

A person can become easily overwhelmed by the vast scholarly out-
put of addiction theorists and psychotherapists and the great diversity
among them. It's a daunting task, even though I limited my selections,
for the most part, to the narrative psychotherapy and recovery landscape. Narrowing this view of the horizon even further, three narrative
metaphors were found distinctive and brought into focus in this book—
namely, hermeneutics, story, and voice. However, each of these lenses, I
discovered, represents multiple perspectives.

Hermeneutics uses the metaphor of conversation, thus characteriz-
ing therapy as the creation of new meaning arising from dialogues between people rather than deliberate interventions by therapists. Clinicians who apply the analogy of story to people's lives see therapy as a
process of helping people develop alternative narratives to describe their
experience. Using methods borrowed from literary criticism and other

339

disciplines in the humanities, this approach tries to deconstruct some of the grand narratives that shape our lives and color our understanding of how our families and cultural institutions work. The idea of voice as a metaphor for therapy comes out of women's psychology and feminist research, which argue that even social justice models of therapy and social work that try to empower clients leave out the experience of many people. These researchers advocate for therapy in a different voice based on an "ethic of care" and what Virginia Goldner (1989) calls "relational engagement." These models look at how writing can help women find their voices in a world that tends to silence them.

How, when interpreting the meaning of a client's writing or story, do we determine the impact it has had on the life of the problem, the client's therapy, her relationship to herself, and her relationships with others? How do we choose one narrative voice over another? What, borrowing an image from one of Grimm's fairy tales, are we to do with this narrative crowd gathered in front of the psychotherapy mirror—whose ideas about therapy and recovery are "the fairest of them all"?

The great books can help you get the picture. Buber and Frankl, along with the other philosophers, therapists, and authors whose words are found in this text, can help you to see what it is that provides our daily bread of meaning, but no book can help you execute. You have two clients in your office, a husband and wife: one wants you to deal with anxieties suffered from the lack of intimacy and affection in the marriage; the other wants you to bear witness to past hurts and traumas caused by drinking. You can't be a "Thou" to both of them simultaneously. Which one to respond to? A book doesn't tell you that. Even the great spiritual texts just tell you that God is the one who is always Thou, whereas we are sometimes Thou and sometimes out to lunch. And they tell you that God can be a Thou to all beings at once, whereas we live inside our limitations; if we are a Thou to one person, one child, we are not a Thou to others. But how do you decide when you are going to be accessible or present and to whom? No book can tell you that.

What my own sojourn in recovery has taught me about therapy and the way I practice my craft is that the spirit in which you do anything as a therapist is much more important than what you actually do. In the end, I come back to Buber's one word answer for God: Presence.

The story of how AA began is a relational one. The founders went for the everyday miracle of a chance encounter between Bill W. and Dr. Bob to rest their mythology on, rather than the more supernatural moment Bill had with God as he lay alone in his room. This story has colored every aspect of AA from 1935 to the present. Something special happens when one alcoholic reaches out to another. Maybe it can be explained, in part, by the laws that govern Jewish mourning.

In Judaism comforting takes precedence over mourning. A 13th century Hebrew text says, "If there are two mourners, each mourning in his own house, the one should leave his house and visit the other, even during the first three days."[1] In Orthodox Jewish practice a mourner is not supposed to leave his house in the first 3 days, and in our time, during the first week, but as Leon Wieseltier writes in his *Kaddish*:

> the obligation to mourn is here superceded by the obligation to console. . . . It would seem cruel for an individual just back from one funeral to be hustled out to another funeral; but in truth it is not cruel, it is an exercise in social responsibility. The mourner, too, has a social responsibility. His experience has conferred upon him an expertise that others need. Grief must not impede the specialist in grief. (1998, pp. 580–581)

Alcoholics are specialists in mourning. They know what it's like to lose homes, jobs, businesses, marriages, relationships, self-respect, and their faith—in themselves and God. Most of all they know what it's like to fear something more than death. When an alcoholic speaks with a fellow sufferer she knows she is conversing with someone who understands what it's like to experience the world as she has. Dr. Bob echoed this sentiment in his story in *Alcoholics Anonymous* when answering his own question: What did Bill Wilson do or say to him that was so different from what others had done or said? "He was the first living human with whom I have ever talked, who knew what he was talking about in regards to alcoholism from actual experience. In other words he talked my language" (*Alcoholics Anonymous*, 1939/1976, p. 180).

Getting sober is a heroic achievement that often involves facing death, one's own or people you care about. Facing death takes great courage. But while the threat of imminent death is utterly terrifying, the fact of death is extraordinarily uncomplicated. The great challenge is to deal meaningfully with its aftermath and the vagrancy of everyday life. A veteran of the Normandy landings put the point well in his reflections on the significance of the fiftieth anniversary of D-Day. *The New York Times* (June 5, 1994, pp. E1, E5) reported the evolution of his thinking about the glories of war and the routines of peace:

> Having passed three score and ten, I have, I believe, put my participation in the Normandy and Holland jumps and the Battle of the Bulge

in reasonable perspective. A decade ago I wrote that taking part in those campaigns . . . overshadowed all that followed, including love, marriage, career and children. That is no longer true. I have belatedly come to understand that slogging across the plain of everyday life with dignity and . . . honesty . . . calls for as much heroism.*

My sense that dealing with family, work, and society's problems requires more heroism than facing death always intensifies when people find out what I do for a living and say to me, "Jon, you must have such interesting clients." In the sense that they mean exotic and eccentric characters, I've had very few. But I find that all the people I see in therapy are interesting. Each one of us is the protagonist of a life story. Each one of us is a center of consciousness who realizes that "when I die my world dies with me." Each one struggles to make her or his life story turn out well. There's considerable heroism involved in this effort, but people who come for therapy are usually unaware of their heroism. They think of it as something found only in theater, books, movies, or television dramas.

A colleague of mine told me of a couple he'd been seeing who were heavily into drugs and alcohol. For 10 years they'd never been together when both of them were sober. Then one day they decided to get help. They went to hospitals, treatment centers, halfway houses, AA—whatever was available. They had two children, and they were having a very difficult time parenting. Somehow they managed against all odds to stay clean and keep their family together. Yet, they gave themselves no credit. They still looked on themselves as a pair of junkies, but their therapist experienced their heroism. After a while so did they.

When people face their own death, they start to live. Their illness becomes more—it's an edge. It makes them feel more alive. It's a gift. AA is saying that with the opportunity for recovery which alcoholism affords, people start owning their life:

> We are creatures of infinite desires and limited capacities. In response to this we cling to things we value. We don't want to let change happen as when we use mind-altering drugs to preserve a high we experience listening to music. The Buddha tells us that this clinging can't work; it increases our suffering, our frustrations. We can't hold on to

---

*The veteran was paratrooper Nelson Bryant who, following the war, became the outdoors editor for *The New York Times*. His remarks were recalled in an editorial entitled "Reflections When an Old Wound Aches."

things we value, the things we love, because everything is constantly changing, including us. The thing to do is to accept this and let go.[2]

Malcolm Diamond, the philosopher and therapist who wrote this, was looking at what Buddhism has to offer people living with cancer, but he could just as easily have been speaking to people suffering from addiction. The Buddha believed that all life entails suffering, that what matters is how we cope with it and find happiness and tranquillity within it.

There are people in AA with years of sobriety who still cling to early recovery—people who will tell you after 12 or 14 years that they're coming to a meeting pretty much every day, almost doing the "90 in 90" to stay away from a drink. If that were true, as a colleague of mine with 20-plus years of sobriety said, "they should shoot themselves." But I don't think it's true. I believe people continue to use 12-step recovery meetings in this fashion because they're not ready to let go of their suffering and move on. In the meantime, the thing that I remind myself of over and over is that I'd rather have them triturating the process this way than at a bar.

The steps, traditions, and other practices which AA offers its followers are intended to help people stop clinging—to help them live life rather than trying so hard to control it and hold onto it. But people can use recovery and AA, just like anything else, to hide from themselves. Winnicott (1971a) made the same observation about therapy when he courageously declared, "Absence of psychoneurotic illness may be health but it's not living" (p. 100). Therapists hide, too, using our client's lives and problems as a way to avoid showing up for our own.

A large part of this book has been about encouraging therapists not to cling to set rules or universal theories when practicing therapy with people in recovery or any other group. Confession: I don't have rules, but I do have three principles I apply universally in my practice regardless of who the clients are—men, women, teens, children—and regardless of what problems they suffer—addiction, anger, anorexia, anxiety, bulimia, depression, divorce, loss, or trauma. *Be present. Do everything with sacred intent. Laugh.*

Notes

PROLOGUE

1. In fact, White and Epston (1990) credit Burton (1965)—writing in the analytic tradition—as laying the groundwork for much of their narrative project.

INTRODUCTION

1. The professor was Malcolm Diamond, and the story is recounted on page 207 of his biography (1960) of Martin Buber.
2. Jerome Bruner (1986) claims narrative (i.e., human) experience is not modeled on formal logic but on poetics. He separates understanding and knowledge into two different modes of thought: the *paradigmatic*, which is scientific and based on logic (he calls it "logo-scientific"), and the narrative, which is poetic–hermeneutic. Bruner's perspective has become a popular one for therapists looking for a theory and praxis for understanding the narratives and stories that they and the people they seek to help bring to the therapeutic context. For further discussion see Laird (1989).
3. This illustration and explanation was borrowed from a talk delivered at a conference in New York by David Berenson (1986).
4. Ludwig Fleck, in his visionary *The Genesis and Development of a Scientific Fact* (1935/1979), explores the history of medicine, using his quest for an effective treatment for syphilis and the discovery of the Wassermann reaction as illustrative of how these sorts of breakthroughs are produced by science. In the case of syphilis, the seemingly serendipitous "discovery" of its cure (during random screening of 900 compounds) was a collective process that drew on mythology and mysticism—which were once viewed by scientists as legitimate sources of scholarship and knowledge—as well as on the research of the three investigators in Germany, working separately: Fritz Schaudinn, who identified the spirochete *Treponema pallidum* as the causative microbe in 1905; August von Wassermann, who developed the blood test in 1906; and

Paul Ehrlich, who in 1909 found that the arsenic-containing compound "606" (Salvarsan) was the "magic bullet" to treat the disease. (Today penicillin is used instead.)

In a discussion of how scientists arrive at solutions, Fleck observed that there are many "correct" theories for the same problem; to be correct is to be accepted collectively: "Facts are not objectively given but collectively created" (1935/1979, p.157). Or, as Richard Rorty is fond of saying, truth is what our colleagues will let us get away with.

5. See Roud (1994), Siegel (1986), van der Kolk (1987, 1994), and van der Kolk and Greenburg (1987).

6. Medical science and research often produce stories that have what Bruner (1986) calls "literary merit." In other words, stories that help people make sense of their compulsions and contribute to their understanding of what needs to happen to help them heal. For example, treatment centers routinely provide recovering persons information on how drugs work. Patients are informed that cocaine interferes with neurotransmitter activity in the user's brain, thereby causing it to stockpile excess amounts of norepinephrine and dopamine, two compounds produced in those brain areas that control wakefulness and arousal. After a period of time the cocaine user's brain gradually stops producing these essential neurochemicals on its own and relies more and more on the drug for this function. This knowledge may help people addicted to cocaine better understand the intense emotional highs and lows the drug causes, as well as their need for increasing amounts of it to obtain the same results. As a consequence, they may be more willing to try a demanding regimen of physical exercise which can produce a similar type of euphoria and help ward off the severe depression experienced during recovery.

7. Some of the more elegant work in circulation includes Arnold Washton and Mark Gold's (1987) *Cocaine: A Clinician's Handbook*; Roger Weiss's (1993) *Cocaine*; David Smith and Donald Wesson's (1985) *Treating the Cocaine Abuser*; and George E. Vaillant's (1983) watershed work, *The Natural History of Alcoholism*.

8. I'm grateful to Roget Lockard for bringing these concerns to my attention (personal correspondence, July 5, 1999).

CHAPTER 1

1. For further discussion of women's sense of self and the concept of codependency, see Bepko (1991a, 1991b).

2. This technique and concept was first pioneered by Dusty Miller (1991). She locates this idea at the core of a model for working with women, addictions, and trauma that she has been developing for some time, a model which has heavily influenced my thinking and that of many other clinicians exploring this topic. This approach is mapped out in its entirety in her book, *Women Who Hurt Themselves: A Book of Hope and Recovery* (1994).

3. For further discussion see Lockard (1985b).

CHAPTER 2

1. *Hope and Dread in Psychoanalysis* is the title of a book by analyst Stephen Mitchell (1993). He uses this phrase as a metaphor for the first session following a vacation or any other disruption in therapy. I will, on occasion, share with clients the story behind the title of this analyst's book as a way of normalizing and helping people make sense of the curious mix of emotions, expectations, and fears they experience during a first therapy appointment. Therapists, too, often experience this gamut of emotions when sitting for the first time with a new client, although presumably (one would hope) not as intensely.
2. For further discussion of people's subjective experience of suicide see Sanville (1991).
3. Firmly established in the traditionally male disciplines of mathematics and science, these constructs for observing and documenting phenomena undermine other ways of knowing and understanding our world that are historically associated with women and rooted in oral tradition. This discussion will be revisited in Chapter 6; however, this is, in part, what Michael White (White & Epston, 1991) refers to when he talks about using letters and other written productions as "counterdocuments." These practices undermine the dominant culture by taking its techniques and other means of tracking, documenting, and gathering information about people's lives out of the hands of professionals— who are acting on behalf of state agencies and institutions—and placing them into the hands of the clients these organizations are meant to serve.
4. From the words of Israel ben Eliezer, the Baal Shem Tov—"Master of the Good (or Holy) Name"—the founder of Hasidism: "He shall rise eagerly from sleep, he shall seize the quality of fervor with might for he has become another man and has become hallow and is worthy to beget like the Holy One blessed be he who begat worlds."
5. White prefers the description "sole parent" over the description "single parent":

> In our culture, it appears that "single" has so many negative connotations, including of incompleteness, of being unmarried, of failure—of not having made the grade. However, at least to my mind, the word "sole" conjures up something entirely different. It carries a recognition of the extraordinary responsibility that these parents face and of the strength necessary to achieve what they achieve. And as well, a second meaning is not hard to discern— "soul." Soul is about essence, and for persons to refer to themselves as "soul parents" is for them to recognize the "heartfulness" that they provide, that their children depend upon to "see them through." (White, 1991, p. 146)

6. In a discussion characterized by his reluctance to describe his technique, Winnicott raises a number of issues that are at the core of many current debates on narrative, postmodernism, and psychotherapy:

> I have hesitated to describe the technique, which I have used a great deal over a number of years, not only because it is a natural game that any two people

might play, but also, if I begin to describe what I do, then someone will be likely to begin to rewrite what I describe as if it were a set technique with rules and regulations. Then the whole value of the procedure would be lost. If I describe what I do there is a very real danger that others will take it and form it into something that corresponds to a Thematic Apperception Test. The difference between this and a T.A.T. is firstly that it is not a test, and secondly that the consultant contributes from his own ingenuity almost as much as the child does. Naturally, the consultant's contribution drops out, because it is the child not the consultant, who is communicating distress.

The fact that the consultant freely plays his own part in the exchange of drawings certainly has a great importance for the success of the technique; such a procedure does not make the patient feel inferior in any way as, for instance, a patient feels when being examined by a doctor in respect of physical health, or, often, when being given a psychological test (especially a personality test). (1964/1989, pp. 300–301)

CHAPTER 3

1. Pappenheim, subsequent to her analysis, wrote about her concerns about her treatment, her life after analysis, and her struggles to return to health. Her story, told under the pseudonym Anna O., was the first case history in Freud's groundbreaking *Studies in Hysteria* (1895/1953a). The inventor—or at least coauthor—of the "talking cure" in her later life, she became a social worker, reformer, feminist activist, and playwright. For further discussion see Chapter 6 of the present volume and Elaine Showwalter's (1985) *The Female Malady: Women, Madness, and English Culture 1830–1980.*

CHAPTER 4

1. A footnote included in Jung's text reads: "As the hart panteth after the water brooks, so panteth my soul after thee, O God" (Psalm 42:1).
2. Because of Bill's concern, at the time, about how people would understand this experience, very little mention of it is made in the AA literature, and Bill himself downplayed its significance in talks he delivered and in the organizing work he performed in AA's early period. Instead, Bill's trip to Akron, Ohio, where he met AA's cofounder, Dr. Bob, is identified in the folklore of AA as the beginning of the program and its tradition of alcoholics helping "fellow" alcoholics become and remain sober.
3. Al-Anon has a similar story that led to its cofounder, Lois Wilson's (Bill's spouse) spiritual awakening, but one not nearly as sublime. As a result of a life spent devoted to an alcoholic, Lois (*Lois remembers*, 1979) recognized her need for a recovery program of her own. In her book, *Lois Remembers: Memoirs of the Co-founder of Al-Anon and Wife of the Co-founder of Alcoholics Anonymous*, she describes this revelation taking place during an argument

with her husband about how much time in their lives was taken up by Bill's alcoholism and involvement with AA. In a heated moment, she hurled her shoe at
Bill's head and shouted, "Damn your meetings." In retrospect, it seems much
of what was required for the care of Lois's soul (and the millions in Al-Anon
who identify with her plight), she derived from the sole of that flying boot.

4. AA's founders made significant use of William James's *Varieties of Religious
Experience* when creating the program, and its strong connection to the Oxford Group at its beginnings was noted earlier. For more religious perspectives
on AA see Antze (1987), Walle (1992), and Dowling and Shoemaker (1957).

5. Buber's comments took place in an exchange with a questioner during a lecture given at Princeton University in the spring of 1958. The question was
posed to him by the late Professor George Thomas of Princeton's Department of Religion (Malcolm Diamond, personal communication, 1997).

6. It is, as Malcolm Diamond (1960) observed in his biography of Martin
Buber, a tribute to Buber, a thoroughly religious thinker, that he became one
of the leading intellectual figures of our secular age. In fact, as his thoughts
have exerted an ever-increasing influence over a wide range of subjects from
psychology to literary criticism and from political science to education, they
have changed the meaning of the word "religion" itself. However, while the
broad dissemination of Buber's outlook has been a gain for our culture, it
also has sometimes led to misinterpretations of his thought. While Buber
was a sophisticated thinker entirely at home with the cultural avant-garde,
his talk of "God as the eternal Thou" should not be, Diamond admonishes,
interpreted in a way that converts the term into a fashionable intellectual
symbol divorced from the living God of Buber's religious heritage.

I enjoy the distinctly Jewish character of Buber's thought because it is
such a prominent part of my people's religious and social history. However,
what attracts me to Buber's ideas about God and spirituality, and Bateson's
(1991) about the nature of the universe, is the way the two men emphasize
that the properties of all things are ultimately about relationships. I am not as
enamored of Buber's concept of God as the "eternal Thou," because it implies
a universe that is organized by external forces, and I personally prefer theories
that accord with the idea of the universe as self-organized, rather than organized from the outside in, so to speak.

7. The contradictions and misconceptions inherent in the concept of strength
through surrender and powerlessness are explored in greater depth in the
works of family therapists David Berenson (1991), and Claudia Bepko
(1991a; see also Bepko & Krestan, 1985, 1991, 1993). It is a stance that
Gregory Bateson (1972a, 1972b, 1991), when writing about the process of
therapy, viewed as more inviting and familiar ground for clinicians versed in
Eastern philosophy and practices.

CHAPTER 5

1. For further discussion of these concepts see Schafer (1992) and Stern (1985).

CHAPTER 6

1. There have been a number of books published recently that attempt to build bridges between the 12 steps and Buddhist practices as well as Buddhism and psychotherapy, one of the most elegant attempts being Mark Epstein's *Thoughts without a Thinker* (1995).
2. Wallace (1985) makes another important point: when discussing the alcoholic's obsession with others we are talking about self-centeredness, not generosity. Alcoholics are often very generous people, but this trait can sometimes be more about the creation of an inflated sense of self or the need to control others than a genuine desire to meet another person's needs.
3. Unfortunately, in psychoanalytic theory people are often referred to as "objects." What's more, this way of referring to our relationships with people is itself a misapplication of the term, which refers to the mental images we have of other people. Hence, the term "love objects" means the images we have in our minds of the people we care about. The term thus refers to these mental representations and is different from the people themselves. Freud's point is that people without the ability to hold these kinds of images of others in their minds are going to have difficulty being able to consider how their behavior impacts on others (Michael Nichols, personal communication, June 1999).
4. Heinz Kohut (1971) labels these three poles of identity the *grandiose exhibitionistic self, the idealized parent imago,* and the *alternative twinship ego,* respectively. In spite of its many limitations—a complex and obtuse vocabulary, too much emphasis placed on the role of psychic structures and mental processes, and an inadequate framework for looking at individuals in the context of their families and culture—self psychology offers a compassionate way of understanding addicts' unconscious conflicts and attachments to substances. It focuses on real, not just "imagined," relationships and experiences. It also allows the client and the therapist to dialogue with one another and to theorize about the psychic trauma and pain that afflict most addicts in a manner that emphasizes their strengths, rather than the deficits, and without blaming or humiliating the client.

   At their core both self psychology and object relations theory, particularly as expressed in Winnicott's work (e.g., 1965, 1971b, 1989), are based on the belief that all human beings struggle toward health. However disturbing a person's behavior, however outrageous the demand or defended that person is, all actions are viewed as a necessary attempt to preserve and protect the fragile self trying to survive as best it can using whatever resources are at its disposal.
5. A good source for further discussion of this point, and Kohut's theory in general, is Wolmark and Sweezy (1998).
6. For further writing on this topic see David Treadway's chapter "Therapist Heal Thyself" in his *Before It's Too Late* (1992), and a pamphlet from Al-Anon Family Services, *Al-Anon for Professionals* (1987).
7. I'm sad to say that many of my colleagues in the narrative family therapy community will find themselves at odds with this position. They are writing about the "mythologizing stories of addiction" that they feel pathologize clients by encouraging them to view their drinking problems as a disease (a con-

cept I don't personally embrace but understand and have, in the case of addictions, deep respect for). I think this position of my narrative therapy colleagues is unfortunate, if not dangerous. It seems to be a knee-jerk reaction to the fact that alcoholism is recognized by the medical community and is included in the DSM-IV (*Diagnostic and Statistical Manual of Mental Disorders, 4th ed.*, American Psychiatric Association, 1994) as a "legitimate" illness and diagnosis. But the story and culture of alcoholism has a unique history of its own, different than the histories of many of the other diagnoses found in DSM-IV—more akin, for example, to the history of the diagnosis of posttraumatic stress disorder than the recent controversial history of borderline personality disorder (which many clinicians and proponents of trauma theory, including myself, would like to see done away with as a diagnosis completely).

As Judith Herman (1992) documented in her groundbreaking study on trauma, the most common posttraumatic stress disorders are not suffered by men in war but by women in civilian life. In the case of PTSD the women's movement created a political context which recognized that the syndromes seen in survivors of rape, domestic battery, and incest was essentially the same as syndromes of survivors of military battles. It has, as Herman observed, never been possible to advance the study of psychological trauma without the context of a political movement. When this kind of support does not exist, history teaches us that knowledge can disappear (as it did earlier in this century when Freud, pressured by his peers in the medical establishment, abandoned his own trauma theory and betrayed his patient's disclosures of sexual abuse). The history of philosophy, said T. W. Adorno, is the history of forgetting. He could have been talking about therapy. It saddens me that narrative and other kinds of therapies appear to be establishing their own history of forgetting when it comes to understanding the experience and trauma of addiction.

Alcoholism was not recognized as a medical condition until its sufferers organized their own grassroots self-help community and demanded that their plight be heard by doctors and therapists. Prior to that, AA and Al-Anon were among the few supports available. These developments transpired long before the DSM ever came into existence (although for-profit treatment centers clearly capitalized on the market created once addiction, like mental illness, became a major growth industry).

8. The story of Marty Mann, AA's first women member, documents the growing pains AA experienced when it came to recognizing women's need for help and support. Mann was referred to AA by Dr. Harry Tiebout, a friend of Bill Wilson and one of AA's strongest supporters and most influential allies in the medical community. Tiebout was Mann's doctor during her stay at his hospital in Greenwich, Connecticut. Prior to his urging her to go to New York to attend some AA meetings, he asked Mann to read a copy of a manuscript members of the New York group were circulating. This was an early draft of *Alcoholics Anonymous* (i.e., the Big Book). Mann would read portions of the book and then discuss them with Tiebout. Her first impressions were positive, and she describes feeling that these people might understand what she'd been through. Shortly after that she literally threw it out the window (an incident confirmed by a number of sources) because, as she put it, there was too much

mention of God and "nowhere did the book mention women." After 3 months of pleading by Tiebout she agreed to meet with some of the book's authors. This gathering went unexpectedly well and led to a lifetime of involvement with AA and cutting-edge work in the addictions field. She founded the Council on Alcoholism, raised people's consciousness about the "invisible" plight of women and addiction, and her new primer on alcoholism quickly became a classic in the field.

However, Mann's acceptance by the group did not come easily. This was 1939 when there were less then 50 members of AA meeting every Tuesday at Bill's house, and none of them women. Most did not believe women could be alcoholics and saw Mann as a freak exception. A touching vignette that captures the gradual metamorphosis in the group's thinking on this issue is the story of how Bill showed up at Mann's apartment during a low point in her life when she was overcome with depression and wanting to drink. Bill, broke himself at the time, his own house in foreclosure, handed Mann a handful of money the group had collected to pay for her to check herself into Towns Hospital, the only facility at the time in New York that would admit alcoholics. Mann's story is told by one of her sponsees in Sarah Hafner's (1992) book *Nice Girls Don't Drink*, and in her own voice in the second edition of the *Big Book* (published in 1955) in a chapter entitled "Stars Don't Fall."

9. There is a growing trend in 12-step literature to take on more contemporary problems, values, and beliefs related to culture, race, and gender that people face in recovery. Not surprisingly, some of the most forward-looking and progressive-minded thinking on these topics is found in OA. A relative newcomer in the self-help recovering community, OA is best described as a "sisterhood" as opposed to a "fellowship." Like other 12-step programs, OA encourages members to use writing as a tool in their recovery. One of its publications, *The Twelve Steps and Twelve Traditions of Overeaters Anonymous* (1990), describes a writing activity to help members with the often-daunting task of fourth step work ("Made a searching and fearless moral inventory of ourselves"): "One good way to inventory ourselves is to ask ourselves questions about specific characteristics. Then we examine in writing the ways that we've exhibited these characteristics in our lives" (p. 34). A good number of these questions have to do with attitudes about racism and sexism, and they extend to heterosexism as well:

> Are we bigoted? Have we ever denied anyone fair treatment because of race, religion, politics, gender, or disability? Do we tell ethnic, racist, or sexist jokes? If not, are we afraid to say that we don't enjoy such "humor"? (*The Twelve Steps and Twelve Traditions*, 1990, p. 36)

Other questions have to do with our relationship to our fears:

> As we take inventory we also look at our fears. For many of us, fear, worry, and anxiety have played a key role in our lives, robbing us of joy and keeping us from fulfilling our dreams. It is not until we take inventory in step four that we begin to realize that we don't have to live in fear. First we list people, places and things that have caused us fear. Then we look at other ways fear has affected us. (*The Twelve Steps and Twelve Traditions*, 1990, p. 37)

Some examples of these types of questions include queries as to specific types of abusive and self-destructive behavior:

> Do we repeatedly get into relationships with the kind of people who mentally or physically abuse us?
> Are we afraid to end existing relationships which are destructive or inappropriate for us?
> Are we so afraid of conflict that we risk abuse rather than asserting ourselves?
> Have we pursued sex in a way that damaged our self-esteem?
> When has fear held us back from taking other actions we should have pursued? Have we stood by and allowed another person to be hurt when we could have done something to prevent it?
> Have we abused others verbally or physically?
> Have we ever sought to satisfy our sexual impulses at the expense of others?
> Have we ever forced or manipulated anyone to have sexual contact with us?
> Have we ever sexually molested anyone? Have we ever had sexual contact with a child or with anyone who was not fully capable of resisting?
> Have we ever abused a position of trust to get sex from someone who sought our help?
> Have we used intimidation to get sex? Have we abused a position of power? Have we ever threatened or sought revenge against someone if they wouldn't go along with our sexual advances?
> Have we used sex or pregnancy to trap someone in a relationship?
> Have we ever gotten someone pregnant and not taken responsibility for it?
> (*The Twelve Steps and Twelve Traditions*, 1990, pp. 39–41)

Nor does every question in this particular fourth step exercise from OA concern issues of sexual and physical violence and abuse. Many, if not most, on this topic relate to issues of reciprocity and mutuality within couples and between sexual partners:

> In what other ways have we misused our sexual drives? Compulsive eating has made many of us uninterested in sex. Have we been unfair to our partners and ourselves, preferring isolation and food to the risk of physical intimacy? (*The Twelve Steps and Twelve Traditions*, 1990, p. 41)

Class issues are not taken on with the same gusto in OA or any other 12-step program, but people's prejudices toward people who possess less social status, wealth, and power are confronted, as are attempts to achieve happiness and emotional security through the acquisition of material things or by obtaining excessive amounts of money at one's own—or another person's—expense. Like alcohol, what is stressed is people's relationship to the substance or thing, not the quantities they consume or, in the case of money, the amount they make or spend. There are no lines drawn about what is too much or not enough to live securely and comfortably (which differs for each individual, even after a person's basic needs are provided for), and certainly there are very wealthy individuals who use these 12-step programs and wealthy communities where such meetings thrive.

We have in the last several chapters been using alcoholism as a kind of classical archetype for addiction in general and referring to a kind of generic recovery from it. However, these explorations can be used as springboards to other "non-tissue-based" addictive processes such as gambling, compulsively getting into debt, and even obsessive–compulsive behavior tied to a political ideology or dogma. The most recent addition to this growing list of compulsions is the Internet, which at the start of this decade comedian Eddie Murphy prophetically labeled "a crack pipe for smart people." A recent Associated Press article printed in *The Boston Globe* of August 23, 1999, reported on a paper delivered by David Greenfield at the annual meeting of the American Psychological Association on Internet addiction. While this study shows that there is a growing number of users on-line who seem to be participating in obsessive Internet surfing for its own sake, most "surfers" are using it to fuel preexisting compulsions to sex, gambling, consumerism, etc. When it comes to treating addictions of any kind, what AA and other 12-step programs counsel addicts against is letting anything, not just drugs and alcohol, become a personal compulsion or obsession.

CHAPTER 7

1. As an earlier discussion of Judith Herman's research (1981, 1992) revealed, more women's lives have been lost in a gender war of trauma and abuse than in all the military wars combined. When it comes to rape and sexual assault, the connection between male violence and aggression, on the one hand, and alcohol, on the other, is analogous to the billions of dollars worth of guns and weapons manufactured and sold legally that always seem to end up in the wrong hands in the wrong places. No purveyors of alcohol are ever held accountable for this form of "innocent" violence. Moreover, this connection between alcohol and violence, which seems fairly obvious, is rarely made in the media or in studies of these crimes. I do not mean to imply there is an easy solution or that a control mindset like prohibition (an inherently flawed strategy that's been tried and failed) is a viable option, but if we can't talk about the whole problem—or at least name it—then we will only produce partial measures, incomplete answers, and half-baked solutions.
2. I'm referring here to Schafer's (1976b) paper "The Psychoanalytic Vision of Reality."
3. In psychoanalysis, the term "used" does not have the exploitative connotations often associated with it in the larger culture. For a better understanding of how it is applied here and by Bollas, readers should refer to the discussion of D. W. Winnicott's (1971a) ideas about play and a person's object relations presented earlier (in Chapter 2).
4. This was also the result of the growing climate of managed care and profit-driven treatment in the medical community. With insurance companies demanding shorter and shorter lengths of stay, both of us were pessimistic that Sophie would receive the care she needed in an inpatient setting. The strongest argument for Sophie going into the hospital would be to have a safe space where the flood of memories, flashbacks, and urges to cut herself that

she was assaulted by could be managed in a safe and protective setting. If Sophie were forced to leave before she felt ready, her hospitalization would become just another iatrogenic experience for her, where the experience of cure mirrored and contributed further to her original trauma. For a more in-depth discussion of clinical and medical options available to women in Sophie's predicament, see Miller (1994).

5. For further discussion of the role of forgiveness in work with trauma survivors see Bass and Davis (1988/1994), Herman (1992), and D. Miller (1994).

6. See Bateson, Jackson, Haley, and Weakland (1956).

CHAPTER 8

1. In a book by the same title, *When AA's Go to OA*, Judith Hollis (1986) maps out a number of themes found in Cara's story. My account of the challenges Cara and other recovering alcoholics face when using OA to help them overcome a food addiction draws heavily on Hollis's work.

2. For more discussion see Bowlby (1988), D. Miller (1994), Shapiro and Dominiak (1992), and Herman (1992).

3. Survivors of Incest and Sexual Abuse Anonymous (SISA) is a recent addition to the recovery landscape. However, clinicians should use caution when referring people to these meeting rooms. My initial sense is that this program can be beneficial to people who have already had lots of recovery and therapy and are looking for an ongoing support group to discuss trauma issues that come up in their daily lives.

CHAPTER 9

1. For further discussion on the history of these developments see Hoffman (1981).

2. In a moving memoir Treadway (1997) tells the story of his mother's lifelong struggle with her addiction and his family's grief and reckoning with her eventual suicide.

3. Bruner's research on the use of narrative was the intellectual scaffolding that White and Epston (1991) cast their work upon when developing a narrative approach to therapy.

4. I borrowed this technique from David Treadway. It's discussed further in his book *Before It's Too Late: The Family Treatment of Substance Abuse* (1989).

5. In narrative and other family therapy circles the concept of the reflecting team has evolved into the practice of breaking into small groups of witnesses/observers that serve different functions during a consultation with a family. One group or individual engages in a dialogue with the family and asks them questions about their experience, while a larger "outside-witness group" forms a circle around them or to one side of the smaller group (but in the same room) and offers guidance and support. I personally like the intimacy of meeting without using a two-way mirror. A reflecting team does not need this

or any other technology (video cameras, audio equipment, etc.) to function effectively, although I still appreciate the use of these tools for training purposes and feel they can take on a playful—almost magical—presence in work with children and adolescents. Although organizing ourselves into small groups based on the principles of creating safety; honoring people's stories and keeping confidences; respecting differences; sharing our strengths, hopes, and truths; and believing that generous sharing is contagious all may be new to the psychotherapy community—such an approach is a long-standing tradition in AA, Al-Anon, and other 12-step programs.

6. Writing, it should be noted, is only one aspect of the narrative approach. The use of correspondence and client's written productions in therapy does not, by itself, locate a therapist's work in a narrative or postmodern context. Other "narrativizing" techniques developed by Michael White and David Epston (1991) include the use of what they call "relative influence questioning." Inspired by the contributions of the Milan group (Selvini-Palazzoli et al., 1978; Boscolo et al., 1987), I like to think of this process as a form of circular questioning for the masses and find it very useful in my work with families (see White 1989b). White uses this technique to encourage a process in therapy that externalizes and objectifies problems confronting people. He is especially interested in attending to the unique outcomes that contradict the "problem-saturated descriptions" of events people often recount in therapy and replace them with more hopeful descriptions of their experiences. For example, if a person were to describe many failed efforts at sobriety, White might ask her to recall a time when she was able to maintain abstinence in the face of adverse circumstances regardless of how long she was able to remain sober or whether she was able to repeat it. He then would ask her a series of questions meant to "historicize" this unique event (i.e., plot its growth and development across time) and connect it to other acts of resistance to alcohol she has experienced any success with. In this way the client would be invited to systematically review and reappraise her relationship to drinking, to others, and to recovery. Examples of relative influence questions directed at people's experience with alcoholism might include the following:

Can you recall an occasion when you could have given into the alcohol but didn't?

Can you think of a time when your sobriety was facing adversity and could have caved in to alcohol, when instead, you rallied and warded off relapse?

Can you recognize an occasion when your determination to get sober was such that you nearly managed to free yourself from alcohol's hold on you?

What does your successful departure from your old course of drinking tell you about your relationship to yourself that you can admire?

How are these new realizations about yourself and your recovery affecting your capacity to respect yourself?

What effect does appreciating your resolve not to cooperate with alcohol's plan for you have on your attitude toward yourself?

Has this new picture of yourself changed how you treat yourself as a person?

What difference will knowing this about yourself make to your next steps in recovery?

While many of my conversations with clients are informed by White's and many others' interviewing techniques, I have not emphasized this method in this chapter. In practice, I find this style of questioning more therapist driven than client centered. In other words, it feels too scripted. However, the same can be said of any technique once it becomes too familiar, routine, or rote. When I first began trying to apply some of these ideas in my practice, I spent many sessions with a clipboard or legal pad in my lap with a copy of White and Epston's questions to refer to during the interview.

Many talented therapists have extended narrative ideas and concepts, including the use of relative influence questions, to many other populations and problems. Some of the more well-known advocates of these practices include the following: Sally Ann Roth and Kathy Weingarten at the Cambridge Family Institute in Massachusetts; Vicky Dickerson and Jeff Zimmerman of Bay Area Family Therapy Training Associates in San Francisco; and Jill Freedman and Gene Combs of the Evanston Family Therapy Center in Evanston, Illinois. While all of these practitioners draw upon White and Epston's use of the narrative approach to therapy, all are innovators in their own right who have added their own signatures to this work. Collectively, this body of literature represents a more formal narrative therapy approach to which the present book makes no claim. Readers interested in gaining a more complete picture of these developments in family therapy would be wise to explore these authors' work and to participate in training or institutes with them if possible. Although I too owe a great intellectual debt to Michael White and David Epston, this book represents my own rendition of narrative therapy and its application to addiction and trauma. Because of the analytic thread in particular that runs through the text, one could argue that this book is only distantly, if at all, related to White and Epston's narrative project and the writing and therapy it has inspired. Readers looking to connect the present work to the work of other narrative therapists might, more appropriately, situate it under the tent term "social constructionist therapy." This designation and its parent label "social constructionism," most often associated with the work of Kenneth and Mary Gergen, refers to a loose-knit collection of researchers and therapists whose work emphasizes the cultural and political consequences of therapy. An excellent reader, *Therapy as Social Construction*, edited by Sheila McNamee and Kenneth Gergen offers more background on these ideas.

CHAPTER 10

1. For further discussion, see Winnicott (1964/1987) Chapter 13, "Further Thoughts on Babies as Persons."
2. I first encountered addiction described this way in an edited summary of three unpublished talks given by José Arguelles at Karme-Choling, a Buddhist meditation retreat in Barnet, Vermont, on November 9–11, 1984. The notes were compiled by Joseph Crane and edited by Roget Lockard.
3. The international monthly magazine of Overeaters Anonymous (OA).

CHAPTER 11

1. Personal communication (April 26, 1998).
2. If you are a therapist who has not had any personal experience in a 12-step program yourself and you have difficulty, or have become impatient, with people's hedging in these places, you should try an exercise: make a commitment to yourself or a colleague to find out more about 12-step meetings in your own community. Once you have done this, keep a journal and track (1) the amount of time it takes you to actually get to a meeting; (2) the reasons and excuses you had for not going sooner; and (3) the thoughts and feelings that come up for you once you actually start attending—especially the ones prior to and during your first meeting.
3. Roget Lockard (personal communication, April 26, 1998).
4. The sponsor relationship, while not a professional one, comes closest to conferring that kind of authority to one member over another. For this reason, to avoid potential abuses of power, members are strongly encouraged to choose sponsors of the same sex, or in some cases (e.g., gay or lesbian members) the opposite sex.
5. There is no psychoanalytic literature, to my knowledge, on analysts in recovery, never mind negotiating boundaries between analysts and patients at 12-step meetings. Clearly though this is and would be considered a "dual relationship." Articles on dual relationships in therapy are more plentiful and the issues complex. The largest discussion in the analytic literature has to do with sexual relations between therapists and clients (see Gabbard and Lester, 1995). Even in situations that do not involve overt acts of therapist abuse or misconduct—for example, in cases where relationships were not started until well after treatment ended—the boundary violations and transgressions that can result from this type of contact can be very damaging and harmful to clients. The reader should be clear that the only types of "dual relationships" being addressed here are the kind of overlaps that result when the client and therapist are both in recovery and/or members of the same 12-step program.
6. For further discussion see Pearlman and Saakvitne (1995, p. 363).
7. The work that influenced White's thinking about this was Sharon Welch's *A Feminist Ethic of Risk* (1990).
8. See White (1992, 1997). Mitchell (1993) observes how psychotherapy has a history of privileging language and words over silence. Interpretations and other speech acts that speak to the absences in people's lives are viewed as more healing than commentary on the significance of the people who have been present for them, or the healing tendencies that the actual presence of the therapist produces in the clients. He also discusses the ways in which psychoanalysis has put greater emphasis on conversations about anger and sex, and how the assumption that anger or arousal is more authentic than curiosity about other aspects of people's stories is a holdover from classical theory and 19th-century romanticism.
    Narrative therapy, despite its use of written productions, and family therapy have also replicated this emphasis on talk and conversation. However, says Mitchell, there are situations in which language itself becomes an obstacle and seems to block off new avenues of experience. Can we, asks

Mitchell, "tolerate being with clients without words that can take us some place?" (1993, p. 225).

CHAPTER 12

1. White and Epston (1990) have mapped out some specific kinds of documents they have found useful in the therapy setting over the years. These authors observe that letters can reinforce the process of transformation in therapy by serving as a wider audience to honor the changes a person has made or by helping clients identify and recruit other audiences to perform this function. White (1989c, p. 16) offers a brief summary of these practices:

   1. Celebrations, prize-giving and awards, attended by significant persons, including those who may not have attended therapy;
   2. Purposeful "news releases" whereby pertinent information as to the person's arrival at a new status is made available to various significant persons and agencies;
   3. Personal declarations, and letters of reference.

   The third category includes "declarations of independence," "letters of retirement," and "discharge letters" dismissing the influence of anorexia, bulimia, or addiction in a person's life; letters of encouragement or support from family members and therapists; and letters that help people get unstuck from the "redundant" roles they play in life, such as "parent watcher" or "marriage counselor." While I haven't used the antibulimia leagues that Epston (1989) writes about, I have used awards and certificates of achievement in my work with children and adolescents. Also, while I haven't organized the letters I draft in as systematic fashion as White and Epston do, I certainly recycle my ideas and thinking about addiction, borrowing themes used in one correspondence for use in another.

2. Gloria Jean Watkins was bell hooks's given name.
3. These insights into Sophie's and hook's experience were informed by Stolorow, Atwood, and Brandehaft (1994). In this book, the authors present their work with a young woman named Anna and their observations about the "psychological functions of masochistic behavior" (p. 124), what I prefer to think of as the conditions of warrant that result in a person seeking pain and the subjugation of the self.

POSTSCRIPT

1. From the Talmudic rulings of Rabbi Hayyim ben Isaac in the late 13th century, as quoted in Wieseltier (1998, p. 580).
2. From Malcolm Diamond (1994a, p. 17).

References and Selected Bibliography

AA comes of age. (1985). New York: Alcoholics Anonymous World Services.

Ackerman, R. (1986). *Growing in the shadow*. Pompano Beach, FL: Heath Communications.

Addison R. B., & Packer, M. J. (Eds.). (1989). *Entering the circle: Hermeneutic investigations in psychology*. Albany: State University of New York Press.

Al-Anon for professionals. (1987). New York: Al-Anon Family Services.

Alcoholics Anonymous. (1976). New York: Alcoholics Anonymous World Services. (Original work published 1939)

Alexander, C. (1979). *The timeless way of being*. New York: Oxford University Press.

Allen, J., & Laird, J. (1990). Men and story: Constructing new narratives in therapy. *Journal of Feminist Family Therapy, 2*(3/4), 75–99.

American Psychiatric Association. (1994). *Diagnostic and statistical manual of mental disorders* (4th ed.). Washington, DC: Author.

Andersen, T. (1987). The reflecting team: Dialogue and meta-dialogue in clinical work. *Family Process, 26*, 415–428.

Andersen, T. (Ed.). (1991). *The reflecting team: Dialogues and dialogues about the dialogues*. New York: Norton.

Andersen, T. (1992). Reflections on reflecting with families. In S. McNamee & K. Gergen (Eds.), *Therapy as social construction* (pp. 54–68). Newbury Park, CA: Sage.

Andersen, T. (1993). See and hear, and be seen and heard. In S. Friedman (Ed.), *The new language of change: Constructive collaboration in psychotherapy* (pp. 303–322). New York: Guilford Press.

Anderson, H. (1991). Thinking about multi-agency work with substance abusers and their families: A language systems approach. *Journal of Strategic and Systemic Therapies, 10*, 20–35.

Anderson, H. (1993). On a roller coaster: A collaborative language systems approach to therapy. In S. Friedman (Ed.), *The new language of change: Con-*

structive collaboration in psychotherapy (pp. 323–344). New York: Guilford Press.

Anderson, H., & Goolishian, H. A. (1988). Human systems as linguistic systems: Preliminary and evolving ideas about the implications for clinical theory. *Family Process, 27*(4), 371–393.

Anderson, H., & Goolishian, H. A. (1992). The client is the expert: A not-knowing position for family therapy. In S. McNamee & K. Gergen (Eds.), *Therapy as social construction* (pp. 25–39). Newbury Park, CA: Sage.

Antze, P. (1987). Symbolic action in Alcoholics Anonymous. In *Constructive drinking: Perspectives on drink from anthropology.* Cambridge, UK: Cambridge University Press.

Aponte, H. (1976). Underorganization in the poor family. In P. Guerin, Jr. (Ed.), *Family therapy: Theory and practice.* New York: Gardner Press.

Armstrong, K. (1993). *A history of God: The 4,000 year quest of Judaism, Christianity and Islam.* New York: Ballantine Press.

Aronowitz, S. (1993). *Dead artists: Live theories.* New York: Routledge.

As Bill sees it. (1967). New York: Alcoholics Anonymous World Services.

Bakhtin, M. (1981). *The dialogic imagination: Four essays.* Austin: University of Texas Press.

Balint, E. (1993). *Before I was I: Psychoanalysis and the imagination.* (J. Mitchell & M. Parsons, Eds.). New York: Guilford Press.

Balint, M. (1968). *The basic fault: Therapeutic aspects of regression.* London: Tavistock.

Bambara, T. (1970). *Salteaters.* New York: New American Library.

Barret, M. J., & Trepper, T. (1991). Treating women drug abusers who were victims of childhood sexual abuse. In C. Bepko (Ed.), *Feminism and addiction* (pp. 127–146). New York: Hawthorn Press.

Bass, E., & Davis, L. (1994). *The courage to heal.* New York: Harper Perennial. (Original work published 1988)

Bateson, C. (1989). *Composing a life.* New York: Penguin Books.

Bateson, G. (1972a). The cybernetics of "self": A theory of alcoholism. In *Steps to an ecology of mind* (pp. 309–337). New York: Ballantine Books.

Bateson, G. (1972b). *Steps to an ecology of mind.* London: Aronson.

Bateson, G. (1991). *A sacred unity: Further steps to an ecology of mind.* New York: HarperCollins/"A Cornelia and Michael Bessie Book."

Bateson, G., Jackson, D., Haley, J., & Weakland, J. (1956). Toward a theory of schizophrenia. *Behavioral Science, 1,* 251–264.

Bean, M. (1975a). Alcoholics Anonymous I. *Psychiatric Annals, 5*(2), 7–61.

Bean, M. (1975b). Alcoholics Anonymous II. *Psychiatric Annals, 5*(3), 7–57.

Belenky, M., Clinchy, B., Goldberger, N., & Tarule, J. (1986). *Women's ways of knowing: The development of self, voice and mind.* New York: Basic Books.

Benjamin, J. (1988). *The bonds of love.* New York: Pantheon Books.

Benjamin, J. (1995). *Like subjects, love objects: Essays on recognition and sexual difference.* New Haven, CT: Yale University Press.

Bepko, C. (1991a). Disorders of power: Women and addiction in the family. In M.

McGoldrick, C. Anderson, & F. Walsh (Eds.), *Women in families* (pp. 406–426). New York: Norton.

Bepko, C. (Ed.). (1991b). *Feminism and addiction.* New York: Hawthorn Press.

Bepko, C., & Krestan, J. (1985). *The responsibility trap: A blueprint for treating the alcoholic family.* New York: Free Press.

Bepko, C., & Krestan, J. (1991). Codependency and the social reconstruction of female experience. In C. Bepko (Ed.), *Feminism and addiction* (pp. 49–66). New York: Hawthorn Press.

Bepko, C., & Krestan, J. (1993). On lies, secrets, and silence: The multiple levels of denial in addictive families. In E. Black (Ed.), *Secrets and families and family therapy* (pp. 141–159). New York: Norton.

Berenson, D. (1976). Alcohol and the family system. In P. Guerin, Jr. (Ed.), *Family therapy: Theory and practice.* New York: Gardner Press.

Berenson, D. (1979). The therapist's relationship with couples with an alcoholic member. In E. Kaufman & P. Kaufman (Eds.), *Family therapy of drug and alcohol abuse* (pp. 233–242). New York: Gardner Press.

Berenson, D. (1985). Foreword. In C. Bepko & J. Krestan. *The responsibility trap: A blueprint for treating the alcoholic family* (pp. ix–xi). New York: Free Press.

Berenson, D. (1986, September 11–12). *Workshop presented at the Lifecycles Conference,* New York.

Berenson, D. (1987). Alcoholics Anonymous: From surrender to transformation. *Family Therapy Networker, 11*(4), 24–33.

Berenson, D. (1991). Powerlessness—liberating or enslaving? Responding to the feminist critique of the twelve steps. In C. Bepko (Ed.), *Feminism and addiction* (pp. 67–86). New York: Hawthorn Press.

Berger, P. & Luckman T. (1966). *The social construction of reality.* New York: Doubleday.

Bernstein, H., & Fortune, J. (1998). *Muddling through: Pursuing science and truths in the 21st century.* Washington DC: Counterpoint.

Bernstein, H., & Raskin, M. (1987). *New ways of knowing: The sciences, society, and reconstructive knowledge.* Totowa, NJ: Rowman & Littlefield.

Best of the grapevine. (1985). New York: Alcoholics Anonymous World Services.

Black, C. (1985). *It will never happen to me.* Denver, CO: MAC.

Black, C. (1986). *My dad loves me, my dad has a disease: A child's view of living with addiction.* Boulder, CO: MGC.

Blume, S. (1983). The disease concept of alcoholism. *Journal of Psychiatric Treatment and Evaluation, 5,* 471–478.

Bollas, C. (1983). Expressive uses of countertransference. *Contemporary Psychoanalysis, 19*(1), 1–34.

Bollas, C. (1987). *The shadow of the object.* London: Free Association.

Bollas, C. (1989). *Forces of destiny: Psychoanalysis and the human idiom.* London: Free Association.

Bollas, C. (1992). *On being a character.* New York: Hill & Wang.

Bollas, C. (1995). *Cracking up: The work of unconscious experience.* New York: Hill & Wang.

Boscolo, L., Cecchin, G., Hoffman, L., & Penn, P. (1987). *Milan systemic family therapy*. New York: Basic Books.

Bourdieu, P. (1992). *An invitation to reflexive sociology*. Chicago: University of Chicago Press.

Bowen, M. (1978). *Family therapy in clinical practice*. New York: Aronson.

Bowlby, J. (1988). *A secure base: Clinical applications of attachment theory*. London: Routledge.

Brechner, S. (1997, February 23). Seeking a theater varied as a rainbow. *The New York Times*, s. 2, p. 5.

Briere, J. (1989). *Therapy for adults molested as children*. New York: Springer.

Brown, S. (1985). *Treating the alcoholic: A developmental model of recovery*. New York: Wiley.

Bruner, J. (1986). *Actual minds, possible worlds*. Cambridge, MA: Harvard University Press.

Buber, M. (1955). *Tales of the Hasidim: The early masters*. New York: Schocken Books. (Original work published 1947)

Buber, M. (1958). *I and thou* (2nd ed. with a postscript by the author). New York: Scribner. (Original English edition, published 1937; Edinburgh)

Burton, A. (1965). *The use of written communications in psychotherapy*. Springfield, IL: Charles C Thomas.

Cameron, J. (1992). *The artist's way: A spiritual path to creativity*. New York: Putnam.

Carter, E. (1994). *Writing as a therapeutic act: Women writing as a means of gaining identity and sense of self*. Unpublished master's thesis, Smith College School for Social Work, Northampton, MA.

Cecchin, G. (1987). Hypothesizing, circularity, and neutrality revisited: An invitation to curiosity. *Family Process, 26*(4), 405–413.

Chatwin, B. (1987). *The songlines*. New York: Viking Press.

Chodorow, N. (1978). *The reproduction of mothering: Psychoanalysis and the sociology of gender*. Berkeley: University of California Press.

Chu, J. (1992). The therapeutic roller coaster: Dilemmas in the treatment of childhood abuse survivors. *Journal of Psychotherapy Practice and Research, 2*.

Clifford, J., & Marcus, G. E. (Eds.). (1986). *Writing culture: The poetics and politics of ethnography*. Berkeley: University of California Press.

Covington, S. (1988). *Leaving the enchanted forest*. Minneapolis, MN: Hazelden.

Cushman, P. (1991). Ideology obscured: Political uses of the self in Daniel Stern's infant. *American Psychologist, 46*, 206–219.

Cushman, P. (1995). *Constructing the self, constructing America: A cultural history of psychotherapy*. New York: Addison-Wesley.

Das, V. (1997). Language and body: Transactions in the construction of pain. In A. Kirenman, V. Das, & M. Lock (Eds.), *Social suffering*. Berkeley: University of California Press.

Davidson, J., Lax, W., & Lussardi, D. (1991). Use of the reflecting team in the initial interview and in supervision and training. In T. Andersen (Ed.), *Dialogues and dialogues about the dialogues* (pp. 143–154). New York: Norton.

Davies, J., & Frawley, M. (1994) *Treating the adult survivor of childhood sexual abuse: A psychoanalytic perspective.* New York: Basic Books.

Derrida, J. (1978). *Writing and difference.* London: Routledge & Kegan Paul.

de Saint-Exupéry, A. (1943). *The little prince* (K. Woods, Trans.). New York: Reynal & Hitchcock.

Diamond, M. (1960). *Martin Buber: Jewish existentialist.* New York: Oxford University Press.

Diamond, M. (1994a). *Buddhism and cancer: The challenges of change.* Unpublished manuscript.

Diamond, M. (1994b). Reflections on therapy while coping with cancer. *Princeton Alumni Weekly, 94*(13), 13–16.

Dickerson, V., & Zimmerman, J. (1993). A narrative approach to families with adolescents. In S. Friedman (Ed.), *The new language of change: Constructive collaboration in psychotherapy* (pp. 226–250). New York: Guilford Press.

Douglas, M. (1982). *In the active voice.* London: Routledge & Kegan Paul.

Dowling, E., & Shoemaker, Rev. S. (1957). Religion looks at Alcoholics Anonymous. Chapter 5 in *Alcoholics Anonymous comes of age: A brief history of AA.* New York: Alcoholics Anonymous World Service.

Dreyfus, H., & Rabinow, P. (Eds.). (1982). *Michel Foucault: Beyond structuralism and hermeneutics.* Chicago: University of Chicago Press.

Durrant, M., & White, C. (1991). *Ideas for therapy with sexual abuse.* Adelaide, Australia: Dulwich Centre Publications.

Edelman, H. (1994). *Motherless daughters: The legacy of loss.* Weston, MA: Addison-Wesley.

Efran, J. (1991). Constructivism in the inner city. *Family Therapy Networker, 15*(5), 51–52.

Efran, J., Hefner, K., & Lukens, R. (1987). Alcoholism as an opinion. *Family Therapy Networker, 11*(4), 43–46.

Efran, J., Lukens, R., & Lukens, R. (1990). *Language structure and change.* New York: Norton.

Eliot, T. S. (1962a). Burnt Norton (first of the "Four Quartets"). In *The complete poems and plays* (pp. 117–122). New York: Harcourt, Brace & World. (Poem originally published 1943)

Eliot, T. S. (1962b). Little Gidding (fourth of the "Four Quartets"). In *The complete poems and plays* (pp. 138–145). New York: Harcourt, Brace & World. (Poem originally published 1943)

Epstein, E., & Loos, V. (1989). Some irreverent thoughts on the limits of family therapy. *Journal of Family Psychology, 14*(3) 225–236.

Epstein, M. (1995). *Thoughts without a thinker.* New York: Basic Books.

Epston, D. (1989). *Collected papers.* Adelaide, Australia: Dulwich Centre Publications.

Epston, D. (1994). Extending the conversation. *Family Therapy Networker, 18*(6), 30–39, 62–63.

Epston, D., White, M., & Murray, K. (1992). A proposal for re-authoring therapy: Rose's revisioning of her life and a commentary. In S. McNamee & K. Gergen

(Eds.), *Therapy as social construction* (pp. 96–117). Newbury Park, CA: Sage.

Erickson, G. D. (1988). Against the grain: Decentering family therapy. *American Journal of Marital and Family Therapy, 14,* 225–236.

Erikson, E. H. (1950). *Childhood and society.* New York: Norton.

Fanon, F. (1978). *The wretched of the earth.* New York: Grove Press. (Original work published 1961)

Felman, S. (1985). *Writing and madness (Literature/philosophy/psychoanalysis).* Ithaca, NY: Cornell University Press.

Feyerabend, P. (1975). *Against method.* New York: Routledge.

Flax, J. (1990). *Thinking fragments: Feminism and postmodernism in the contemporary west.* New York: Routledge & Kegan Paul.

Flax, J. (1993). *Disputed subjects: Essays on psychoanalysis, politics, and philosophy.* New York: Routledge.

Fleck, L. (1979). *Genesis and development of a scientific fact.* Chicago: University of Chicago Press. (Original work published 1935)

Foucault, M. (1977). *Language, counter-memory, practice.* Ithaca, NY: Cornell University Press.

Foucault, M. (1978). *The history of sexuality.* New York: Vintage Books.

Foucault, M. (1980). *Power/knowledge: Selected interviews and other writings.* New York: Pantheon Books.

Freedman, J., & Combs, G. (1996). *Narrative therapy: The social construction of preferred realities.* New York: Norton.

Freeman, L., & Lobovits, D. (1993). The turtle with wings. In S. Friedman (Ed.), *The new language of change: Constructive collaboration in psychotherapy* (pp. 188–227). New York: Guilford Press.

Freud, S. (1953a). Studies in hysteria. In J. Strachey (Ed. & Trans.), *The standard edition of the complete psychological works of Sigmund Freud* (Vol. 3, pp. 1–306). London: Hogarth Press. (Original work published 1895)

Freud, S. (1953b). The interpretation of dreams. In J. Strachey (Ed. & Trans.), *The standard edition of the complete psychological works of Sigmund Freud* (Vol. 4, pp. 1–623). London: Hogarth Press. (Original work published 1900)

Freud, S. (1953c). Three essays on the theory of sexuality. In J. Strachey (Ed. & Trans.), *The standard edition of the complete psychological works of Sigmund Freud* (Vol. 5, pp. 125–245). London: Hogarth Press. (Original work published 1905)

Freud, S. (1953d). Creative writing and day-dreaming. In J. Strachey (Ed. & Trans.), *The standard edition of the complete psychological works of Sigmund Freud* (Vol. 9, pp. 141–153). London: Hogarth Press. (Original work published 1907)

Freud, S. (1958). Remembering, repeating, and working through. In J. Strachey (Ed. & Trans.), *The standard edition of the complete psychological works of Sigmund Freud* (Vol. 12, pp. 155). London: Hogarth Press. (Original work published 1914)

Friedman, S. (Ed.). (1993). *The new language of change: Constructive collaboration in psychotherapy.* New York: Guilford Press.

Gabbard, G. (1996). *Love and hate in the analytic setting*. Northvale, NJ: Aronson.

Gabbard, G., & Lester, E. R. (1995). *Boundaries and boundary violations in psychoanalysis*. New York: Basic Books.

Gadamer, H. (1975). *Philosophical hermeneutics*. Berkeley: University of California Press. (Original work published 1960)

Geertz, C. (1973). *The interpretation of cultures*. New York: Basic Books.

Geertz, C. (1983). *Local knowledge: Further essays in interpretive anthropology*. New York: Basic Books.

Gelinas, D. (1983). The persisting negative effects of incest. *Psychiatry, 46,* 312–322.

Gergen, K. (1982). *Toward transformation in social knowledge*. New York: Springer-Verlag.

Gergen, K. (1985). The social constructionist movement in modern psychology. *American Psychologist, 40,* 266–275.

Gergen, K. (1988). If persons are texts. In S. B. Messer, L. A. Sass, & R. L. Woolfolk, *Hermeneutics and psychological theory* (pp. 28–51). New Brunswick, NJ: Rutgers University Press.

Gergen, K. (1989). Warranting voice and the elaboration of self. In J. Shotter & K. J. Gergen (Eds.), *Texts of identity*. London: Sage.

Gergen, K. (1991). *The saturated self*. New York: Basics Books.

Gilligan, C. (1982). *In a different voice*. Cambridge, MA: Harvard University Press.

Gluck, L. (1994). *Proofs and theories*. Hopewell, NJ: Ecco Press.

Goldner, V. (1989). Generation and gender. In M. McGoldrick, C. Anderson, & F. Walsh (Eds.), *Women in families* (pp. 42–60). New York: Norton.

Goodman, N. (1978). *Ways of worldmaking*. Hassocks, Sussex, UK: Harvester Press.

Grosz, E. (1990). Contemporary theories of power and subjectivity. In S. Gunew (Ed.), *Feminist knowledge: Critique and construct* (pp. 59–120). London: Routledge & Kegan Paul.

Gunew, S. (Ed.). (1990). *Feminist knowledge: Critique and construct*. London: Routledge & Kegan Paul.

Hafner, S. (1992). *Nice girls don't drink: Stories of recovery*. New York: Bergin & Garvey.

Hastings, J., & Typpo, M. (1984). *An elephant in the living room*. Minneapolis: CompCare.

Herman, J. (1981). *Father–daughter incest*. New York: Basic Books.

Herman, J. (1992). *Trauma and recovery*. New York: Basic Books.

Hillman, J. (1972). *The myth of analysis*. Chicago: Northwestern University Press.

Hoffman, L. (1981). *Foundations of family therapy*. New York: Basic Books.

Hoffman, L. (1990). Constructing realities: An art of lenses. *Family Process, 29*(1), 1–12.

Hoffman, L. (1993). *Exchanging voices: A collaborative approach to family therapy*. London: Karnac Books.

Hoffman, L. (1994, July 19–20). *The narrative therapy of Michael White.* Workshop presented at Smith College School for Social Work, Northampton, MA.

Hollis, J. (1986). *When AA's go to OA.* Minneapolis, MN: Hazelden.

hooks, b. (1984). *Feminist theory: From margin to center.* Boston: South End Press.

hooks, b. (1989). *Talking back: Thinking feminist, thinking black.* Boston: South End Press.

hooks, b. (1990). *Yearning: Race, gender and cultural politics.* Boston: South End Press.

hooks, b. (1993). *Sisters of the yam: Black women and self recovery.* Boston: South End Press.

hooks, b., & West, C. (1991). *Breaking bread: Insurgent black intellectual life.* Boston: South End Press.

Imber-Black, E., Roberts, J., & Whiting, R. (Eds.). (1988). *Rituals in families and family therapy.* New York: Norton.

Jacoby, R. (1975). *Social amnesia.* Boston: Beacon Press.

Jamison, K. R. (1995). *An unquiet mind.* New York: Knopf.

Jenkins, A. (1990). *Invitations to responsibility: The therapeutic engagement of men who are violent and abusive.* Adelaide, Australia: Dulwich Centre Publications.

Jones, J. (1991). *Contemporary psychoanalysis and religion.* New Haven, CT: Yale University Press.

Jones, J. (1992a). Knowledge in transition: Toward a Winnicottian epistemology. *Psychoanalytic Review, 79*(2), 223–237.

Jones, J. (1992b). Psychoanalysis, feminism and religion. *Pastoral Psychology, 40*(6), 355–367.

Jones, J. (1995). *Religion and psychology in transition.* New Haven: Yale University Press.

Kabat-Zinn, J. (1994). *Wherever you go there you are.* New York: Hyperion.

Kaplan, L. (1995). *No voice is ever wholly lost.* New York: Simon & Schuster.

Kasl, C. D. (1989). *Women, sex, and addiction: A search for love and power.* New York: Harper & Row.

Kasl, C. D. (1992). *Many roads, one journey: Moving beyond the 12 steps.* New York: HarperCollins.

Kaufmann, E. (1979). The application of the basic principles of family therapy to the treatment of drug and alcohol abusers. In E. Kaufmann & P. Kaufmann (Eds.), *Family therapy of drug and alcohol abuse.* New York: Gardner Press.

Kaufmann, E., & Kaufmann, P. (1979). Family therapy with adolescent substance abusers. In E. Kaufmann & P. Kaufmann (Eds.), *Family therapy of drug and alcohol abuse.* New York: Gardner Press.

Keillor, G. (1991). A short story: Al Denny. *Family Therapy Networker, 15*(5), 66–68.

Keller, E. F. (1992). *Secrets of life and death: Essays on language, gender and science.* New York: Routledge.

Keller, E. F., & Flax, J. (1988). A feminist critique of psychoanalysis. In S. B.

Messer, L. A. Sass, & R. L. Woolfolk (Eds.), *Hermeneutics and psychological theory* (pp. 334–366). New Brunswick, NJ: Rutgers University Press.

Kerr, M., & Bowen, M. (1988). *Family evaluation*. New York: Norton.

Kestenberg, J. (1972). Psychoanalytic contributions to the problems of children of survivors from Nazi persecution. *Israel Annals of Psychiatry and Related Disciplines, 10,* 249–265.

Kestenberg, J. (1989). Transpositions revisited: Clinical therapeutic and developmental considerations. In P. Marcus & A. Rosenberg (Eds.), *Healing their wounds*. New York: Praeger.

Klein, M. (1984). *Love, guilt, and reparation and other works 1921–1945*. New York: Free Press.

Knapp, C. (1996). *Drinking: A love story*. New York: Dial Press.

Kohut, H. (1971). *The analysis of the self*. New York: International Universities Press.

Kohut, H. (1977). *The restoration of the self*. New York: International Universities Press.

Kohut, H. (1984). *How does analysis cure?* Chicago: University of Chicago Press.

Kramer, P. (1993). *Listening to prozac*. New York: Penguin Books.

Kramer, W. (1992). *I'm dysfunctional, you're dysfunctional: The recovery movement and other self-help fashions*. New York: Vintage Books.

Kuhn, T. (1962). *The structure of scientific revolutions*. Chicago: University of Chicago Press.

Kurtz, E. (1979). *Not God: A history of Alcoholics Anonymous*. Minneapolis, MN: Hazelden.

Kurtz, E. (1988). *AA: The story*. San Francisco: Harper & Row [a revised edition of the same author's *Not God: A history of Alcoholics Anonymous*].

Laird, J. (1989). Women and stories: Restorying women's self-constructions. In M. McGoldrick, C. Anderson, & F. Walsh (Eds.), *Women in families* (pp. 427–450). New York: Norton.

Laird, J. (1993a). Women's secrets, women's silences. In E. Black (Ed.), *Secrets and families and family therapy* (pp. 243–267). New York: Norton.

Laird, J. (1993b). Lesbians and lesbian families: Multiple reflections [Special issue]. *Smith College Studies in Social Work, 63*(3).

Laird, J. (1995). *Postmodern feminist family therapy*. Workshop presented at the Franklin Medical Center, Greenfield, MA.

Lax, B. (1992). Postmodern thinking in clinical practice. In *Therapy as social construction* (pp. 69–87). Newbury Park, CA: Sage.

Lerner, H. (1985). *The dance of anger*. San Francisco: Harper & Row.

Levin, S. (1988). *Hearing the unheard: Stories of women who have been battered*. Unpublished master's thesis, The Union Institute, New York.

Levine, S. (1987). *Healing into life and death*. New York: Doubleday.

Lew, M. (1991). *Victims no longer: Men recovering from childhood sexual abuse*. San Francisco: Harper & Row.

Lockard, R. (1985a). *Epistemological issues in treating alcoholism in families*. Unpublished manuscript.

Lockard, R. (1985b). *The discovery process: An approach to alcoholism.* Unpublished manuscript.

Lockard, R. (1993). Self-will run riot: The earth as an alcoholic. Unpublished paper adapted from a talk at the public symposium: *Is the Earth a Living Organism?* University of Massachussets at Amherst, August 3, 1985.

Lockard, R. (1999). *Another voice: A handbook on addiction, recovery, and the survival of the human species.* Manuscript in preparation.

Loewald, H. (1980). *Papers on psychoanalysis.* New Haven, CT: Yale University Press.

Lois remembers: Memoirs of the co-founder of Al-Anon and wife of the co-founder of Alcoholics Anonymous. (1979). Al-Anon Family Group.

Lorde, A. (1978). School note [poem]. In *The black unicorn.* New York: Norton.

Lorde, A. (1982). *Zami: A new spelling of my name.* Watertown, MA: Persephone Press.

Lorde, A. (1984). *Sister outsider.* Freedom, CA: Crossing Press.

Luepnitz, D. A. (1988). *The family interpreted.* New York: Basic Books.

Luepnitz, D. A. (1992). Nothing in common but their first names: The case of Foucault and White. *Journal of Family Therapy, 14*(3), 281–284.

Lussardi, D. J., & Miller, D. (1991). A reflecting team approach to adolescent substance abuse. In T. Todd & M. Selekman (Eds.), *Family therapy approaches with adolescent substance abuse* (pp. 143–161). Needham Heights, MA: Allyn & Bacon.

Lyotard, J. F. (1979). *The postmodern condition: A report on knowledge.* Minneapolis: University of Minnesota Press.

Masson, J. (1984). *The assault on truth.* New York: HarperCollins.

Maturana, H., & Vareia, F. (1987). *The tree of knowledge.* Boston: New Science Library.

McGoldrick, M., Giordano, J., & Pearce, J. K. (1996). *Ethnicity and family therapy* (2nd ed.). New York: Guilford Press.

McKinnon, L., & Miller, D. (1987). The new epistemology and the Milan approach: Feminist and socio-political considerations. *American Journal of Marital and Family Therapy, 13,* 139–155.

McNamee, S., & Gergen, K., (1992). *Therapy as social construction.* Newbury Park, CA: Sage.

Messer, S. B., Sass, L. A., & Woolfolk, R. L. (1988). *Hermeneutics and psychological theory.* New Brunswick, NJ: Rutgers University Press.

Metzger, D. (1992). *Writing for your life: A guide and companion to the inner worlds.* San Francisco: HarperCollins.

Miller, D. (1990). Women in pain: Substance abuse/self-medication. In M. Mirkin (Ed.), *Social and political contexts of family therapy.* Boston: Allyn & Bacon.

Miller, D. (1991). Are we keeping up with Oprah?: A treatment and training model for addictions and interpersonal violence. In C. Bepko (Ed.), *Feminism and addiction* (pp. 103–126). New York: Hawthorn Press.

Miller, D. (1993). Incest: The heart of darkness. In E. Black (Ed.), *Secrets and families and family therapy* (pp. 181–197). New York: Norton.

Miller, D. (1994). *Women who hurt themselves: A book of hope and recovery.* New York: Basic Books.

Miller, D., & Lax, W. D. (1988). Interrupting deadly struggles: A reflecting team model for working with couples. *Journal of Strategic and Systemic Therapies, 7*(3), 16–22.

Miller, J. B. (1976). *Toward a new psychology of women.* Boston: Beacon Press.

Miller, J. B. (1988). *Connections, disconnections and violations.* Wellesley, MA: Stone Center Working Papers Series (No. 33).

Milne, A. A. (1926). *Winnie the Pooh.* London: Metheun.

Milner, M. (1957). *On not being able to paint.* London: Heinemann.

Minuchin, S. (1974). *Families and family therapy.* Cambridge, MA: Harvard University Press.

Minuchin, S. (1979). Constructing a therapeutic reality. In E. Kaufmann & P. Kaufmann (Eds.), *Family therapy of drug and alcohol abuse.* New York: Gardner Press.

Mitchell, S. (1987). *Relational concepts in psychoanalysis: An integration.* New York: Basic Books.

Mitchell, S. (1993). *Hope and dread in psychoanalysis.* New York: Basic Books.

Mitchell, S., & Black, M. (1995). *Freud and beyond.* New York: Basic Books.

Moore, T. (1992). *Care of the soul.* New York: HarperCollins.

Morrison, T. (1987). *Beloved.* New York: New American Library.

Muller, J. (1996). *Beyond the psychoanalytic dyad: Developmental semiotics in Freud, Pierce, and Lacan.* New York: Routledge.

Myerhoff, B. (1982a). Life history among the elderly. In J. B. Ruby (Ed.), *A crack in the mirror: Reflexive perspectives in anthropology* (pp. 305–340). Philadelphia: University of Pennsylvania Press.

Myerhoff, B. (1982b). The journal as activity and genre. In J. B. Ruby (Ed.), *A crack in the mirror: Reflexive perspectives in anthropology* (pp. 341–360). Philadelphia: University of Pennsylvania Press.

Napier, A., & Whitaker, C. (1978). *The family crucible.* New York: Harper & Row.

Norris, K. (1998). *Amazing grace: A vocabulary of faith.* New York: Riverhead Books.

O'Hanlon, W. (1994). The third wave. *Family Therapy Networker, 18*(6), 19–29.

Olson, M. (1995). Conversation and writing: A collaborative approach to bulimia. *Journal of Feminist Family Therapy, 6*(4), 21–44.

Olson, T. (1978). *Silences.* New York: Delacorte Press.

O'Neil, M., & Stockwell, G. (1991). Worthy of discussion: Collaborative group therapy. *Australian and New Zealand Journal of Family Therapy, 12*(4), 201–206.

Ong, W. (1982). *Orality and literacy.* New York: Norton.

Parry, A. (1991). A universe of stories. *Family Process, 30,* 37–54.

Parry, A. (1993). Preparations for postmodern living. In S. Friedman (Ed.), *The new language of change: Constructive collaboration in psychotherapy* (pp. 428–459). New York: Guilford Press.

Pearlman, L., & Saakvitne, K. (1995). *Trauma and the therapist.* New York: Norton.

Penelope, J., Lorde, A., & Rich, A. (1991). *The transformation of silence into language and action.* San Francisco: Sinister Wisdom Press.

Penn, P. (1985). Feed-forward: Future questions, future maps. *Family Process, 24,* 299–311.

Penn, P. (1991). Letters to ourselves. *Family Therapy Networker, 15*(5), 43–45.

Penn, P., & Schienberg, M. (1991). Stories and conversations. *Journal of Strategic and Systemic Therapies, 10*(3/4), 30–37.

Phillips, A. (1993). *On kissing, tickling, and being bored.* Cambridge, MA: Harvard University Press.

Rabinow, P. (Ed.). (1984). *The Foucault reader.* New York: Pantheon Books.

Rich, A. (1979). *On lies, secrets and silence: Selected prose, 1966–1978.* New York: Norton.

Ricour, P. (1970). *Freud and philosophy: An essay on interpretation.* New Haven, CT: Yale University Press.

Ricour, P. (1980, Autumn). Narrative time. *Critical Inquiry, 171,* 169–190.

Riessman, C. (1993). *Narrative Analysis.* Newbury Park, CA: Sage.

Roberts, J. (1988). Use of ritual in "redocumenting" psychiatric history. In E. Imber-Black, J. Roberts, & R. Whiting (Eds.), *Rituals in families and family therapy* (pp. 307–330). New York: Norton.

Roberts, J. (1994). *Tales of transformation: Stories in families and family therapy.* New York: Norton.

Rorty, R. (1979). *Philosophy and the mirror of nature.* Princeton, NJ: Princeton University Press.

Rorty, R. (1982a). *Philosophical papers* (Vol. 1). Princeton, NJ: Princeton University Press.

Rorty, R. (1982b). *Philosophical papers* (Vol. 2). Princeton, NJ: Princeton University Press.

Rorty, R. (1989). *Contingency, irony, and solidarity.* Cambridge, UK: Cambridge University Press.

Rorty, R. (1994). Feminism and pragmatism. In J. Smith & A. Mahfouz (Eds.), *Psychoanalysis feminism and the future of gender* (pp. 42–69). Baltimore: Johns Hopkins University Press.

Rosen, H., & Kuehlwein, K. T. (Eds.). (1996). *Constructing realities: Meaning-making perspectives for psychotherapists.* San Francisco: Jossey-Bass.

Roth, G. (1991). *When food is love.* New York: Dutton.

Roth, S. A. (1989). Psychotherapy with lesbian couples: Individual issues, female socialization and the social context. In M. McGoldrick, C. Anderson, & F. Walsh (Eds.), *Women in families* (pp. 286–307). New York: Norton.

Roud, P. (1994). *Making miracles.* New York: Harper & Row.

Rowe, R. (1992). Postmodern studies. In S. Greenblatt & G. Gunn (Eds.), *Redrawing the boundaries* (pp. 179–208). New York: Modern Language Association of America/Rowman & Littlefield.

Rowley, H., & Grosz, E. (1990). Psychoanalysis and feminism. In S. Gunew (Ed.),

Feminist knowledge: Critique and construct. London: Routledge & Kegan Paul.

Ruby, J. B. (Ed.). (1982). *A crack in the mirror: Reflexive perspectives in anthropology.* Philadelphia: University of Pennsylvania Press.

Sanville, J. (1991). *The playground of psychoanalytic therapy.* London: Analytic Press.

Sarton, M. (1975). *Letters from Maine.* New York: Norton.

Satir, V. (1964). *Conjoint family therapy.* Palo Alto, CA: Science and Behavior Books.

Satir, V. (1972). *Peoplemaking.* Palo Alto, CA: Science and Behavior Books.

Schafe, A. W. (1987). *When society becomes an addict.* New York: Harper & Row.

Schafer, R. (1976a). *A new language for psychoanalysis.* New Haven, CT: Yale University Press.

Schafer, R. (1976b). The psychoanalytic vision of reality. In *A new language for psychoanalysis* (pp. 22–56). New Haven, CT: Yale University Press.

Schafer, R. (1980). Narration in the psychoanalytic dialogue. *Critical Inquiry, 7*(1), 29–54.

Schafer, R. (1981). *Narrative actions in psychoanalysis.* Worcester, MA: Clark University Press.

Schafer, R. (1983). *The analytic attitude.* New York: Basic Books.

Schafer, R. (1992). *Retelling a life: Narration and dialogue in psychoanalysis.* New York: Basic Books.

Selvini Palazzoli, M., Boscolo, L., Cecchin, G., & Prata, G. (1978). *Paradox and counterparadox.* New York: Aronson.

Shapiro, S., & Dominiak, G. (1992). *Sexual trauma and psychopathology: Clinical intervention with adult survivors.* New York: Lexington Books.

Shotter, J. (1993). *The cultural politics of everyday life.* Toronto: University of Toronto Press.

Showwalter, E. (1985). *The female malady: Women, madness, and English culture 1830–1980.* New York: Pantheon Books.

Siegel, B. (1986). *Love, medicine, and miracles.* Boston: Hall.

Siegel, B. (1990). Foreword. In P. Roud, *Making miracles.* New York: Harper & Row.

Simon, R. (1988). Like a friendly editor (An interview with Lynn Hoffman). *Family Therapy Networker, 12*(5), 55–58, 74–75.

Simonds, W. (1992). *Women and self-help culture: Reading between the lines.* New Brunswich, NJ: Rutgers University Press.

Smith, D., & Wesson, D. (1985). *Treating the cocaine abuser.* Minneapolis, MN: Hazelden.

Spence, D. (1982). *Narrative truth, historical truth.* New York: Norton.

Spence, D. (1987). *The Freudian metaphor: Toward paradigmatic change in psychoanalysis.* New York: Norton.

Starhawk. (1987). *Truth or dare: Encounters with power, authority and mystery.* San Francisco: Harper & Row

Starhawk. (1989). *The spiral dance.* New York: Harper & Row.

Steier, F. (1991). *Research and reflexivity.* Newbury Park, CA: Sage.

Stern, D. (1985). *The interpersonal world of the infant.* New York: Basic Books.

Stierlin, H. (1986a). Family therapy with adolescents and the process of intergenerational reconciliation. In M. Sugarman (Ed.), *The adolescent in group and family therapy.* Chicago: University of Chicago Press.

Stierlin, H. (1986b). Countertransference in family therapy with adolescents. In M. Sugarman (Ed.), *The adolescent in group and family therapy.* Chicago: University of Chicago Press.

Stiver, I. (1992). *A relational approach to therapeutic impasse.* Wellesley, MA: Stone Center Working Paper Series (No. 58).

Stolorow, R., Atwood, G., & Brandehaft, B. (1994). *The intersubjective perspective.* Northvale, NJ: Aronson.

Sugarman, M. (1986a). Office network therapy with adolescents. In M. Sugarman (Ed.), *The adolescent in group and family therapy.* Chicago: University of Chicago Press.

Sugarman, M. (1986b). Transference in adolescent group therapy. In M. Sugarman (Ed.), *The adolescent in group and family therapy.* Chicago: University of Chicago Press.

Tapping, C. (1993a). In search of a just therapy. *Dulwich Centre Newsletter, 1,* 15–17.

Tapping, C. (1993b). Gender: The impact of western definitions of womenhood on other cultures. *Dulwich Centre Newsletter, 1,* 23–25.

Todd, C. (1979). Structural family therapy with drug addicts. In E. Kaufmann & P. Kaufmann (Eds.), *Family therapy of drug and alcohol abuse.* New York: Gardner Press.

Tomm, K., Suzuki, K., & Suzuki, K. (1990). The *Ka-No-Mushi:* An inner externalization that enables compromise? *Journal of Australian and New Zealand Family Therapy, 11*(2), 104–107.

Treadway, D. (1987). The ties that bind. *Family Therapy Networker, 11*(4), 16–23.

Treadway, D. (1989). *Before it's too late: The family treatment of substance abuse.* New York: Norton.

Treadway, D. (1990). Codependency: Disease, metaphor, or fad? *Family Therapy Networker, 14*(1), 38–42.

Treadway, D. (1992). Therapist heal thyself. In *Before it's too late.* New York: Basic Books.

Treadway, D. (1997). *Dead reckoning: A therapist confronts his own grief.* New York: Basic Books.

The twelve steps and twelve traditions of overeaters anonymous. (1990). Torrance, CA: Overeaters Anonymous.

Vaillant, G. E. (1983). *The natural history of alcoholism.* Cambridge, MA: Harvard University Press.

van der Kolk, B. A. (Ed.). (1987). *Psychological trauma.* Washington, DC: American Psychiatric Press.

van der Kolk, B. A. (1994). The body keeps the score: Memory and the evolving psychobiology of posttraumatic stress. *Harvard Review of Psychiatry, 1,* 253–265.

van der Kolk, B. A., & Greenburg, M. (1987). The psychobiology of the trauma response: Hyperarousal, constriction, and addiction to traumatic reexposure. In B. A.van der Kolk (Ed.), *Psychological trauma*. Washington, DC: American Psychiatric Press.

van Gennep, A. (1960). *The rites of passage*. Chicago: Chicago University Press. (Original work published 1908)

Waldegrave, C. (1990). Just therapy. *Dulwich Centre Newsletter, 1,* 6–46.

Wallace, J. (1985). Working with the preferred defense structure of the recovering alcoholic. In S. Zimberg, J. Wallace, & S. Blume (Eds.), *Practical approaches to alcoholism psychotherapy* (2nd ed., pp. 23–36). New York: Plenum Press.

Wallace, J. (1986). *Alcoholism: New light on the disease*. Salisbury, NC: Lexis Press.

Walle, A. H. (1992). William James' legacy to Alcoholics Anonymous: An analysis and a critique. *Journal of Addictive Diseases, 11*(3), 91–99.

Walters, M., Carter, B., Papp, P., & Silverstein, O. (1988). *The invisible web: Gender patterns in family relationships*. New York: Guilford Press.

Washton, A., & Gold, M. (Eds.). (1987). *Cocaine: A clinician's handbook*. New York: Guilford Press.

Watzlawick, P., Weakland, J. H., & Fisch, R. (1974). *Change: Principles of problem formation and problem resolution*. New York: Norton.

Wegscheider, S. (1981). *Another chance: Hope and health for the alcoholic*. Palo Alto, CA: Science and Behavior Books.

Weiss, R. (1993). *Cocaine*. Washington, DC: American Psychiatric Press.

Welch, S. (1990). *A feminist ethic of risk*. Minneapolis, MN: Fortress Press.

Wellisch, P., De Angelis, G., & Bond, D. (1979). Family treatment of the homosexual adolescent drug abuser: On being gay in a sad family. In E. Kaufmann & P. Kaufmann (Eds.), *Family therapy of drug and alcohol abuse*. New York: Gardner Press.

West, C. (1996). Black strivings in a twilight civilization. In L. Gates & C. West. *The future of the race*. New York: Knopf.

Whitaker, C. (1976). The hindrances of theory in clinical work. In P. Guerin, Jr. (Ed.), *Family therapy: Theory and practice*. New York: Gardner Press.

Whitaker, C. (1981). *The roots of psychotherapy* (2nd ed.). New York: Brunner/Mazel.

Whitaker, C. (1986). The symptomatic adolescent: An AWOL family member. In M. Sugarman (Ed.), *The adolescent in group and family therapy*. Chicago: University of Chicago Press.

White, M. (1989a). Saying hello again. In *Selected papers* (pp. 29–36). Adelaide, Australia: Dulwich Centre Publications.

White, M. (1989b). The process of questioning: A therapy of literary merit. In *Selected papers* (pp. 37–46). Adelaide, Australia: Dulwich Centre Publications.

White, M. (1989c).The externalizing of the problem and the re-authoring of lives and relationships. In *Selected papers* (pp. 5–28). Adelaide, Australia: Dulwich Centre Publications.

White, M. (1989d). The conjoint therapy of men who batter. In *Selected papers* (pp. 101–106). Adelaide, Australia: Dulwich Centre Publications.

White, M. (1989e). Family therapy and schizophrenia: Adressing the "in the corner lifestyle." In *Selected papers* (pp. 47–58). Adelaide, Australia: Dulwich Centre Publications.

White, M. (1989f). Anorexia nervosa: A cybernetic perspective. In *Selected papers* (pp. 65–76). Adelaide, Australia: Dulwich Centre Publications.

White, M. (1989g). *Selected papers.* Adelaide, Australia: Dulwich Centre Publications.

White, M. (1991). Deconstruction and therapy. In M. White & D. Epston, *Experience, contradiction, narrative and imagination: Selected papers of Michael White and David Epston.* Adelaide, Australia: Dulwich Centre Publications.

White, M. (1992, October 11–12). Workshop presented at the Family Therapy Center of Burlington, Burlington, VT.

White, M. (1997). *Narratives of therapists' lives.* Adelaide, Australia: Dulwich Centre Publications.

White, M., & Epston, D. (1990). *Narrative means to therapeutic ends.* London: Norton.

White, M., & Epston, D. (1991). *Experience, contradiction, narrative and imagination: Selected papers of Michael White and David Epston.* Adelaide, Australia: Dulwich Centre Publications.

Whitfield, C. (1987). *Healing the child within.* Pompano Beach, FL: Health Communications.

Wieseltier, L. (1998). *Kaddish.* New York: Knopf.

Winnicott, D. W. (1949). Hate in the countertransference. *International Journal of Psychoanalysis, 30*(2), 69–74.

Winnicott, D. W. (1965). *The maturational process and the facilitating environment.* New York: Basic Books.

Winnicott, D. W. (1971a). *Playing and reality.* London: Tavistock.

Winnicott, D. W. (1971b). *Therapeutic consultations in child psychiatry.* New York Basic Books.

Winnicott, D. W. (1987). *The child, the family and the outside world.* Reading, MA: Addison Wesley. (Original work published 1964)

Winnicott, D. W. (1989). *Psychoanalytic explorations.* Cambridge, MA: Harvard University Press. (Original work published 1964)

Wolmark, A., & Sweezy, M. (1998). Kohut's self psychology. In R. Dorfman (Ed.), *Paradigms of clinical social work: Vol. 2.* New York: Brunner/Mazel.

Woolf, V. (1954). *Women and writing.* New York: Harcourt Brace Jovanovich.

Woolf, V. (1957). *A room of one's own.* New York: Harcourt, Brace, Jovanovich.

Zinberg, W., & Blume, S. (1985). *Practical approaches to alcoholism psychotherapy.* New York: Plenum Press.

Index

n indicates a note